Occupational Therapy with Older People

GAIL A. MOUNTAIN PhD, MPhil, DipCoT

Sheffield Hallam University

Consulting Editors in Occupational Therapy
Clephane Hume and Jennifer Creek

W
WHURR PUBLISHERS
LONDON AND PHILADELPHIA

© 2004 Whurr Publishers Ltd
First published 2004
by Whurr Publishers Ltd
19b Compton Terrace
London N1 2UN England and
325 Chestnut Street, Philadelphia PA 19106 USA

British Library Cataloguing in Publication Data

A catalogue record for this book
is available from the British Library.

ISBN 1 86156 376 0

Typeset by Adrian McLaughlin, a@microguides.net
Printed and bound in the UK by Athenæum Press Ltd, Gateshead,
Tyne & Wear.

Contents

Preface

This book is about older people, and the contribution that occupational therapy can make towards the maintenance of health and appropriate provision of rehabilitation and care. It is a reflection of current and future practice in light of current and anticipated demand.

Older people are increasingly at the centre of public policy and individual concern, and particularly so when they become incapacitated. A minority of older people will succumb to a cocktail of physical frailty, physical ill health and sometimes mental ill health. This in turn can result in decreased mobility and difficulties with daily living, leading to the likelihood of falls, other accidents and self-neglect. The consequence is usually a need for assistance from both health and social care services, as well as demands being placed upon family, friends and neighbours.

It goes without saying that the effective treatment of the complexity of problems older people can present with requires a skilled approach. Occupational therapists are acknowledged as being established practitioners with older people who have complex needs. Their contribution is in demand, particularly in light of the recent resurgence of interest in the part that occupation can play in promoting and maintaining a healthy lifestyle. As a consequence, the majority of occupational therapy practitioners will find themselves working with older people at some time during their career.

A goal common to many health and social care interventions with older people is the prevention of further disability and dependency and ultimate admission to long-term care. Demographic trends and consequent needs for services, shifting societal expectations of older age, the increasing use of technology in society, and the imperative to make best use of limited publicly provided resources are all factors which will ensure that the skills of occupational therapists continue to be required. Therefore, those concerned with the delivery of occupational therapy services have to ensure continued responsiveness to new and in some cases enhanced demands. It follows that maintenance of the correct blend of skill and experience to benefit older people and their carers cannot be taken for granted. It is essential that occupational therapy personnel, in common with others working with older people, constantly reflect upon how their skills can be developed and utilized to produce the best outcomes for older people and their carers.

The aim of this book is to help occupational therapists, and those involved in the commissioning of occupational therapy services for older people, to target their efforts both sensitively and effectively, and to anticipate the demands which will shape service provision in the future.

CHAPTER 1
Older people in society

Introduction

This book explores how occupational therapy can most appropriately respond to the needs of older people by truly focusing upon their needs, and those of their carers. The description of a portfolio of service responses and prescriptive interventions cannot meet this aim. To present solutions in this manner would be a gross oversimplification, both of the needs of people in older age and of the responses necessary to bring about optimum outcomes for them and for their carers. It would also fail to acknowledge and explore why some services do not operate in the best interests of older people even though they are adequately resourced, whereas others are able to deliver quality provision despite various limitations. More fundamentally, a sterile 'cookbook approach' listing a series of actions deemed to be necessary from a professional perspective depersonalizes a topic which ultimately impacts upon each and every one of us, either through our personal experiences of old age or through those of relatives and friends. The workers of today are the future generation of older people. It is therefore in our own interest to consider the services provided for older people, and how they should be run, both now and in the future. We need to question the contribution of occupational therapy from a personal as well as professional perspective. What are the constituents of services for older people and their carers which meet the expectations of what we would like for our families and for ourselves?

Working with older people demands a sensitive and expert approach towards their needs. To achieve this the following must be developed by commissioners of services, managers and individual practitioners:

1. Insight into our personal belief systems about older age and how these beliefs shape the responses made to the needs of older people.
2. Informed views of the lifestyles and expectations of people after their retirement.

1

3. The contributions older people can make within communities, and the changing expectations of older people in society. These factors set the wider context within which services for older people (including occupational therapy) are determined.
4. Knowledge of the impact of ill health and frailty upon the quality of life of older people, and the ways in which a reasonable lifestyle can be maintained despite difficulties.
5. The ability to keep questioning and aiming for services that are personally acceptable.

The above are all fundamental requirements for occupational therapists working with older people. How they underpin and impact upon the development and maintenance of quality practice are explored in this and forthcoming chapters.

The opinions of older people interviewed during several research projects undertaken by the author (details of which are given in Appendix 1) are quoted at relevant points in this book. (Views of older people attributable to the work of other authors are specifically cited.) While these quotations cannot be taken to be representative of the opinions of all older people, they serve as a reminder of the voice of those for whom we would aim to provide quality services.

Other sources of evidence used to underpin the recommendations for practice cited in this book are drawn from research and from documented examples of practice innovation. The search strategy employed to identify relevant literature to inform the views and suggestions for practice presented in this work is described in Appendix 2.

This first chapter will consider the view Western society has of older people, taking into account the implications of recent policies. This forms a backdrop for individual experiences of older age, and service responses to needs, described in forthcoming chapters.

Who are older people?

At what point in our lives do we consider ourselves to be old, and what are our attitudes to age and the ageing process? How do personal perceptions affect our expectations of our own lifestyle post-retirement, and that of others during this phase of life? The social and cultural meaning of older age is being constantly shaped and reshaped by the expectations of society, as well as being located in our individual experiences of older people as relatives, friends, neighbours and work colleagues. What then are the most significant factors that contribute towards our understanding of older age? Chronological age is the most obvious but not the most important indicator of the ageing process, which it is agreed encompasses a complex mix of physical, medical and social functioning (Scrutton, 1992). Perceptions of self are associated with attitude and physical abilities as much as with age. Mountain and Moore (1995) found that fit retired people interpreted individuals in need of care as being old but did not consider that the term 'old' could also be applied to them.

> You'll find that some people are not able to handle life, especially if they're on their own. ... You'll find that people like that would rather be in a residential home and there are others who would rather have a small bungalow or something, looked after by wardens.

The observed lives of older people in our society continually undermine the significance of age in years. A study of risk-taking behaviour in older age (Wynne-Hartley, 1991) included examples of older people who continued to participate in risky occupations such as skiing, water sports, marathon running, and arts and crafts activities which use potentially dangerous equipment. Some celebrities and politicians continue to work well beyond the established retirement age. A list provided by Carlson et al. (1998) named men and women who have achieved significance beyond the age of 65 years, including heads of state, parachutists and musicians. Despite these challenges to traditional stereotypes, the extent of negative imagery of older age still outweighs positive messages, leading to a tendency for people to restrict their expectations of this phase of their lives (Scrutton, 1992).

One of the problems of the term 'older people' is that it is applied indiscriminately to all those who have reached retirement age. This exacerbates problems of understanding who older people are and what they can be expected to contribute. Given that increasing numbers of people are retiring early, older people as a group potentially include those aged from between 50 and 100-plus years, and consequently several generations! This view is confirmed by the Cabinet Office, who have been consulting with people aged 50 and over regarding services for older people (Cabinet Office, 2000a). Confusion over who older people are is being exacerbated by the policy aim of maintaining people in work for as long as they are able to contribute. Therefore the notion of retirement marking the beginning of old age is no longer viable. This fit and well older person observed the irony of our desire to categorize people:

> We sound as though they [frail older people] are different from the human race. We all get there.

Individuals whose ages range from 50 to over 100 years will have very different stories to tell of the community, societal and environmental conditions they will have lived through. Such experiences have a profound effect upon expectations of services. People who in the year 2003 live in Europe and are over the age of 75 years experienced the deprivation of the war years. In the UK, they were also recipients of health care prior to the introduction of the National Health Service in 1947. Consequently, they grew up in a culture of lower expectations, relative material and nutritional deprivation and poorer public health. Some of the older people interviewed about their quality of life by Mountain and Moore (1995) agreed that their quality of life was better than it had been for their parents, and recalled living with very little money in their earlier life. It had also made them resilient.

There's a lot of things that you couldn't afford that you did yourself.

Those now in their sixties grew up in the post-war years when material goods became more plentiful and health services were provided by the state. Additionally, a number are relatively affluent due to workplace pension schemes and property inheritance.

As well as being a diverse population with respect to age and social mix, increasing numbers of older people in our society are from different ethnic groups. The United Kingdom is now multicultural, with a rich mix of people whose origins were in other countries. Those who immigrated to this country in the 1950s from Afro-Caribbean states and from Asia at our invitation to fill gaps in the job market are now joining the ranks of older people. Another example is the people from Eastern European countries like Poland who were not able to return to their homeland after the Second World War. These different groups of older people have different needs and expectations of services. Problems are exacerbated by the acknowledged fact that access to both health and social care by minority ethnic groups can be limited.

One model developed to make sense of the different experiences of life post-retirement is to divide the human lifespan into four phases, the first being childhood, the second adulthood, and the third a healthy and fulfilling retirement. The fourth and final age is associated with disability and dependence. The fourth group therefore includes those who will be heavy users of health and social services. This can provide a useful framework when projecting extent of future service need (MRC CFAS, 2000). Within the sociological literature, a differentiation has been drawn between those people aged 75 years and over and those aged between 65 and 74 years. This is located in the premise that as a person becomes older, their ability to adapt to changing life circumstances is a major factor in continuing life satisfaction (Hunt, 1978; Abrams, 1980). It has already been observed that older people themselves tend to make this distinction, with those who are younger referring to those who are older in the context of needs for care. While the differentiation has proved useful in the past for policy-makers, service commissioners and providers, it is questionable whether this will remain the case given the improved health of the population overall and the changing policy focus, described in this and forthcoming chapters. Most recently, the National Service Framework for Older People (DoH, 2001a) placed older people within three broad groups, making reference to the fact that groupings might be influenced by age but not necessarily so:

- those *entering old age*, defined as such by the cessation of paid employment; they are generally active and independent and can be as young as 50;
- those in the *transitional phase*, between independent life and vulnerability and dependence;
- those who are *frail* due to health problems.

Even this latest definition has its problems, given the rapidly changing perceptions of what marks the beginning of retirement.

Increased lifespan

Much has been written about the consequences of the increasing numbers of older people in our society. Therefore, to avoid repetition of what are well-known facts, this section is brief. Ageing is a global phenomenon, the speed of demographic change varying from country to country; for example in Germany, Italy and Japan it is progressing more rapidly than in the UK. A study of population projections to 2066 for the UK (Khaw, 1999) found that the number of people aged 60 years and over is projected to increase from 20 per cent of the total size of the population in 2001, to 30 per cent by the year 2031. The Cabinet Office (2000b) estimated that between 1995 and 2025, the number of those aged 85 years and over will double and of those aged 90 years and over will treble. By the year 2040, 25 per cent of the population of the UK will be aged 60 years or over.

One of the most striking features of the population characteristics of people aged 65 years and over is the greater numbers of women. In 1995, Grundy observed that women made up 60 per cent of all older people, and 74 per cent of those aged 85 years and over. The reasons for this are multifactorial and not completely understood. Therefore society has to adjust to the needs of an older population containing a greater proportion of women. Rather than quoting various statistics, what is required is an examination of the consequences and benefits of the increasing numbers of older people in our society as described in the forthcoming sections of this chapter.

Conflicting views of the societal value of older people

Older people are often the focus of two parallel policy concerns. The first is associated with increased lifespan as discussed in the previous section. This is resulting in greater numbers of very old people in society, a proportion of whom will have needs for care. The second, associated debate stems from the lowered birth rate which, as the previous section described, is leading to proportional increases in the numbers of older people – as opposed to younger, economically active individuals. Consequently the government is concerned with how to support the increasing numbers who may not be economically active as well as taking account of the high costs of health and social care provision to the few with complex needs.

The need to look creatively at ways of sustaining economic viability is forcing policy-makers to take a fresh look at the contributions older people can continue to make to their communities, and how they might be encouraged to support themselves beyond the age of 65 years. However, long-standing beliefs and attitudes of the established role of older people within society, in contrast with more positive perceptions, mean that this is not an easy matter in the UK or in other developed countries.

In the past the impact of the growing numbers of older people, particularly upon health services, was presented in pessimistic terms in various policy documents, for example in *The Rising Tide* (Health Advisory Service, 1982). This and other reports emphasized the increasing drain upon societal resources if the needs of an ageing population were to be met.

> Medical advances and the increasing conquest of disabilities associated with the second half of life mean that more and more people are reaching a great old age. Very old people need a lot of care in their final years, much of it because of the greatly increased incidence of mental illness and intellectual failure in old age. Unless challenges are met, the flood is likely to overwhelm the entire health care system. (Health Advisory Service, 1982, p. 1)

The contents of earlier documents like *The Rising Tide* contrast sharply with more recent thinking that is promoting the opportunities older people present to society (DTI, 2000a; DTI, 2000b). Policy-makers are now acknowledging the previous neglect of older people and the undervaluing of their contribution. A commitment has been made towards appraising all areas of policy from the viewpoint of older people; for example:

> It would be wrong to assume that older people would not be affected by changes in childcare policy or that they would not want to take part in

activities which some might consider generally the preserve of younger people. (Cabinet Office, 2000b)

Various policy initiatives have been introduced globally to try to promote the value of older people. The year 1999 was designated by the United Nations as the International Year of Older Persons, with the aims of promoting UN principles on ageing; namely independence, care, self-fulfilment and dignity. The response in the UK was to introduce an inter-ministerial group for older people, and promote a series of activities and events with the aim of challenging negative stereotypes of ageing, identifying gaps in provision and making recommendations for the future.

However, society's attitude towards older people has always been fickle. The expressed views of policy-makers and of individuals can all too easily switch from a sympathetic mode to an impatient and dismissive attitude. Older people are aware of how they are often portrayed by society and blamed for being a burden.

> They always try and blame the old for living long ... It's always 'And they're living longer' you know! And you feel as if they are getting at you all the time because you're living longer.

Throughout history, the prevailing approach towards older people by Western society has been patronizing, suggesting that as a group they require care and protection. (The services that were developed in line with this belief system are discussed in Chapter 5.) Workplace pension schemes, early retirement and property inheritance are now questioning this understanding. There has been a recent and radical increase in the numbers of comparatively affluent 'younger older' people with the time, physical ability and resources to enjoy life. Minkler and Estes (2000) noted a significant shift in American attitudes towards their older population.

> One perceived as a deserving subgroup of poor, frail and politically powerless individuals, the elderly increasingly are being portrayed by the mass media, policy makers and others as greedy geezers ... (Minkler and Estes, 2000, p. 65)

In the UK, the future impact of this younger, more empowered group of older people has been described in relation to the work market:

> The number of Mature Entrepreneurs will rise sharply as more older individuals strike out on their own: 'Generation M'. Not only will there be an increasing number of people entering older age-brackets, their aspirations are also more likely to be more entrepreneurial than previous generations. (DTI, 2000b, p. 16)

Some of the older people interviewed during the study on quality of life in older age by Mountain and Moore (1995) felt disadvantaged by having to retire. They felt that they still had something to offer society and felt irritated by societal norms that they perceived fostered the segregation of older people.

Even now, use of the negative term 'bed blockers' by politicians to describe older people who are unable to leave hospital, most often due to lack of residential care provision, helps to perpetuate a view of older people as being problematic for society.

So, on the one hand older people are seen as being an increasingly affluent, active group, a potential workforce which might be drawn upon to sustain the economy and a group which politicians would do well to persuade. On the other they are considered to be frail, in need of care and a drain upon resources. The conflicting views of society are illustrated in Table 1.1.

Table 1.1 Polarized views of abilities and contributions in older age

Positive perceptions	Negative perceptions
Physically fit	Physically frail
Independent	Dependent/in need of care
Worker/contributor	Drain on resources
Engaged with society	Increasingly disengaged
Able to learn new skills	Learning ability restricted
Able to adapt to changing circumstances	Resistant to change

Some of the many issues challenging policy-makers and our society that are of specific relevance to occupational therapy practice are now discussed in more detail.

Funding long-term care

Policy-makers are clearly struggling to reach viable solutions regarding how funding for long-term care can be most satisfactorily met for those of us who become too frail to live an independent life at home. This was evidenced through the length of time the government took to respond to the recommendations of the Royal Commission on Long Term Care (1999). The solution reached in England is to request payment for all care which is not deemed to be nursing, thus including personal care within the umbrella of services for which charges will be levied (DoH, 2003). The devolved Scottish Parliament have taken a different approach, providing all types of care free. A poll of public opinion to identify what the public thought about these policies was undertaken by the King's Fund in 2001 (Deeming, 2001). The poll found that most people did not agree with the policy decision regarding means testing of people who need help with personal care, irrespective of where it is provided. Most supported free personal care. The King's Fund suggested that this indicated the need for a rethink of this policy. It is not surprising that there is anger on the part of older people about the expectation of payment for care which they were always led to believe would be funded by the state.

Underlying economic dilemmas like payment for long-term care is the realization on the part of policy-makers that the sheer numbers of older people living in democracies like the UK make their vote a powerful influence, which can make or break governments. Therefore politicians are aware that they tread a precarious path if they antagonize older people.

Extending working life

The economic pressures contained by a society where, in the future, it is anticipated that there will be more unproductive than productive individuals, are leading to a reconsideration of the merits of retaining the established retirement age. Debates regarding the duration of working life are strongly interwoven with the question of how society can afford to support those on a pension. The demographic support ratio is the number of people of working age (20–64) to older people (65-plus). In the UK this is 4 to 1. By the year 2030, it will have fallen to 2.5 to 1. In Italy and Germany, by the year 2035 it will have fallen to below 2 to 1. It is therefore not surprising that well-grounded concerns across Europe about economic sustainability in light of there being more retired people than workers in the future is leading to an examination of factors which might encourage people to continue working past the age of 65 years. Most recently it has been suggested that normal working life should continue to the age of 70 years. There are also urgent questions about the problems resulting from early retirement. The proportion of men between 50 years and 65 years who are not working has doubled over the last 20 years. The Cabinet Office (2000a) attributed this to the following reasons:

* prejudices within society, employers and older people themselves that they have less to offer;
* perverse occupational pension schemes that have encouraged people to retire early;
* the possession of skills that are no longer needed by society;

- barriers to work, paid or unpaid, perpetuated by beliefs about the benefits system and lack of information.

The requirement to extend working life is not confined to the UK. An examination of the patterns of employment in Finland, and how they relate to overall patterns in Europe, demonstrated an urgent need for new strategies to reduce early retirement and extend the length of working life (Sihto, 1999). One problem to be overcome is the mismatch between the skills contained within the older workforce and those required by society, particularly in light of increased globalization, together with reliance upon technology (Sihto, 1999). Nevertheless, a comprehensive portfolio of work is being undertaken in Europe to examine how technology can enhance the lives of older people, including home working (DTI, 2000b). The extension of working life has specific implications for occupational therapists. Vocational rehabilitation will extend to meet the needs of older people as well as being confined to those aged under 60 years, and a different emphasis may be required during the rehabilitation process to take account of the needs of the older worker. This is discussed further in Chapter 7.

Age discrimination

Age discrimination can manifest itself in a number of ways, including access to paid and unpaid work. Established societal norms have marginalized the continued involvement of the majority of older people. One woman interviewed by Mountain and Moore (1995) saw that being retired had disadvantaged her in that although she had been a lifelong member of the Guide movement and remained fit and well, she was no longer allowed to go on camps once she reached 60 years of age. Another described being 'finished' at 40 when she had been unable to find employment after her husband had died.

Most recently, the UK government has stated that it is wrong for employers to discriminate against individuals upon the basis of their age, and are looking towards ways of legislating against age discrimination. This is being driven by the adoption of an EC Directive requiring that age discrimination be banned by 2006. An examination of the experiences of other countries to inform the steps that should be taken in the UK found that the behaviour of employers has not shifted in relation to older people as much as with other marginalized groups (Hornstein, 2001). Legislation has had a positive effect upon older people retaining employment for longer, but removal of the statutory retirement age may also have made employers less likely to take on older workers.

As well as age discrimination occurring in paid and unpaid work, it can also be manifested in other ways, for example availability of financial services and access to health care. Discriminatory access to health care is considered further in Chapter 5.

The pension debate

One of the premises underpinning the requirement to extend working life is the UK government's desire to withdraw compulsory retirement, and therefore reduce the extent of obligation to provide state funding for pensions. This is in stark contrast to the compulsory retirement packages of past decades. The present goal is to provide individuals with choice about whether they remain in work or not, but, given the prevailing economic imperatives, there are questions about whether the notion of choice will remain the main driver. Recently reported research has indicated that being provided with choice about when retirement commences is a powerful factor in maintaining quality of life (Gaber, 2003).

Traditionally there has been a clear message about the duration of working life in Western society. Retirement at the age of 65 years and the granting of a retirement pension have been the accepted norm, thus enabling the younger generation to take their place as 'worker members' of society. The initial reasons for enforced retirement in the UK stem from the industrial revolution, when it was deemed that older workers were no longer able to fulfil the demands of factory life (Mulley, 1995). The history of statutory pension provision in the UK commenced with implementation of the recommendations of the Beveridge report in 1942. These were based upon the notion of the employee being male and in full-time work (Tinker, 1997). Clearly, there have been substantial societal shifts since 1942. Recognition of the need to equalize benefits for men and women in the 1990s led to the 1995 Pensions Act. Implementation is leading to a phased introduction of an increase in the state pension age for women from 60 to 65 years. However, there is little doubt that in the foreseeable future, state pension support will have to be removed to meet financial imperatives. Debates continue regarding the best way of withdrawing the state pension while guaranteeing individuals a minimum income. This is further complicated by problems surrounding the current performance of workplace pension schemes.

Income and poverty in older age

As has previously been stated, today's generation of younger old people tend to be wealthier than their predecessors. This can largely be attributed to home ownership, promoted in the post-war years. In the future, finances may also be increased by a flexible retirement age, with benefits being balanced by the need to finance a longer lifespan (particularly as people may expect to spend thirty or more years in retirement). Policy debate continues over how to help older people to capitalize upon the equity some of them will have accumulated over the years and to plan for their needs over time. The Foresight Panel (DTI, 2000b) identified that more use could be made of the capital tied up in housing, with a need for government to work with the financial sector to ensure that financial products are both fair and trusted by customers. There are also concerns that younger people are not adequately preparing financially for retirement, and as a consequence the difficulties associated with supporting an older population will continue well into the future.

Given these debates about increasing affluence in older age and the anticipated extension of working life, it is easy to overlook the topic of poverty in older age. However, for some older people living on nothing more than the basic pension, and therefore on a minimum income, it is a way of life. A study commissioned by the Foresight Panel (DTI, 2000b) found that those people who had had interrupted work histories and on low incomes were likely to find that their pension is at the minimum guaranteed by the government. Overall, older people are more likely than the rest of the population to be living in poverty, in poor housing and without adequate transport (DoH, 1999b). Care and Repair England compiled a number of facts on their web site illustrating the poverty that exists among a substantial minority of older people in our society; for example:

- Older women are most affected by poverty in older age. A study by Help the Aged found that 25 per cent were found to be living on incomes of less than £80 per week or less. Sixty per cent were worried about paying bills.
- Pensioners in a household headed by someone from an ethnic minority are more likely to be managing on a low income.
- In 1996, at least three-quarters of those living in unfit housing or housing in serious disrepair had annual incomes below £12,000.

Incidences of hypothermia in cold weather are one indicator of poverty, where older people are fearful of incurring bills if they turn on their heating. Much of the illness and mortality in older people is related to socioeconomic factors. The Department of Health (1999b) raised the complex question of whether this is due to a lifetime of relative deprivation or if it is a syndrome of older age.

The growing voice of older people in society

A variety of drivers are leading to the greater empowerment of older people. These include a desire for recognition and inclusion on the part of older people themselves, changing perceptions on the part of society and a continuing number of government initiatives.

The Foresight programme (DTI, 2000a; DTI, 2000b) made a number of recommendations to improve the status of older people in society and value what they can offer; for example:

- helping businesses to meet the challenges of the age shift by introducing flexible working patterns for older people, and looking at the new market opportunities created by ageing consumers and products to improve quality of life for frail older people;
- the introduction of inclusive policies across employment, health, social care and businesses, fostered by the inter-ministerial group for older people;
- improving the images of older people presented by advertising and by the media;
- promoting inclusive design and application, and access to information technology;
- information and education to promote healthy ageing;
- prioritizing the integration of health and social services.

Citizenship and social inclusion

In the UK, as in other countries, there are a growing number of older people who are not satisfied with the role carved out for them by society, and who wish to have greater influence and control over their lives. A number of groups and forums are having an increasingly powerful voice within a developing culture of social inclusion, which is promoting full participation in every aspect of community life by all members, and particularly those who have previously been marginalized. Intertwined with social inclusion is the desire for full citizenship on the part of older people. The concept of people as citizens encompasses the notions of status, duties and rights. It is an ideal that began to gain favour in the 1990s (Barnes M, 1997). Minkler and Estes (2000) suggested that the increased affluence of those most recently retired, together with their life experience, has resulted in a more assertive group of older people who are not averse to complaining if services they receive do not reach their expectations.

The impetus for social inclusion and citizenship can be traced back to the demands of older people as well as awareness on the part of government. Organized groups of older people who are promoting and in some cases demanding citizenship for older people permeate all aspects of political, academic and community life. The Pensioners' Parliament is one example of a forum that is enabling older people to have a greater political profile in society and debate the issues of particular importance to them as a group. This group has a national network, and links with other international groups. During the Annual National Pensioners' Parliament at Blackpool in May 1999, 2000 pensioners gathered with a common aim of presenting concrete demands to government. This quote from veteran campaigner Jack Jones, provided in the press release, summed up the atmosphere:

> Politicians need to listen to what older people are telling them – and act on it. Pensioners want better state pensions as a matter of justice – at least £75 per week this year for a single pensioner, with future increases linked to average earnings. Pensioners want a national minimum concessionary fare scheme for transport. And they want to see the recommendations of the Royal Commission on Long Term Care implemented without delay.

This older person interviewed by Mountain and Moore in 1995 expressed a similar view:

> You've got to be counted nowadays when there's more of the elderly than not – they're going to have a bigger say in politics and everything.

The increasing voice of older people in our society is being fostered by a number of organizations, for example Help the Aged, Age Concern and the Alzheimer's Society. As well as providing information and support and speaking on behalf of older people, they assist individuals and groups to add their voice to the growing numbers willing to speak out. Age Concern actively seeks participation (particularly by older people) in their mission to improve the lives of older people. This includes influencing government legislation, raising awareness through the media and working in partnership with other organizations to improve services. Combating age discrimination is an example of a targeted Age Concern campaign. Views were actively sought up to the end of March 2002 on whether legislation is required to end age discrimination in health care, training and financial products and services.

Other initiatives with political undertones continue to be introduced to raise the current profile of older people in society and examine how society will successfully accommodate increasing numbers of older people. One example is The Debate of the Age, a high-profile project launched in 1996 by Age Concern, England. The explicit aims were to discuss the future of an ageing society with people from all generations and walks of life, raising awareness and making recommendations for public policy. Over a period of 20 months, the initiative ran over 1500 events, debates, research programmes and surveys. One way in which the conveners tried to fully consult with people was through citizens' juries, a method by which members of the general public can be actively involved in policy-making. The focus of the debate was the following five areas:

1. the future of the built environment;
2. the future of health and care;

3. paying for care;
4. values and attitudes in an ageing society;
5. future work and lifestyles.

The conclusions drawn from the Debate are provided in a number of documents containing clear recommendations for government (Henwood, 1999; Gilchrist, 1999).

Policy-led consultation and participation

The concept of citizenship of older people is leading to a burgeoning number of policy-led recommendations and initiatives to increase the involvement of those who are well and readily able to engage. However, questions remain about the extent of participation of those who are less able and vocal. There are also lingering doubts regarding the speed with which expressed aims are being put into practice.

Better Government for Older People was introduced in 1998 with the aim of increasing the participation of older people in local government. It initially involved 28 pilot programmes in local authorities across the UK. All pilots were subjected to an evaluation with the aim of spreading and maintaining good practice. Results showed that the participating authorities involved older people and developed more integrated strategies to improve the quality of life of older people. The evaluation (BGOP, 2000) made 28 recommendations in the following four key areas:

1. combating age discrimination so that older people are positively portrayed by the media;
2. engaging with older people so that they are able to advise on issues that affect them;
3. improving decision-making so that difficult issues like poverty among older people and the consequences of the ageing population are confronted;
4. meeting older people's needs through better care services.

Another government-led initiative, the People's Panel, involved contributions from a total of 5,064 people aged 16 and over, of which 2,145 were 50 years and over (Cabinet Office, 2000a). Individuals were recruited from a random sample of postal addresses in 1998. Face to face and telephone interviews were conducted, with the results from older respondents being as follows.

Public services: Older people overall have lower expectations of services. However, nearly half of older people in full-time work said that public services did not meet their expectations. With respect to complaints about services, 85 per cent thought that getting something done requires great determination.

Health concerns: Taking into account a range of health concerns spanning subjects like air pollution, poverty, unemployment and education, older people were more likely to prioritize air pollution than other age groups.

Care in the community: More older people were critical than other age groups, particularly those who were carers.

GPs, the NHS and social care: Older respondents stated that they were happy with the service they were getting.

Homes and neighbourhoods: Older people were more likely to be happy with where they lived, but they were also more likely to say that things had got worse. They were more likely to be critical of the consequences of traffic congestion. They want better, more reliable, less costly bus services. Train travel was less likely to be criticized, apart from the cost. This finding was attributed to the fact that older people were more likely to use trains for leisure than for work.

Community involvement: Certain groups of older people were more likely to feel socially excluded. These were those in older age groups, in lower social classes or tenants of social housing.

Technological society: Fear of new technology is a major concern for older people. Concerns spanned usage and confidentiality.

Improving information-giving and access

The Service Action team (DoH, 1999f) has been established to ensure that citizens can both identify and access the help they require from public services. Examples of their work include the guide to help people who need long-term care, and their relatives, and the bereavement action team, concerned with improving information provision to the bereaved.

Involvement in health services

Greater involvement in public sector health and social care provision by all sectors of society is a relatively long-standing political aim. However, there are a number of recent policy initiatives of specific relevance to older people. One example is the concept of the Expert Patient (DoH, 2001b). This is based in the premise that people with chronic health problems have expert knowledge regarding the management of their condition. As up to 75 per cent of all people over the age of 75 years experience chronic ill health, the Expert Patient initiative should impact upon older people. The stated intention is to establish self-management training programmes for people with chronic illness over a six-year timescale. This programme is being integrated into existing health care provision, thus requiring partnership with professionals. Exploration is also ongoing regarding the implementation of Patients' Forums to represent the views of users of health services. Interviews with a sample of individuals from socially excluded groups (Opinion Leader Research, 2001) raised the issue of how confidentiality might be maintained, but also recognized that a speedy resolution of any difficulties might be more likely. The conclusion drawn from this research was that people encounter a number of problems with health services. These include those stemming from service usage, for example waiting times, by being a member of a certain population such as an older person, and through prejudice towards certain marginalized groups of people like gypsies.

Volunteering by older people

Volunteers are long-standing members of the mixed economy of social and community care, made up of paid work provided by the statutory and voluntary sectors alongside unpaid contributions. The government is currently promoting volunteering by older people. A report by the Cabinet Office (2000b) stated that one of the government's aims should be helping older people to make use of their skills and experience for the benefit of the wider community. They suggest two ways of achieving this: by increasing opportunities for volunteering generally and by targeting older people specifically. This suggests that volunteering by older people is a new concept whereas in reality it is long-standing practice. Older people have traditionally contributed to society in this capacity following retirement. Advocacy on the part of other older people, particularly when negotiating services, is a more recent development of the volunteering role.

A number of older people interviewed by Mountain and Moore (1995) were actively engaged in voluntary work in their communities. This included helping in schools, membership of various committees and visiting housebound older people. One lady was assisting her sons with their business and another worked as a childminder. It was observed that, while fit for voluntary work, prevailing attitudes made them unfit for paid work.

> They want you quickly, though, when you do voluntary work. I did plenty of voluntary jobs because I wasn't getting paid. They want you then ...

Chapter 4 looks at the role of carers in maintaining older and disabled people in their own homes. These arrangements differ from organized voluntary work in that they are informal, personal, can form part of agreed family duties and are more likely to change over time (Hoad, 2002).

Lifelong learning

Lifelong learning is a policy initiative introduced by the Labour government in the UK (DfEE, 1998), located in the desirability of continuing education throughout the life course. Some sectors of the older population were practising lifelong learning well before the introduction of this initiative. The University of the Third Age (U3A) is an international voluntary movement run by older people, with around 130 local branches in the UK. The aims of U3A are to organize and maintain a cooperative learning community for retired and semi-retired people on a not-for-profit basis, to encourage the pursuit of learning and to exchange ideas with other groups both nationally and internationally. However, this organization does not readily provide access to learning to older people if they were not professionals in their previous working life. The access and use of lifelong learning by older people has recently been investigated by the EPSRC as part of the "growing older" programme of research (see Appendix 3 for web address).

Accommodating an older population

The embedding of more positive societal values towards older people has to be demonstrated through changes to the fabric of our environment and provision of services.

Housing and environment have a direct impact upon the ability of older people to maintain an independent lifestyle. It is also well known that effective transport systems are vital for minimizing social isolation and fostering engagement with the community, including with health and social care provision. The importance of these external factors and how they can enhance, or alternatively contribute towards loss of, independence is raised in Chapters 2 and 3. Some of the policies and initiatives shaping the external environment in light of the needs of an ageing population are described below.

Inclusive design

One of the aspirations of the government-led Foresight programme was the adoption of a fresh approach to design on all levels. The goal should

be to build and adapt environments in a manner that makes th~
ing to all age groups, thereby mainstreaming access for disabled and o~
people rather than making it exceptional. The priorities for inclusive
design are given in Table 1.2. This demonstrates an acknowledgement of
the importance of external factors upon independence.

Table 1.2 Three priorities for inclusive design (Source: DTI, 2000b, p.21)

(1) Flexibility	(2) Independence	(3) Social interaction
Adaptable for different users and uses	Choice	Family and friends
	Control	Neighbourhood and wider communities
Responsive to age-related change		Work opportunities
		Democratic participation as citizens

The philosophy of inclusive design extends beyond buildings to transport and other aspects of life. It is an approach to creating everyday
environments, products and technologies that can be used by all members
of the population, irrespective of age and disability (Mynatt and Rogers,
2001/2002). It therefore promotes participation and involvement. The new
London taxi is one example of inclusive design. It is said to be the most
accessible in the world, with the design being based upon research and
consultation with disability groups. Mynatt and Rogers (2001/2002) suggested that interviewing people about their preferences regarding design
of technological solutions is a crucial part of the design process, bearing in
mind that the design has to meet needs as individuals become older.

Housing for older people

The Housing Green Paper and subsequent implementation document
(DTLR, 2000, 2001) stressed the need for both quality and choice in housing for older people. The challenges of planning adequate provision to
meet the needs of a population that is living longer were also highlighted. The policy goal is to enable everyone to have a decent, affordable and
appropriate home to promote the wider goals of well-being, independence and social inclusion. The Green Paper suggested that the optimal
approach should be:

- *Integrated*: operating across all sectors;
- *Holistic*: considering a spectrum of needs over time;

- *Inclusive*: meeting the needs of specific groups like ethnic minorities, older women and people with physical and/or mental frailty;
- *Involving*: ensures the participation of older people in delivering and reviewing housing programmes;
- *Preventive*: enabling older people to retain their independence and quality of life.

There are a number of approaches being taken towards housing provision to meet the needs of an ageing population.

An external development group, including older people, is working with the DoH and DTLR to encourage the joint actions and joint approach promoted by the Green Paper. Current strategies include an exploration of the key housing issues affecting older people and development of initiatives to ensure that appropriate policies are in place to address them.

A study of the type and nature of housing that older people want in older age, undertaken to inform the commissioning of a proposed retirement village in York, reinforced the need for consultation with older people regarding the design of homes and communities (Appleton, 2002). Houses for older people and the environment in which they are sited should match the lifestyle requirements of older people. The study found that older people wish to retain car ownership for as long as possible and that, in contrast to a commonly held belief, space requirement changed in older age rather than diminished. Access to community facilities like the post office and GP surgeries were an important requirement. For those people from black and ethnic minorities, the importance of being able to access family and places of worship was emphasized. Another study that involved interviewing older people about satisfaction with housing found that the physical quality of the house was extremely important for all older people (Wilson et al., 1995). With increasing age, the design of the kitchen and bathroom commanded more importance. This study also confirmed the need for access to public transport and shopping facilities.

Some of the current developments in housing for older people are raised below.

1. Segregation or integration

The benefits of retirement villages of the sort first developed in the USA continue to be debated (Jeffrys, 1996). Such housing provides increasing levels of care as a person becomes more dependent. The Joseph Rowntree Foundation has built one of these villages in North Yorkshire. Anchor Housing are currently planning a development in the south of England, incorporating necessary wiring so that technology for care and surveillance can be introduced for the resident when it is required.

The wider discussions regarding whether older people should be segregated in any form of specialist housing away from mainstream society continue. Some older people prefer to live alongside different age groups whereas others can see the benefits of some segregation. This older lady had very definite views about the negative impact of sheltered housing schemes:

> I'm 81 ... There's one 90, there's one 94 in the place where we are, but ... I don't like to be with old people.

Another individual expressed a similar negative view about segregation:

> You go down an ordinary suburban street and you'll get all age groups whereas when you get older people of a similar age will all be together. I think that it is better to be mixed.

> I find that if I can go and sometimes mix with some of the young ... forty year olds and coming up to fifties ... it's nice I find to go and talk to them or be with them ... I feel that there's more looking forward in that sense ... We've started looking backwards all the time and looking a little bit forwards but only in the sense of well, how long? But young people have got more vision.

Discussions of benefit tended to be expressed in the context of other, more needy individuals rather than from a personal perspective.

> I think if we could get more homes built for elderly people who really need to go into them and be looked after, or some old people's complexes built, then I feel that it would help each area.

The option of enhanced sheltered housing provision or 'very sheltered housing' as an alternative to residential care was explored by Oldman (2000). She concluded that:

> There are some major policy obstacles to be addressed before the concept of 'your own front door' can become a reality for older people living in every type of communal setting. (Oldman, 2000, p. 2)

2. Lifetime homes

Demand for new homes will change in the future, in line with technological advances and the increasing number of single households.

The concept of lifetime homes is that of housing that can be adapted over time and will therefore be suitable for people for life. They therefore negate the need for specialist, segregated provision. These houses are being developed with the aim of being adaptable to meet changing needs as a person becomes older, for example having space for wheelchair use and a stairlift (Metz, 2000). They incorporate 16 design features including easy access, space for further installations like lifts and fixtures, and fittings that are easy to reach. Sopp (2001) interviewed 300 residents of lifetime homes to ascertain their views. Significantly, many did not realize that they were living in a lifetime home. Most, however, thought that they were a good idea and without prompting mentioned positive design features such as widened doorways and a downstairs toilet.

3. Smart homes

Engineers, designers and health and social care providers are beginning to realize the potential of technology in helping older people to remain living in the community. Smart homes include technologies for care and surveillance. The technology is wired into the infrastructure of the building and can include an ever-increasing number of possibilities. This technology is being developed with the needs of vulnerable older people in mind. However, the concept of buildings that incorporate the necessary wiring for use (should it be necessary) is increasing in popularity, therefore overlapping with the notion of lifetime homes. Smart homes are discussed in some depth in Chapter 9.

Implications for occupational therapy

This chapter has drawn out some of the many implications for society of our increasing numbers of older people. The contents of this chapter also indicate the requirement for the adoption of certain approaches by occupational therapists if practice is to meet the expectations of different populations of older people within our society.

Improve policy awareness

Societal attitudes and government policy are intertwined. These factors have far-reaching consequences for how older people are both perceived and treated by society, including whether they work and where they live. It is therefore essential that those working with older people understand current policy initiatives and their consequences. This awareness has to extend across all aspects of the lives of older people and all sectors of older people in society. It is important that we do not confine ourselves to those who have become vulnerable. This awareness can assist occupational therapists to become champions of older people, challenging views when they are not in the interest of older people and their families. It can also promote a proactive rather than reactive stance to current policy.

View older people as a resource

Consideration of the contributions of older people who are well is a timely reminder of the many contributions they make to society. It is all too easy to set aside the contributions of the majority when working with older people who are frail and ill. Only a small proportion of older people are in receipt of services compared with the overall population aged 60 years and over. It is also easy to forget that older people who are now in need of services will have lived full lives in the past. Appreciating the current and previous potential of older people irrespective of their current circumstances, rather than seeing them as problematic, can also help workers to maintain positive rather than negative perceptions, which translates into a positive attitude.

Get involved in initiatives to improve the lives of older people

In the past occupational therapists have tended to confine their work to those who have been referred to health and social care services. However, current interest in how the quality of life of older people can be improved and maintained through inclusive design and preventive strategies is leading to new demands for occupational therapy involvement. This is leading to partnerships between occupational therapists and professionals from what might have previously been considered to be disparate professions, including architects, designers, artists and engineers. Examples of current projects include a reconsideration of the housing needs of older people, improving the design of household items so that they are both acceptable and meet the needs of older users, and redesigning transport systems.

Pointers for practice

- Examine your own personal attitudes towards ageing, and consider their origins.
- Become aware of the various living situations of older people within your own community.
- Become alert to policy-led initiatives aimed at older people and track how they are being translated locally.
- Observe the contributions made by older people towards community life, and the impact of any policy-led initiatives to increase involvement.
- Consider the policy, community and societal contexts within which services are developed.
- Take opportunities to work with other professions and disciplines to improve the quality of life of all older people in our society.

CHAPTER 2

Growing older: an individual experience

New societal attitudes suggest that older age can be a time of new experiences and growth for the individual, and that in turn older people can continue to contribute to society. However, this change in thinking and emphasis demands commitment from all sectors of society, including older people themselves.

> A great challenge for health care providers, researchers and elders is how to ensure that the quality of individual and family life can be maintained during the extended lifespan. (Jackson et al., 2001, p. 5)

Continued involvement in society demands that older people remain actively engaged. This chapter considers the individual experiences of older people in our society, putting the policies and initiatives described in Chapter 1 into a personal context. Theories and research concerning quality of life are used as well as the experiences of older people themselves. Quality of life in older age is then considered in the context of the part played by occupation in maintaining and sustaining independence and lifestyle choices.

The heterogeneity of older people

Chapter 1 briefly described the various generations that, within our society, all fall within the rubric of older people. Aside from age, a range of other factors also results in difference between individuals, for example culture, gender, religious orientation and previous and current life roles. These factors continually shape alternative lifestyles, beliefs and expectations for human beings at all stages of the life course. Given the long-standing tendency within Western society to herd older people together in homogeneous groups and negate this diversity, this difference is worth underscoring. In her work on living a meaningful existence in older age, Jackson (1996) discussed the need to value the 'richness of a lifetime's experiences' of older age as well as placing appropriate recognition upon physical limitations that inevitably accompany increasing years. White (1998) reported an ethnographic study to explore the health practices, attitudes and beliefs of older people in good health from different ethnic groups living in America. These were black, Hispanic, Vietnamese and white rural and city groups. Drawing upon the highly individual perspectives raised during this small study, White made the following statement:

> As we grow older we become more diverse, rather than more alike. ... Knowing the range of diversity that exists among old people, therapists can seek this information when engaged in treatment planning so that decisions that can be made are the most relevant to individual needs and cultural heritage. (White, 1998, p. 12)

The above point is an important one given that the denial of individuality in older age is often pronounced when people become consumers of health and social care services.

As described in Chapter 1, the numbers of older people from ethnic minorities resident in Great Britain are small but growing, as the population who emigrated in the 1950s and 1960s age (DoH and SSI, 1998). Mountain and Moore (1995) found that cultural influences shaped both expectations and experiences of quality of life. This group can find the British way of life difficult, as illustrated by the observation of an older woman, recounting her perceptions of the differences between Sikh and English methods of child rearing:

> Their thinking is different because during childhood their children start to go out, they receive their pocket money ... whereas our children don't. Here give and take is too much.

Therefore the experience of older age is an individual one. This understanding is at the heart of forthcoming discussions about how to maintain a full and fulfilled life in old age.

Life and health expectancy

Much has been written about the consequences of the increasing numbers of older people in our society. A less recognized reality is that medical advances are leading to the numbers of older people in good health also being larger than ever before. The previous chapter described the current emphasis being placed upon the citizenship of older people and the contributions that older people in good health can make. Government policies are encouraging the perception of older people as a resource to be drawn upon by society. A population study of older people in nine European countries by de Jong-Gierveld and van Solinge (1995) contradicted the commonly held belief that old age inevitably leads to infirmity. Most people are expected to live a well older age due to improvements in health care, which have eradicated or lessened the prevalence of acute infectious diseases. However, de Jong-Gierveld and van Solinge (1995) also projected an increased demand for services based upon the shift from acute infectious diseases to chronic conditions.

There is an ongoing debate about the effects upon individuals of increasing average life expectancy. Will it lead to improvements in life quality and shortening of the period of illness and disability before death, or an extended period of debility and dependency? In other words will *life* expectancy equate with *health* expectancy? Khaw (1997) raised another consideration in balancing life expectancy and health expectancy. He observed that the majority of chronic disabling conditions, which limit healthy life expectancy, could be postponed or prevented, citing cardiovascular disease and osteoporosis as examples. Therefore if the full potential of preventive strategies could be realized, the increase in chronic conditions in older people projected by de Jong-Gierveld and van Solinge (1995) would be lessened. Khaw emphasized the need for a greater focus upon health promotion and prevention, taking into account factors like environment and income.

The views of this person emphasized the importance of maintaining health in older age.

> It's all right when you get older and your health is all right. You've no problems. Then old age is good and you can enjoy it.

The term 'compression of morbidity' means that life expectancy will have an upper limit, but that the onset of illness and disability can be prevented (Fries, 1980, quoted in Henwood, 1999). Therefore improvement of health in older age and compression of morbidity should be a health policy goal. (Health promotion and prevention is an increasingly important aspect of the work of occupational therapists working with older people, and is considered in depth in Chapter 8.)

Another aspect contributing to the experience of health in older age is the effect of age upon psychological well-being. We are all aware of the effects of physical factors like brain degeneration upon cognitive ability, but do other factors come into play to affect personality and attitude? Through a consideration of the evidence concerned with the psychology of human ageing, Coleman (1990) concluded that biological ageing has limited effect upon psychological functioning, with social and environmental factors, attitudes and interests being more influential. Thus older age for many of us can be a productive, enjoyable period of our life.

Quality of life

For the majority of older people, hopes and plans for the future will be closely related to their perceptions of how quality of life can be sustained following retirement, and hopefully enhanced. Because it means different things to different people, quality of life is a difficult concept to explain and measure. While workers struggle to reach agreement about how to define and measure quality of life, there is consensus regarding contributory factors in older age. These include health, disability, environment, involvement in meaningful occupations, income, extent of social contact and personality.

> It is the minutiae of life which form the major component of life experience and play the central role in determining the individual's life character and quality. (Wenger, 1984, p. 11)

It has been said that quality of life is the modern counterpart of the *good life*. Powell Lawton (1983) looked at the factors in older age that contribute to a good life. He identified the following three dimensions:

1. psychological well-being;
2. perceived quality of life, including housing and neighbourhood, use of time and family and friends;
3. the objective environment, as distinct from the way that a person perceives their environment.

Sinclair et al. (1990) used the following three dimensions to explore quality of life:

1. ability to solve practical problems;
2. involvement in a social life and the extent to which the individual is lonely;
3. overall satisfaction with life, together with mental health.

It is also generally agreed that dimensions of quality of life are a combination of life experiences and the conditions within which those experiences took place (George and Bearon, 1980). Therefore the past lifestyle of a person cannot be divorced from expectations of quality of life. Meaningful leisure is essential to quality of life (Csikszentmihalyi, 1993). Occupations that are demanding and enjoyable are of far greater value than passive recreation like watching television. Csikszentmihalyi (1993) also suggested that problems could arise from the extent of unstructured, as opposed to structured, leisure time.

Research into the quality of life of older people (Mountain and Moore, 1995) revealed a number of common themes. Those interviewed ranged from those who were physically well and involved in the community to those who were housebound and reliant on others for a once-a-week outing, as well as a group who had got together because they were all bereaved. The composition of the groups is given in more detail in Appendix 1.

One important issue that emerged was that growing older could have some benefits.

You've got more sense when you get older.

As you get older you get more and more damned independent. You don't care what other people think!

... you can also express yourself a lot more because you've learnt a lot in the course of your life.

However, this was contingent upon maintenance of health and having sufficient income.

You can please yourself what you do if you are well enough.

Research conducted by Clark et al. (1996) identified the following ten quality-of-life domains for 29 older people in good health, living in a low-income area of Los Angeles, with the importance of the areas being those attributed by the older people interviewed:

1. activities of daily living;
2. adaptations to a multi-cultural environment;
3. use of free time;
4. spirituality;
5. maintenance of health;
6. maintenance of mobility;
7. personal finances;
8. personal safety;
9. psychological well-being and happiness;
10. relationships with others.

The authors pointed out that these domains were specific to the situations of the group of older people interviewed and therefore could not be generalized to other settings.

However, a review of the practical application of this typology to occupational therapy with older adults undertaken by Wood (1996) demonstrated its value in helping practitioners to move away from an approach confined to promotion of activities of daily living and mobility.

Research by Lau et al. (1998) examined perceptions of quality of life of a small group of older Chinese people living in Hong Kong through focus group interviews. It was significant that those interviewed were not familiar with the term 'quality of life' but related to the expression 'a good life'. In other respects the findings mirrored the multi-dimensional construct of quality of life uncovered in studies of older people from Western societies. Differences were found in the relative importance of the factors, for example the significance attributed to social relationships (including social eating) and economic well-being.

Some of the factors that Mountain and Moore (1995) found to be influential in the actual and perceived quality of life of older people living in a UK urban setting also echoed many of the domains identified by Clarke et al. (1996). They included the following.

Transport

The availability of cheap public transport was a key factor in enabling a social life as well as helping people to undertake necessary tasks like shopping. Some people stated that the infrequent public transport system prevented them from getting out and about. Others were more resourceful.

> Well nowadays there's an Access bus and anybody that can't go to town, they can get on the Access bus and it's free and they wait for you and bring you back, so that's not so bad.

Finances

The past lifestyle of the individual could not be separated from prevailing expectations. Thus, if a person had never had money to spend, then surviving on a pension did not predominate in determining quality of life. Some of the older people interviewed were financially comfortable whereas others were coping on a minimal income. Those without much money were determined to cope. There was general agreement that money was not as important as having health and happiness, but on the other hand, it can give the individual more choice. Regret was expressed over leisure and social occupations that had to be abandoned because of lack of adequate finance.

> Probably a lot more people would be more adventurous if they could afford to do what they wanted to do.

> By the time you've paid your way there's very little left to do the other things that make life worth while. And that's where I feel people are being deprived.

For more disabled participants, the cost of paid help like gardening was an issue.

Housing

Some of the older people interviewed had moved house. One person interviewed had moved into sheltered housing from a house where she had spent all her married life. Her family arranged the move, and although she was aware of the reasons why it had been necessary, she was not happy with it.

> I didn't want to go. I didn't want to move. When you can't walk and you've a lot of steps you have to move.

Those who had moved into sheltered housing could appreciate both the benefits, like the on-call warden, alarm system and lack of stairs, as well as the drawbacks like restrictions upon pet ownership.

Use of leisure time

Sedentary occupations within the home like television and reading were the most commonly cited leisure interests. Some women went to bingo, one of the few social activities that it was perceived that a woman could attend alone. Knitting, crocheting, reading and telephoning friends were also mentioned. For some women, being able to continue with household tasks was a pleasure. Some older people felt that lack of opportunities to carry out leisure interests in earlier life was one reason for current limitations.

> I think the important thing is to have an interest, a pastime that we can spend more time with now than when we could in our working lives. But many of us I'm afraid do not have an interest like that.

Crime and fear of crime

One of the most striking and consistent features of the interviews with older people living in a big city was fear of crime and the self-enforcement of a night-time curfew, particularly for those without their own transport. The predominant view was that going out in the evening was risky, even in the summer.

> You daren't go out at night ... we get a taxi. We daren't walk, not round where we live.

It was unusual to set aside this fear of crime. Sometimes, however, the choice was made to balance perceived risks with quality of life.

> I wouldn't go to town and be there at ten o'clock at night. I do go out at night if I have to be somewhere, because I'm starting a class next Wednesday so I will go out.

The experiences of older people living in an area of high crime illustrated the importance of social and care networks in trying to offset both the fear and reality of crime.

> I mean on an estate like this you know all the villains there are!

However, living in an area with a high crime rate ultimately had an adverse effect upon life quality. Limitations were described variously, for example refusing invitations, not being able to go on holiday and giving up car ownership due to continual vandalism. The general view of these older people was that the situation was continuing to deteriorate and continual vigilance was necessary.

> At one time they used to rob you but they wouldn't hurt you but now they hurt you so you're best letting them take what they want and go.

Life circumstances

Those interviewed described a number of life circumstances that could impact upon quality of life. Bereavement and its consequences were frequently raised.

> Retirement's good, isn't it … if you've got your partner retirement's good. But otherwise then you're lonely when you lose them.

> I think that when you go in and you close that door, the fact that you know that nobody is coming in after you makes a difference.

Empty weekends could be a problem:

> At the weekend there isn't much to do, when you've to stop in on a Saturday and Sunday.

Others raised the impact of ill health within marriage:

> It depends upon your luck doesn't it – whether it's companionship or disablement.

The effects of life circumstances, though still apparent, were less dominant in those individuals with a more active lifestyle who had greater expectations of life quality. However, as individuals became disabled, extraneous circumstances could have a big impact upon quality of life. Ultimately, increased disability led to lowered expectations and resignation, for example acceptance of the wait for community equipment to assist with showering or bathing.

Spirituality

The Sikh women were the only group to speak about religious beliefs in any depth. The importance of the temple was strongly expressed in several contexts. The temple is the place where an older person can go at any time. However, strong religious beliefs stay with an individual whether or not they are able to get to the temple. This was also the only group to talk philosophically about the life course and mortality. Death was discussed openly and without fear.

> Now I have passed so many days ... you never know when you will fall asleep. Breath will leave you any time.

Lack of fear of death was related to strong religious beliefs, with attendance at the Gurdwara being seen as preparation for death.

> I only want that God should take me for worshipping in the Gurdwara.

More recently, Coleman (2002) has reported research on spiritual beliefs in later life. Through the exploration of the experiences of 28 recently bereaved older people over a two-year period he concluded that those with a strong sense of spiritual belief were less likely to experience depression and other mental health problems following the death of their spouse.

Fears for the future

Those older people interviewed by Mountain and Moore who were fit and well expressed fears for the future when faculties would begin to deteriorate.

> I think well at least if I've got my mind still able to cope then I've got something. I know I'm not just going to sit there and vegetate.

It was also recognized that increasing disability would incur cost, for example paying for transport and paying for care.

> But very soon I won't be able to walk because it's uphill ... so then I'll have to start worrying about transport. When you worry about transport, finance comes into it.

Additionally, given the greater numbers of older women than men, issues specifically affecting women were expressed in some of the groups.

> Wherever you go there's always more women than men. I mean it's a fact of life that women reach old age and men don't. You go anywhere and there's always more women than men.

Relationships

Continued close and intimate relationships in older age are undeniably as important a constituent of quality of life for older people as they are for the rest of the adult population. However, this aspect was not captured during focus group interviews with older people (Mountain and Moore, 1995). The reasons for this can only be postulated. First, a group discussion is less likely to lead to discussions of topics perceived to be personal in nature. Secondly, an older person having sexual relations does not equate with popular societal images even though it is recognized as being a central part of the adult human experience. Common negative stereotypes are encapsulated through ageist humour and the notion that sex is the province of younger generations. One reason put forward is the childish social status often given to older people (Hockey and James, 1993). A paper by Marshall (1997) describing the incidence of HIV and AIDS in older people also put paid to the myth that older people are asexual. There has been a dramatic increase in the incidence of sexually transmitted disease in older people. As well as correcting inaccurate perceptions on the part of society that sexual activity ceases at the age of 60, health and social care professionals should provide information to older people (Pointon, 1997). Marshall (1997) also identified the need for a more proactive, rational approach, concluding that ageist attitudes were preventing homosexual older people from receiving adequate medical care, information and education, and thereby putting them at risk. An earlier paper by Rickard (1995) drew attention to the same problems faced by homosexual older men, and referred to a 1993 Age Concern profile to raise attention to the problem termed 'a crisis of silence'. This campaign serves as a reminder of the fact that homosexuality used to be a crime in the eyes of the law. More recently Age Concern have developed a practice guide based upon this work. 'Opening Doors' aims both to challenge stereotypes and provide guidelines for best practice when working with homosexual older people.

Normal adaptations in older age

All of us continue to make adaptations throughout our lifetime in line with changing circumstances. In older age, this requirement becomes more pronounced. Some of the adaptations that people may expect to make in older age are given below. It must be emphasized that the sectioning of different types of adaptation is to aid clarity. However, in reality the individual may well be coping with a number of adaptive processes concurrently, for example increasing disability alongside bereavement.

Adapting to loss of employment

The structure of Western society confers certain benefits to the employed. These include personal identity, status and respect, financial reward and a structure to daily life. If it were possible most people would choose to retain these benefits in retirement. Furthermore, unemployment can have adverse effects upon health and relationships (Kendall, 1996). Therefore the extent of personal resource required to manage loss of employment is usually significant.

Adaptation to the change brought about by the cessation of employment usually starts well before the event. Studies have been conducted to examine the occupational transitions arising from retirement. A qualitative study conducted in Sweden by Jonsson et al. (2000) explored the views of 15 men and 14 women who were nearing or had just reached retirement. Analysis showed that retirement had a substantial impact upon the lives of those interviewed. The majority enjoyed the freedom offered by retirement but also expressed a desire to continue to be productive in their lives. Aspects of work that would be missed included social contacts and belonging, being part of a larger whole, use of one's knowledge and capabilities, income, being productive and having an external structure to life. Negative aspects were boring work and routines, undesirable changes to the workplace and workforce, stress and responsibility. Lack of freedom was the most frequently mentioned negative factor regarding employment. The preparedness of the person to cope is a further factor; hence the existence of courses to help people plan for retirement with the aim of easing the transition from a life of work and regular income to that of pensions and leisure. The work of Jonsson et al. (1997) emphasized the uniqueness of each individual's work experience and perceptions of that experience. In 1995, in discussions with older people about their quality of life, Mountain and Moore found that regret was also expressed at no longer being able to be part of the job market. Certain individuals still felt that they had something to offer and would have liked the opportunity to enhance their income. The lack of preparation for retirement was also raised.

> I mean what they could do to me, with a lot of people, you know this cut-off point, they could say at 60 or 65 or even before, they could start easing people off, you know instead of doing a full week. Like maybe doing only half a week and winding them down to retirement age instead of having them work full time one day and the next day that's it, they're finished, or even let them go part-time after they've retired, if they feel up to it.

Adapting to retirement

The cessation of paid employment is associated with retirement. This is a landmark in a person's life and a time of occupational adjustment. Whenever it occurs in a person's life it is a significant event, both for the individual and their family, heralding a time of great change.

After a lifetime of employment, retirement can be eagerly anticipated or it can be dreaded. It gives rise to increased leisure time while at the same time it results in a greatly reduced income for some. It is also accompanied by having to relinquish the status of worker. For the wives of men who have retired, there may need to be a realigning of the long-standing division of labour in the home. However, there is no direct causal relationship between certain predisposing factors and smooth transition from worker to retiree (Kendall, 1996). Jeffers (1995) examined how previously employed people structured their days immediately following retirement. Observations suggested that retirement did not lead to any significant changes to daily routine. However, the types of activity being carried out during certain times of the day were work-like in origin. Voluntary work can also substitute for work:

> You feel that at least you're doing something when you've stopped work. I think it's more noticeable if you've had a job up to retiring. You just need to be doing something to keep yourself going.

Underlying the life course and the events that shape it, are the expectations we all have of our own retirement. We may plan to travel, undertake pastimes denied to us due to the demands of paid work, share interests with our partner, care for our grandchildren, or undertake voluntary work. Alternatively, there are people who do not plan ahead in this way, perhaps because they wish life to continue in the same manner as before, or because they have set aside the consequences of their older age.

Adapting to loss

It is often said that older age and loss are synonymous, for example role loss, the loss of lifelong partners, the loss of income, loss of health or loss of independence. Some types of loss are also subjected to personal interpretation; for example, some women who have spent most of their lives looking after others enjoy their newly found freedom when at last released from the caring role. In comparison, others are overwhelmed by this change and do not know how to spend their time.

Mountain and Moore (1995) found that a substantial number of the older people they interviewed mentioned the devastating effects of bereavement upon life quality. Being left without a partner in retirement was a life event that was not anticipated. Death of a lifelong partner results in loss at different levels, extending from love and companionship to the more practical aspects of life. Some people described long marriages where the practical and companionship needs of husband and wife had been inextricably linked. Therefore loss of a spouse resulted in a completely changed lifestyle. The consequences included feelings of isolation, loneliness and an inability to mix socially. Not having anyone to describe the events of the day to was an illustration of the long-term, continuing effects of an enforced single life. The importance of companionship provided through marriage was described thus:

> You've got to have a person to share your life with, to enjoy even the garden. When you've done the garden, you've nobody to share it with. There's no sharing.

A frequently reiterated point was that, once bereaved, everyone else appeared to be enjoying their retirement with their partners. For many of those left alone, taking holidays alone was too problematic to contemplate and therefore did not occur. Even trips out from home were a great challenge. The views of the women with whom we spoke indicated that their experiences differed from that of men. In more than one group it was said that it is more difficult for them to develop a new social life; they cannot go to a public house alone or out in the evening.

> My lifestyle has altered since I lost my husband, definitely.

Chambers (1994) used the life history interview to explore the lives of five older women who had been widowed. This research method is closely allied to the Occupational Performance Interview described by Kielhofner et al. (1989) (see Chapter 6 on assessment). The life history interview involves allowing the respondent to tell the story of their life on their own terms. This method of enquiry has great value when used with older people. It can enable the person to describe their past and current lives and present coping strategies. This can throw light upon why and how an individual copes, or alternatively fails to manage significant events like the death of a spouse. Chambers (1994) concluded that the portrayal of widows as lonely and vulnerable could result in the perpetuation of negative attitudes towards this phase of life. This can prevent the individual from exploring their new state and adopting a positive approach. Nevertheless, some of the statements made by older bereaved people in the study by Mountain and Moore (1995) underscored the real difficulties that widowhood brings.

Bereavement also has financial implications, particularly for women who have never worked:

First of all when I retired I was really angry when I saw that it's considered that a woman only needs about half what a man does to live on to start with even though you've been paying your stamps. Secondly, now as a widow you find that your standard of life has gone down completely in money terms.

Adapting to lowered physical abilities

I think that you still expect to be able to do, and carry on, the same as you did when you were younger. I think you forget.

Clark et al. (1996) raised the use of adaptive strategies as a means of maintaining control. Therefore if an older person is no longer able to undertake certain activities of daily living themselves, strategies to enable them to remain in control can help to maintain independence and feelings of satisfaction. The example used by Clark et al. was that of shopping where control might be maintained through use of the Internet and catalogues or by asking friends to help. Other examples quoted elsewhere in this book include the use of technology to assist with independence around the home and implementation of direct payments to frail older people by social services whereby they are able to purchase their own care. Mountain and Moore (1995) found that people made adjustments so that participation in certain occupations could be maintained, for example using large-print books, shopping little and often, using equipment to assist with activities of daily living, and taking more care with mobility.

You've got to sit down and do things whereas normally you would have just stood up to do it.

Older people in good health interviewed by Mountain and Moore (1995) mentioned having hobbies in reserve for a less active time of life.

I have a strong interest in old Leeds and old Bramley and I collect pictures, articles about it. There's loads and loads of those things I've stored away that I haven't read yet.

One man who had been a keen gardener had adapted his interest from working on other people's gardens to providing plant cuttings for people as he became older.

For the more able, health problems were linked to being prevented from carrying out leisure and DIY occupations like recreational walking, gardening and home maintenance.

One of the biggest problems of growing older is the frustration of not being able to do ordinary things. I used to decorate my house and do all the

> repairs ... I'm having a man in to decorate my front room and I'm so frustrated at having to pay him quite a sum of money to do something that five or six years ago I could have done myself.

Occupational adaptations included doing shopping more frequently and compromising on previous standards around the home and garden. It might also require a realignment of long-standing tasks between spouses:

> Well he used to do a lot of my carrying but he can't do much now. I have to give him a bag with just a few light things in and I'm stuck with two heavy bags myself.

Physical frailty can lead to certain recreational activities having to be relinquished altogether.

> I used to be a big dancer but I can't dance now because my legs won't let me – otherwise I would be the first up.

Housebound older people interviewed by Mountain and Moore (1995) explained how they had learnt to adapt to their lowered abilities, for example sitting down to tasks like personal washing, ironing and baking, and using mobility equipment around the home.

> A lot of elderly people, if they can't get in the bath they'll just have a wash down, they adapt. Although they don't like it but that's the best they can do if they don't have a shower.

As physical abilities diminish, increasing cost can be a factor.

> When you've got deteriorating health as well, it means that things that you want to do cost more.

For many older people, the implications of diminishing physical skills on their ability to maintain their homes can result in considerations of whether they are able to stay there or move to different accommodation. For some the need to move can be a natural progression whereas for others the emotional ties of their house can make such a decision extremely painful.

Jackson (1996) explored the occupational adaptations made by 20 community-living, disabled, older people in America who had formed themselves into a group of health care advocates. All were white with varying degrees of physical, cognitive and emotional impairment. They therefore had to manage the ageing process alongside disability. Data collection methods included observation of the group, and individual semi-structured taped interviews with a sample of the group selected on the basis of different living situations. Jackson described their adaptation as frequently being:

a subtle and continuous challenge, requiring constant negotiations between resources and limitations against a background of personal meaning. (Jackson, 1996, p. 345)

Jackson found that themes of meaning underpinned strategies for organizing both present and past events by participants, and for shaping present patterns of activity. Religion was a commonly expressed underpinning theme. Others included care giving, generosity, creativity and family bonds. Despite their disabilities, regular opportunities were sought by individuals to express their personal themes. All participants expressed a desire to remain engaged and all wished from time to time to rise to the challenge of being involved in a new activity. More time had to be allowed for established routines to be undertaken, and in particular to accommodate any new occupations.

Occupation in older age

The previously described interviews with older people about their quality of life confirmed that how they occupied their time was very important. The adaptations people make in older age to enable continued participation in occupation illustrate the centrality of what people do and how this translates to perceptions of self. Nelson observed this relationship thus:

The human being can attain enhanced health and quality of life by actively doing things that are personally meaningful and purposeful. (Nelson, 1997, p. 11)

Nelson pointed out that the strength of this purpose is that it is so fundamental.

Occupation or purposeful activity is a central aspect of the human experience (Wilcock, 1993). Occupation has been interpreted as what people do in their everyday lives (AOTA, 1995); therefore work, leisure and play are within the domain of occupation. The complexity of the construct, and its purpose and meaning for the individual, distinguish occupation from activity, which according to Golledge (1998) does not have personal meaning for the individual. Another interpretation was provided by Wilcock (1999), who described occupation as the fundamental process of being and doing and becoming in everyday life, and as such is essential.

Nelson (1988) postulated that occupation embraces occupational form, occupational structure and occupational performance. Occupational form describes the setting within which occupation takes place and includes the physical environment as well as interpretations made by the individual of the actions that might be taken within the setting. Occupational structure is the person's abilities, skills, attributes, emotional state and cognitive abilities, with these factors being dynamic rather than static over time. Occupational performance is the process of undertaking an occupation. The importance of Nelson's work for occupational therapists and other professionals working with older people is the description of the complexity underpinning the observable actions.

Occupational balance was defined by Wilcock (1993) as a state of well-being in which the individual fully exercises their mental, physical and spiritual capacities so that mind, body and spirit also have time for sufficient reflection and rest. Well-being is achieved through choice of occupation and the experience of meeting occupational challenges incurred in the process.

Occupation is a common thread running through different aspects of maintenance of, anticipation of, and adaptations to, lifestyle in older age. Some theorists previously promoted the notion of disengagement in older age whereby people voluntarily relinquish occupations and responsibilities while still experiencing a satisfying older age. The original research leading to disengagement theory by Cumming and Henry (1961) involved research on 279 people aged between 50 and 90 years. They used the data to argue that social disengagement is a natural outcome of older age, with the consequence that new roles for older people following retirement are neither sought nor required. Critics of this theory are extremely vocal in their condemnation.

> It provided a scientific rationale for the new twentieth century practice of retirement from the labour force. It justified a rocking chair lifestyle, and placement of housing schemes for older people on the periphery of towns and cities, away in the peace and quiet ... It was a peculiarly dangerous form of theory because of its potential of becoming a self-fulfilling prophecy. If we expect and demand less of people because they are old, they are likely to conform to this expectation. (Coleman, 1990, pp. 77–8)

The activity theory posed by Havighurst and Albrecht in 1953 suggested that the more active older people continue to be, the greater their life satisfaction, and that people seek replacement occupations for work in retirement. Fontana (1977) introduced a classification of retired people by their levels and type of activity, identifying the following groups:

- *Relaxers*: people who choose activity because of the enjoyment it will give them.
- *Do-gooders*: those who undertake unpaid work, which can be likened to paid work from the perspective of the time and effort involved.
- *Joiners*: those who seek organized activity in group settings.
- *Waiters*: people who have given up and either do little or fill their time with minor tasks.

The simplistic nature of both disengagement theory and activity theory fails to address the true complexities that exist, illustrated through the later work of Wilcock, Nelson and other academics. Stanley (1995) used the literature to discuss the validity of the activity theory, describing two of the arguments against the theory. First, both activity levels and life satisfaction tend to be greater for those in good health. Second, decreased activity in older age can also be attributed to external factors like income.

What then are the factors that enable some to cope successfully with the process of growing older, and continue to engage in a range of occupations, while others experience continued difficulty and limit their involvement? The cessation of paid work or a role caring for others can offer opportunities for increased leisure. Alternatively, the continuance of life interests may become impossible due to infirmity, which for some will accompany increasing age. However, the reasons why some people remain fulfilled cannot be explained by physical well-being alone. Attitude and mental well-being also play a significant part. Why a person chooses to continue with certain occupations in older age, engage in certain new occupations or, alternatively, disengage is complex and poorly understood. Nevertheless, the importance of occupation as a central contributor towards quality of life is evident.

The current focus upon the fundamental and curative effects of occupation has been shaped by factors within the profession of occupational therapy as well as external to it (Whiteford et al., 2000). Academic interest in occupation has developed into the discipline of occupational science. This was defined by Yerxa et al. (1990) as being located in the understanding that humans are occupational beings, with the drive to be occupied being a fundamental one with evolutionary, psychological, social and symbolic origins. The comparatively early work of Nelson in describing the meaning and purpose of occupation, and the relationships with environment, is clearly related to some of the more recent thinking underpinning occupational science.

Jackson (1996) unpacked the concept of occupational science thus:

1. People do not make occupational choices in isolation. Choices are based upon a complex range of individual and society-driven values.
2. Occupations have symbolic significance for the individual. This is illustrated through a paper on tea drinking by Hannan (1997) in which she identifies six shared meanings for tea drinking which extend far beyond the occupation itself.
3. The human being is able to adapt in response to new occupational challenges.

Occupational justice and occupational deprivation are two further concepts developed by Wilcock, which are of particular relevance to older people. Occupational justice is concerned with the distribution of services, resources and opportunities in recognition of the diversity of people's occupational needs. Occupational deprivation describes external circumstances that prevent a person from acquiring, using or enjoying something, with limitations sometimes being imposed by external agencies. While occupational deprivation has been most frequently described in the context of prison life (Whiteford, 1997), it can also occur in treatment and care settings for older people.

An ever-increasing number of academic papers examining dimensions of occupation and describing theories of occupation is evidence of the resurgence of interest in occupation, both as an important concept underpinning occupational science and as a topic for theory and practice development. A few examples of the literature are given in Table 2.1 to illustrate the diversity that exists.

The acknowledged importance of occupation for human beings and the interplay between occupation and other factors like quality of life has led to a number of theories. Theory development has in turn resulted in

Table 2.1 Examples of academic papers and research into occupation

Authors	Paper and year of publication	Contribution
Whiteford, Townsend, Hocking	2000: Reflections upon a renaissance of occupation	Influence of occupation on post-modernism and occupational therapy
Wilcock	1999: Reflections on doing, being and becoming	The relationship between occupation and health and well-being
Hannan	1997: More than a cup of tea: meaning construction in an everyday activity	The meanings and values underlying the everyday occupations like that of tea making
Kielhofner, Forsyth	1997: The model of human occupation: an overview of current concepts	Overview of concepts to explain how human occupation is motivated, organized, performed and influenced by the environment
Jackson	1996: Living a meaningful existence in old age	Occupational adaptation in older age

Table 2.1 (contd)

Authors	Paper and year of publication	Contribution
Stanley	1995: An investigation into the relationship between engagement in valued occupations and life satisfaction for elderly South Africans	An exploration of the relationship between occupation and well-being in older age
Christiansen	1994: Classification and study in occupation: a review and discussion of taxonomies	Builds taxonomies of occupation drawn from the psychological, sociological and vocational literature as a means of increasing understanding
Yerxa et al.	1990: An introduction to occupational science: a foundation for occupational therapy in the 21st century	Describes how occupational science can support the practice of occupational therapy
Nelson	1988: Occupation: form and performance	Describes the relationship between occupational form (the context within which occupation takes place) and occupational performance

research to explore their validity as well as leading to the development of practical applications. However, the complexity of occupation has limited the extent of research undertaken to date. The theory of human occupation (Kielhofner, 1985) described the human being as an open system which interacts constantly with the external environment. The theory suggested that there are three overarching subsystems within the human, namely: volition, which is responsible for choice; habituation, which is concerned with roles and habits; and performance or occupational skills.

Burton (1989) applied the model of human occupation to an examination of the evidence base concerned with normal ageing, and drew a number of conclusions, some of which do not conform with the stereotypic picture of abilities in older age. The conclusions drawn from the literature are shown in Table 2.2.

The most interesting implications concern the evidence regarding performance. The body of evidence reviewed suggests that communication skills remain intact except when disrupted by illness. The picture painted by Burton is therefore one of continued ability to be able to learn and adapt to changing circumstances. The fact that older people are the most

Table 2.2 Summary of findings of a review of evidence on normal ageing

Subsystem	Research evidence concerned with normal ageing
Volition	• Little evidence of lowered self-esteem except following sudden loss • A desire for more control than there is perceived to be • A tendency to both underestimate and overestimate abilities • Dwelling on the past is common in depression • Occupational tasks have different values for individuals • Leisure interests positively correlate with life satisfaction
Habituation	• Role loss increases the importance of leisure and social roles • Institutional routines disrupt the balance of work, rest and leisure • Maintenance of routines by the individual is important, but there is also evidence of adaptation in response to changing circumstances
Performance	• Communication skills remain intact except when disrupted by illness • Perceptual motor skills can slow down • Learning is important and while it takes longer, it is not impaired • Problem-solving is good if within the context of familiar situations

rapidly increasing group of users of the Internet demonstrates this ability to learn and develop new skills.

Lifestyle, well-being and occupation

Occupation and lifestyle are broadly similar processes, including regular participation in activities, habits and social interactions. Lambert (1998) defined lifestyle thus:

> The pattern of life adopted by the individual, or group which is influenced by the resources available to them ... specific elements include fluid intake, diet, physical exercise and rest. (Lambert, 1998, p. 194)

Wellness has been described as a lifestyle for well-being, or leading to optimal well-being (White, 1998). There is increasing acknowledgement of the importance of maintaining a healthy balance between work, rest and play. Intuitive links between occupation, health and well-being are being acknowledged despite the limitations of the current evidence base (Ilott and Mounter, 2000). The role of occupation in promoting health was acknowledged within the Ottowa Charter for Health Promotion (WHO et al., 1986), referred to further in Chapter 8.

Research by Stanley (1995) examined the relationship between occupation and well-being in a sample of older people living in South Africa. Results supported the complexity of the interplay between different factors in determining involvement in occupations; for example, the involvement in necessary activities of daily living may not give great satisfaction and yet not being able to perform them emphasized the importance of the activity. Her study did not support the existence of a relationship between participation in certain social occupations and increasing life satisfaction.

Routines in older age can make the occurrence of certain occupations more likely, particularly if others are involved. Ludwig (1997) examined the importance of routine for seven middle-class white older women, who were all well at the time of study. Data collection methods included in-depth interviews, autobiographies and observation. Results found that the women had all adapted their routines over time and had willingly given up some of their previous routines when they could no longer be conducted to a personally acceptable standard. In particular, helping older people to link their past to their current lifestyle is important for continuity and to promote a sense of well-being. Significantly, Ludwig found that the demands of health interventions could replace or interrupt long-standing occupation, leading to loss of meaning and ultimately depressed mood.

Several studies undertaken in different countries have demonstrated the existence of links between the extent of activity a person engages in and their survival, but they have been focused upon physical activities only. One exception is a longitudinal study to look at the links between social and productive occupations and survival, reported by Glass et al. (1999). The research commenced in 1982 with the recruitment of 2761 men and women aged over 65 years living in America. Baseline data included socio-demographic information, health status and participation in 14 occupations during the previous month. These were grouped into social activities like church attendance, going to restaurants and bingo; productive activities like gardening, shopping and unpaid work; and physical activities like walking and other forms of physical exercise. Results of a complex analysis showed that those who were least active overall were more likely to die than those who were more active. However, it also revealed that participation in occupations to promote social engagement was also strongly associated with survival, supporting the notion that this aspect is at least of equal importance to physical exercise. Chapters 7 and 8 take the important themes identified in this and previous sections forward into occupational therapy practice.

A framework for making decisions about involvement in occupations

A complex mix of intrinsic and extrinsic factors will determine whether or not an older person engages in an occupation. They include perceived and actual physical and mental abilities, habits and routines, the restrictions imposed due to living on a pension, transport, previous education experiences and expectations. Additionally, involvement will be shaped by what the individual perceives to be the right responses within any given setting. Christiansen (1994) discussed the value of developing a taxonomy of occupation, describing a number of such classifications from different bodies of literature. His paper confirms that a simple paradigm cannot reflect the complexity of occupation. However, it can begin to help us to make sense of some of the factors that shape the decisions taken by older people. Involvement will be influenced to some extent by the following:

1. *What we have to do*: Occupations which the individual must engage in to manage their daily life independently, for example personal care, shopping and cooking, financial and household management.
2. *What we choose to do*: Occupations that a person chooses to be involved in rather than being essential to maintain independent life, for example social activities, hobbies and leisure, travel, religious activities.
3. *Maintaining our roles*: Occupations which stem from the adoption of specific roles of recognized societal value, for example worker, carer and volunteer.

What we have to do

If we do not have help from others, engagement in this group of occupations is essential for the maintenance of an independent lifestyle. While these occupations may not directly contribute towards a fulfilling life in themselves, inability to undertake them can severely impair quality of life and will result in admission to a setting where others can take over the undertaking of these occupations on behalf of the person. Paradoxically, admission to acute hospital settings, or to residential or nursing care, often requires the older person to relinquish many activities within this category that they might still be capable of performing.

What we choose to do

This second grouping includes the occupations stimulated by skills, interests and aspirations which, though not directly essential for maintenance of independence, are arguably essential if quality of life is to be maintained.

Some fit older people interviewed by Mountain and Moore (1995) chose to participate in lifelong learning, even though it could take courage to try a new activity:

> Well when I went on my computer course I was very hesitant at first ... I didn't feel confident at all ... I just thought 'I'm not a machine person'.

Other, less active individuals enjoyed the social atmosphere and activities offered at a day centre. An added benefit was the allaying of loneliness.

> They might come here to play bridge, but it's really the loneliness that makes them come here to play bridge ... it's to be with other people.

> I come here to lunch not because I can't make my own lunch but it's because I'm with people. At home I'm sitting on my own.

At home, television, radio and calling friends were important recreational activities for some.

> I watch television quite a lot. I read quite a lot. I go to the library for books.

> I phone friends long distance. One weekend it's one lot; another weekend it's another. And they phone me. Sometimes they go on for an hour and a quarter and the phone bill goes up but I don't mind.

There was general agreement about the benefits of keeping pets. However, it was also acknowledged that pets were not viable for those who lived in flats, or if the person could not manage the extra responsibility they demanded.

Holidays could be important. However, some older people interviewed had stopped taking holidays for a variety of reasons including being alone and not having adequate financial resources.

Maintaining our roles

The third group includes occupations undertaken to fulfil certain roles, like that of a worker, and as such can confer status in society as well as a sense of personal achievement. Mountain and Moore (1995) found that older people involved in unpaid work tended to have several interests, volunteering for a number of organizations.

> I'm a governor on two schools ... I'm also president of Horsforth Royal British Legion and I'm chairman of Bramley pensioners and I've been nominated as chairman here [another voluntary organization].

> I've got a dining room that's an office ... I'm secretary to so much.

> There are quite a lot of retired people getting involved in voluntary work.

No matter what sort of voluntary work it is, whether it's Help the Aged or Age Concern shops or something like that, you go in there and it's nearly all retired women.

The benefits of voluntary work included 'keeping your mind going' and maintaining confidence. Those involved in volunteering also acknowledged that they had more time to give than people still in work. They did not identify with vulnerable older people, viewing themselves as carers rather than cared for:

When you go to visit old people you can't just rush in and out, can you? You've got to sit down and talk to them and give them time.

Contributing towards the family life of grown-up children including caring for grandchildren and family pets was an important role for some fit older people.

I'm pretty committed to my daughter and her children ... I look after them and bring them home from school for her.

Therefore, taking into account existing academic work into the meanings of occupation, it is postulated that decisions about participation in certain occupations will be assisted by a number of nested factors. This is illustrated by Figure 2.1.

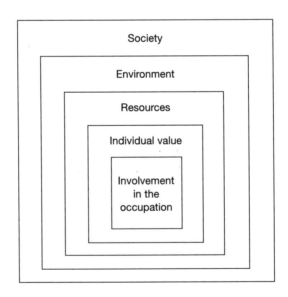

Figure 2.1 A framework within which decisions are taken about involvement in occupations.

The centre of Figure 2.1 is the occupation itself. Available evidence supports the view that the value the individual places upon different occupations, and their importance for the continuance of an independent lifestyle, provide one important context for decisions about involvement. However, participation also has to be reliant upon resources. These can be physical, like stamina and mobility, can be personal, like having the confidence to try something new or alone, or can be practical, like the availability of finance and personal assistance. Even with the necessary resources to undertake the occupation, the environment has to enable participation. The built environment can facilitate or discourage participation, as can the availability of certain conditions like good transport and recreational facilities. The perceived expectations within a certain setting will also shape the nature of involvement. If the older person wishes to embark upon an occupation not normally perceived to be within their role, it can take a great deal of personal resilience to overcome prevailing community and societal attitudes.

The paradigm is simplistic in that these groupings cannot be mutually exclusive. For some older women, continued ability to undertake household tasks is a central part of their lives, providing them with personal fulfilment. Similarly, for many people the adoption of a useful role improves their quality of life as well as giving status. However, it might assist occupational therapists and other workers to extend beyond the model of independence to one that takes into account the overall lifestyle of an individual as well as what they may aspire to.

Implications for occupational therapy

Chapters 7 and 8 on occupational therapy interventions link the issues highlighted in this chapter to desired practice.

Understand quality of life and what this means for older people

Much of the literature on quality of life of older people lies within sociological texts. Given the interplay between involvement in occupations and quality of life, it is important for this literature to be drawn on by occupational therapy practice. It is also important to talk to older people and understand their perspectives of quality of life and what they consider to be important to them.

Listen to the past lives of older people

All of us have a story to tell of our lives. It is important for us to be able to tell others our experiences, whether they be recent or in the more distant past. We do this for a variety of reasons, for example to validate ourselves, to hear the opinions of others and link our past lives to the present. All too often, this right to be heard is denied to older people, particularly when they become frail, even though they may have lived a varied and interesting life. Furthermore, past experiences make the person what they are today. If we are to understand the person, we have to allow them to express themselves in their own terms.

Link the past to the future

Research has shown that older people seek to maintain connections between their past and future, particularly after major disruptions like the onset of disability. Therefore the occupational therapist needs to be able to build upon what the older person sees as being the possibilities for the future, while drawing upon their past experiences.

Provide new occupational opportunities for older people

The previous chapter showed how the policy climate is emphasizing the contributions older people can continue to make. Occupational therapists must capitalize on these changing perceptions of society to benefit individual older people. We should not be constrained by dated views of what older people might be interested in and can achieve; for example, in the future continued employment will be a real possibility for those who wish to continue working. It is also important to acknowledge the different generations of people who are classified as being older, and their varied life experiences, as this will impact upon their interests and aspirations.

Assist older people to adapt to changing circumstances

This chapter has described the many transitions that can be necessary in older age, and the differing capacities of individuals to be able to manage these adjustments. Even the most resilient people will only be able to cope with a number of changes at the same time. This is one of the many reasons why listening to the older person is essential before any solutions can be agreed. Once the person has been given time to cope with the change, occupational therapists can be instrumental in identifying new strategies in partnership with them.

Pointers for practice

- Develop your understanding of the lifestyles of older people in good health, and the range of occupations that they engage in.

- Take time to listen to accounts of the past and current lifestyles of older people and the importance they place upon different occupations.

- If your work leads you into contact with older people from different ethnic groups, ensure familiarity with the community's expectations of these people and their customs.

- Understand the financial and other limitations constraining involvement in occupations.

- Acknowledge the contributions that older people can continue to make to society, and their lifelong learning needs.

- Extend the remit of work rehabilitation services to meet the needs of an older workforce.

CHAPTER 3

Triggers to vulnerability

The previous chapter looked at the process of normal ageing and the domains that encompass quality of life and life satisfaction for older people. It also illustrated how the process of growing older naturally incorporates a number of losses and adjustments, and the importance of listening to the past and present stories that older people have to tell.

This chapter considers the range of health and associated needs that can emerge in older age. The full and accurate interpretation of those needs in light of the individual's coping abilities and strategies can be instrumental in helping a person to get the services they need in a timely manner. This sets the scene for the description of responses from both formal and informal carers, service systems and specifically from occupational therapists within forthcoming chapters.

Concepts of vulnerability

The interplay between illness and/or disability, environment and quality of life is at the heart of occupational therapy practice with older people. Illness in older age can signal the onset of general decline. However, overall problems with coping are usually due to the consequences of illness accompanied by a number of other causal factors; for example, Sinclair et al. (1990) identified the onset of difficulties as being ill health or bereavement, leading to enforced withdrawal from life and subsequent reduction in life quality. Verbrugge (1990) quoted in Clark et al. (1996) postulated that disability equates to the gap between the capability of a person (including their coping strategies), and the demands placed upon them by their environment. Consequently a person can manage to retain a level of independence in the face of severe disability if they have good coping strategies and they live in an environment that facilitates their coping. In comparison relatively mild problems can severely impair a person with less developed strategies for coping. Living in an environment that presents barriers to continued independence will also compromise coping abilities.

The previous chapter discussed the loss that can occur in older age. If several losses are experienced in a relatively short time period, coping strategies are severely tested, and erosion of independence is more likely. It is not surprising that older people in good health tend to express fears for the future when their faculties could begin to deteriorate. This was illustrated in the quotes from older people cited in the previous chapter. This man was clearly in transition between health and frailty.

> I don't meet with many people except with this particular group and our own pensioners' group and I'm in the house a lot. I don't say that I get depressed but I get worried about stuff.

The relative significance of a number of factors in triggering or exacerbating vulnerability in older people was highlighted through interviews with older women with mental health problems (Mountain, 1998a). They were all challenged in their attempts to maintain independence in the face of mental ill health severe enough to warrant hospital admission, combined with co-existing physical illness and frailty. However, this combination of mental and physical ill health only formed part of a spectrum of difficulties that they described. Mrs KA had cancer;

> Since I've been ill – I had cancer – I haven't been very well with that, and I would say that I've more or less spent about a year in hospital ... in stages. When I came out nobody medically seemed to talk too much about things and I got really depressed and didn't want to go out much at all.

The illness had compromised her confidence as well as her physical stamina. Going out was problematic:

> Sometimes I like to walk to that gate and I change my mind. If somebody's with me I'd probably go further.

In addition to increased difficulties in undertaking activities of daily living, the effects of age and infirmity touched other areas of the women's lives, for example the ability to undertake lifelong interests. For most of the women interviewed during this study, the consequences of mental health problems like loss of confidence and lack of motivation were difficult to reconcile. Respondents used words like 'lazy' and 'guilty' to describe and criticize themselves.

Sinclair et al. (1990) suggested that dependency is interpreted in three ways by older people, namely not being able to do things for yourself, having to depend upon others and not being able to do something when you choose to do it. Dependency is therefore concerned with the nature of relationships rather than being an individual attribute. The same study also revealed that as people become frailer, their life horizons can become limited to a consideration of how to undertake necessary tasks in order to maintain independence. Nevertheless, why some people continue to manage independently in the face of substantial difficulties whereas others who are far less personally challenged find coping with daily life problematic cannot be explained in terms of functional ability alone. Personality and attitudes also influence how older people manage health problems. This in turn affects their perceptions of the levels of support they consider that they need. Research by Chesterman et al. (2000) found that older people with a more independent attitude were more likely to be satisfied with social services they received in comparison with those who coped less well, who were more likely to be dissatisfied.

It is well known that the extent of hidden need among older people in the community remains considerable, even for those already in receipt of services. By the time most older people have come to the attention of the medical profession, it is likely that they have already experienced at least one crisis. Some people who were previously well and managing independently will experience sudden, unexpected trauma, for example a fall or a stroke. This can leave them ill and incapacitated. They may find themselves hospitalized or receiving hospital services at home, with subsequent need for rehabilitation and lifestyle adjustments. Other older people experience a slow insidious decline, which can remain undetected in the community until a crisis occurs and subsequent investigations reveal a whole raft of problems and consequent need for services. Difficulties can often be traced back to a number of often-interwoven sources, for example a single or multiple medical conditions, overall frailty, lack of carer support and an environment that fails to accommodate changing needs. Inevitably, quality of life is severely limited in situations where the person is dependent and has no assistance to draw upon from informal care networks (DoH, 1997a; Barnes M, 1997). The Gospel Oak Project (Cullen et al., 1993) confirmed that users of multiple community services are generally very old, isolated and either physically or mentally unwell. The same studies also found that older people with dementia were more likely to be in contact with social services rather than health provision.

Illness and disability in older age

There is general agreement about the patterns of incidence and prevalence of disability in old age. Khaw (1999) deduced that alongside the 10 per cent increase in numbers of people aged 60 years and over to the year

2031, there will be a two- to threefold increase in the incidence of chronic disease and disability. Although the majority of older people remain fit and active, with advancing years certain problems are more likely to emerge which increase a person's vulnerability and decrease independence. As a consequence, coping with activities of daily living becomes more arduous, mobility decreases and there is an increased incidence of falls. De Jong-Gierveld and van Solinge (1995) found that after the age of 75 years, need for care services increases due to greater frailty and existence of chronic conditions. This finding is echoed by a more recent study of prevalence of disability among people aged 65 years and over (MRC CFAS, 2000). Results confirmed that people aged 85 years and over, and those with cognitive impairment, are large consumers of long-term care and intensive home care. The study also found that a degree of disability is a more important indication of need for services than whether disability is present or absent. The National Service Framework (DoH, 2001a) stated that the most common problems are related to mobility, vision and hearing.

Prevalence of dementia increases as life expectancy extends; Jorm et al. (1987) demonstrated a ratio of incidence doubling every 5.1 years up to the age of 95 years. Twenty per cent of those aged 80 years and over have some form of dementing illness. However, although the evidence confirms that dementia increases with age, statistics can present an exaggerated picture. Only around one-third of those with a diagnosis of dementia are at the severe end of the scale, requiring constant supervision.

A diagnostic approach to needs

Some of the common illnesses of older age are now briefly summarized. This list is by no means inclusive, and while the conditions are common in older age, they are not restricted to later life. Treatment of older people is often similar to that for all age groups, with the rationing of health care for older people now increasingly being challenged.

Coronary heart disease

According to the National Service Framework (DoH, 1999a), coronary heart disease is the biggest cause of premature death in the UK, but it can occur at any age. Moreover, rates vary according to social circumstances, gender and ethnicity. Direct links have been made between the adoption of certain lifestyles and heart disease; for example, smoking, diet, stress and lack of exercise are all common precipitating factors. Heart disease can manifest in a number of ways, including angina, heart failure, hypertension and heart attack. The British Heart Foundation describes these and other associated conditions. Angina pectoris is the medical term for chest pain due to coronary heart disease. It occurs when heart muscle is deprived of oxygen. The classic symptom is heaviness or tightness in the chest. A heart attack or myocardial infarction occurs when one of the coronary arteries which supplies the heart muscle is blocked by a clot, starving the heart, with subsequent damage to the muscle. Thickening of the artery walls, attributable to fatty deposits, encourages clotting of the blood. The National Service Framework (DoH, 1999a) provides standards for the treatment of coronary heart disease. These include the need to provide timely effective treatment as well as health education and rehabilitation.

Stroke is the biggest cause of severe disability in the UK and is one of the biggest killers, being the third most common cause of death (DoH, 2001a). One hundred thousand people each year experience a first stroke, and a further 30,000 have a further stroke (Stroke Association, 2001). Therefore stroke has a large impact upon health and social care provision. Stroke can occur in people of any age, with incidence increasing with age. Consequently, over 90 per cent of strokes occur in people over the age of 55 years. Certain populations are at more risk than others, for example lower socio-economic classes and men of Afro-Caribbean and Asian origins (DoH, 2001a).

There are two main types of stroke: ischaemic, resulting from decreased blood flow to the brain, and haemorrhagic, where the blood vessel bursts and blood leaks into the brain. Transient ischaemic attacks (TIAs) are mini-strokes resulting from minor episodes of reduced blood flow to the brain; they signal the likelihood of a future major ischaemic attack. The effect of the stroke is dependent upon which part of the brain has been damaged. Recovery can continue over a long time. National Clinical Guidelines for Stroke have been developed for the management of stroke (Intercollegiate Working Party for Stroke, 1999). Occupational therapy involvement was integral to the development of the guidelines, with the clear recommendation that rehabilitation should commence as soon as possible after the stroke. Further to this, the specific guidelines of relevance to occupational therapy were identified and produced in a brief booklet for easy reference (NANOT, 2000).

Parkinson's disease

Parkinson's disease is a progressive neurological condition which results in increasing disability over time despite available drug therapies. It is a common cause of admission to institutional care (Baker, 2000). A shuffling gait, involuntary movements and fixed facial expression are typical of people with the disease. People in the later stages of Parkinson's disease can exhibit cognitive impairment and communication problems. Probability of falling is increased as the disease progresses (Ashburn et al., 2001). The impairments experienced by people with Parkinson's disease who fall include reduced stability, use of small frequent steps when walking and difficulty maintaining balance. Depression is another commonly experienced symptom.

Arthritis

This group of conditions is one of the main contributors to disability in older age (DoH, 1999b). According to the Arthritis Research Campaign, osteoarthritis affects over a million people in the UK, these being mainly older people. Approximately 60 per cent of people over the age of 64 years have osteoarthritis in an least one joint. Osteoarthritis is characterized by the thickening and distortion of joints as a result of cartilage degeneration. Obesity and previous injury exacerbate the disease. The consequences of the resulting condition can range in severity from minor aches and pains to excruciating pain. Additionally the affected joints become stiffer and less functional, reducing ability to undertake self-care tasks. Available treatments are palliative only, with joint replacement being the only solution to joints worn out by osteoarthritis. Moderate exercise and retaining physical activity is considered to be beneficial. The Arthritis Research Campaign have suggested that one of the reasons for the poor range of treatment options is the fact that it is perceived to be a chronic, non-life-threatening disease of old age. Rheumatoid arthritis is also prevalent in older people, even though it is not a disease of later years like osteoarthritis. It is characterized by joint inflammation and stiffness.

Osteoporosis

This condition is a loss of bone mass and density. Statistics quoted in the National Service Framework for Older People (DoH, 2001a) demonstrate the high prevalence of the condition. One in three women and one in 12 men over the age of 50 have osteoporosis. The condition increases the likelihood of fracture. Almost half of all women over the age of 70 experience a fracture as a result of osteoporosis (DoH, 2001a). Prevention of osteoporosis in later life is a neglected aspect (DoH, 1999b). While some loss of bone density in older age is inevitable, despite exercise, treatments in the form of hormone replacement therapy, dietary supplements and reducing smoking and alcohol can be beneficial (Gilchrist, 1999).

Diabetes

There are two main types of diabetes: Type 1 and Type 2. In Type 1 diabetes, the pancreas is not able to produce insulin. In Type 2, glucose builds
up in the blood. People over the age of 40 are more likely to develop Type
2 diabetes, with this accounting for 85 per cent of all people with diabetes
(DoH, 2002a). Incidence of Type 2 diabetes rises with age; one in twenty
people over the age of 65 years in the UK have diabetes. The underlying
causes of Type 2 diabetes include diet and lifestyle, with individuals from
ethnic minority, poor and socially excluded communities being at greater
risk of developing the disease. The National Service Framework for older
people (DoH, 2001a) noted that the risk of developing diabetes and the
extent of understanding of the illness varied significantly within the population. It therefore follows that older people from socially excluded groups
will be at very high risk. Symptoms include tiredness, thirst, blurred vision,
frequent urination and infections. The National Service Framework for
Older People (DoH, 2001a) states that diagnosis can be delayed in older
people and they may experience discrimination in the extent of active
management of the condition compared with younger people. This can
lead, among other things, to a high incidence of visual impairment (DoH,
1999b). The National Service Framework for diabetes was recently published (DoH, 2002a). As with the other National Service Frameworks, it
contains a number of targets for services to meet, and emphasizes the
importance of self-management programmes.

Respiratory disease

Chronic obstructive pulmonary disease (COPD) is an umbrella term used
to describe a number of respiratory disorders. These include emphysema,
chronic bronchitis, chronic airflow limitation, chronic obstructive airways
disease and some cases of chronic asthma. Differentiation between the
different disorders can be difficult. People with COPD present with significantly reduced capacity for exercise, difficulty breathing and fatigue,
with the condition being chronic and slowly progressing (British Thoracic
Society, 1997). Most cases are a direct consequence of smoking. It is therefore not surprising that it is a common condition in older people, for
whom the adverse consequences of smoking were revealed too late. It is
also a condition prevalent within certain populations exposed to dust, the
best known example being that of miners. Recommendations from the
British Thoracic Society (1997) include provision of pulmonary rehabilitation programmes (specifically the encouragement of exercise), weight
control, assessment of social circumstances and the person's ability to
cope, and active treatment of depression.

Cancer

Cancer is a disease of the cells of the body, where cells rapidly divide to grow tumours; some tumours are benign or non-invasive and others are malignant. There are over 200 different kinds of cancer, with the cause of some cancers being related to the environment, for example smoking, contact with certain harmful substances like chemicals and asbestos, and exposure to sunlight. Additionally, some people have a genetic predisposition to the disease. Even though cancer is not a disease confined to older age, the likelihood of developing all cancers, apart from testicular cancer and some types of leukaemia and lymphoma, increases with age, with 60–70 per cent of all incidences of cancer occurring in people over the age of 65 years. Certain cancers are more likely to manifest in later years; these include lung cancer (most serious cancer in people under the age of 85 years), prostate cancer (most common cancer in men over 85 years) and stomach cancers (25 per cent occurring in people over the age of 80) (Cancerbacup, 2003). Available treatments depend upon the extent of the disease and the prognosis. Both the disease and some of the treatments can lead to weight loss, fatigue, pain, sickness and nausea. Generalization is very difficult as the progression of the disease and the coping abilities of the individual will vary from person to person. The NHS Cancer Plan (DoH, 2000c) details four aims: to save lives, ensure that people get the right treatment and support, tackle underlying inequalities known to lead to a greater incidence of cancer in some populations, and to invest in research and the workforce. The importance of preventive strategies is emphasized.

Mental health problems

Older people with mental health problems are a highly heterogeneous group. They include the following:

- people with functional mental illness, for example depression;
- people with dementia, for example Alzheimer's disease;
- those with mental health problems caused by physical illness or substance misuse;
- people who have had mental health problems for an extended period of time and have grown older (this includes those with long-term psychotic illness and those with severe depression), as well as those who have spent many years institutionalized in long-stay hospitals.

Additionally, older people can have symptoms that cross over different diagnostic categories; for example, people with dementia can become depressed.

Depression

Depression is the most common mental health problem among older people, with a prevalence of 15 per cent in the community, 25 per cent in general practice patients and 30 per cent in residential homes (MacDonald, 1997). Moreover, its consequences can be severe, with suicide being the ultimate expression of the despair it causes. Older people become depressed as a result of a large number of factors. These include the direct consequences of physical illness like stroke, the erosion of physical capabilities (including fear of falls), and the effects of life events like bereavement and loss of role. Conversely, depressive illness itself can result in decreased activation and interest. Given the interplay between physical and mental ill health, recognition and treatment of physical illness is important. There are also a number of individuals who experience depression throughout their lives, with the illness extending into older age.

Severity is exacerbated by poor rate of detection, even when individuals are already in receipt of health and social care (Banerjee, 1993). The most common form of treatment for depression in older people is drug therapy. MacDonald (1997) identified chances of response to pharmacological treatment being increased if: biological symptoms of the illness are prominent; there is a clear change in the person's mood; there is a history of previous successful treatment; and there is no history of depression, mania or dementia. There is no doubt that, beyond this, professionals and informal carers can struggle to find solutions to the extent and range of problems older people with depression present with. For those with more pervasive, complex problems, their needs may not be satisfied by medicines alone, necessitating referral to a range of other professionals and ongoing support from a wide care network. Anxiety is often accompanied by depression, but can also be a sign of early dementia.

Dementia

Dementia describes loss of cognitive abilities in someone who was previously intellectually intact, to the extent that it interferes with work or social occupations and presents a complex set of needs both physical and psychological. Dementia is an umbrella term for a number of illnesses. The most common type, Alzheimer's disease, can have early onset (before the age of 65 years) where deterioration is rapid, or late onset, usually after the age of 75 years, where deterioration is slower and the main symptom is memory loss. Alzheimer's disease accounts for about 60 per cent of all cases of dementia. Vascular dementia occurs as a result of stroke or cerebrovascular accident and may have a sudden or alternatively a more gradual onset. A third type of dementia is called Lewy Body dementia, characterized by symptoms like those in Parkinson's disease as well as hallucinations and falls (DoH, 2001a).

The different types of dementing illness result in distinct symptom patterns and the illness manifests itself in different ways from person to person. The insidious onset of most types of dementia can make it difficult for family members to acknowledge that their relative is ill. This situation can continue over an extended period of time. According to carers, the most commonly recognized initial signs of the illness are poor memory, confusion and disorientation (Chenoweth and Spencer, 1986).

However, the consequences of the dementia syndrome are the same in that it impacts upon the whole fabric of the person's life, including psychological, intellectual and functional abilities. Research has shown that carers of people with dementia are totally unprepared for the extent of problem behaviours that can result. These include daytime wandering, hiding things, night waking, demanding, critical behaviour, catastrophic reactions and memory disturbance. The most difficult behaviours reported by carers in a study undertaken by Mace (1990) were falls, night disturbance, incontinence and attention-seeking behaviour.

At present, despite strenuous research efforts, there is no cure for dementia. The recently introduced anti-dementia drugs can only arrest some aspects of the condition, not cure it. Occupational therapists are being involved in trials of these drugs to see whether they lead to improved occupational performance.

Substance misuse

A study of the incidence of substance misuse in hospitalized older people aged 65 years and over in Australia found that over 41 per cent used alcohol, tobacco and tranquillizers more than the recommended safe limits (McInnes and Powell, 1994). As the authors pointed out, these problems in older people are likely to be overlooked by professionals. One reason they cited is the belief that older people should not be discouraged from continuing with long-established habits. Given the links between these habits and other health problems, as well as the direct consequences of the behaviour, we should not collude with this belief. Occupational therapists, in common with other health professions, must be alert to the presence of such problems in the older person as well as in the people who care for them.

Delirium

This is a term for a combination of symptoms whereby the person suddenly becomes confused and disturbed. Behaviours include changes in behaviour including increased activity, distress and acute disturbance, disorientation in time, place and person, and sometimes hallucinations. Delirium occurs in 30 per cent of all older people admitted to hospital (MacDonald, 1997). The syndrome can be attributed to dementia, but is more likely to be due to a treatable physical condition, for example infections or cardiac disease.

Psychotic illness

These illnesses are characterized by delusional ideation and/or hallucinations. These may also be accompanied by a number of negative symptoms like lack of energy and interests, and poor self-care. Acute psychosis is rare in older age (MacDonald, 1997). The continuance of a long-standing psychotic illness like chronic schizophrenia is more common. The National Service Framework for Mental Health (DoH, 1999c) should be used to inform the delivery of services to this group.

New problems are emerging due to the ageing of those people who were transferred from institutional to community care during the 1970s and 1980s. Living arrangements like group homes that may have been appropriate decades ago are no longer satisfactory due to the effects of older age and illness.

Learning disabilities in older age

Advances in medicine mean that people with learning disabilities have a longer life expectancy than in the past, with many living in the community rather than being institutionalized. This has led to a new set of challenges for services (Godfrey, 1998), with the needs of older people with learning disabilities being raised within The National Service Framework for Older People (DoH, 2001a).

The needs resulting from growing older with a learning disability require ongoing treatment and care as well as access to rehabilitation. Additionally, older people with learning disabilities are at greater risk of developing dementia in later life than the overall population. Rates of dementia in older people with learning disabilities are around 13 per cent for those aged 50 years and over. This increases to 22 per cent in those aged 65 years and over (Cooper, 1997). For people with Down syndrome, it has been observed that the number with dementia increases over the life course, with prevalence being almost 55 per cent for those aged 60 years and over (Prasher, 1995). In common with other people who develop dementia, management is assisted by early detection.

Limitations of the diagnostic approach

Understanding different diagnostic conditions is important, particularly when interacting with other hospital-based professionals. Furthermore, the observation of certain symptoms on the part of the occupational therapist can help to detect when the health status of the older person has changed. Diagnosis can also inform those interventions that might be contra-indicated. However, the adoption of a medical paradigm alone is not the most helpful approach for occupational therapists to use both during assessment and in planning interventions; for example:

• It can limit early identification of needs in community settings, and a preventive approach.
• It can limit a holistic response.
• It does not promote the contribution of other extrinsic factors in the context of overall need like availability of social support and housing.

Older people are all individuals, with their own lives and circumstances. The following table shows the variance that will exist within a limited number of the many factors that will differ across all older people with dementia. It underscores the limitations of taking only diagnosis into account and confirms the need for an individual approach to needs, taking account of a whole spectrum of factors.

Table 3.1 Older people with dementia: health needs and circumstances

Personal characteristics	Cognitive impairment	Physical health	Living circumstances	Care available
Male or female; younger or older	Mild or moderate or severe	Good or limited or poor	Alone or co-resident household or residential/ nursing home	Primary care and/ or secondary/ tertiary health care; informal care and/or social care; housing; Church

The World Health Organization's *International Classification of Functioning, Disability and Health (ICF-2)* (World Health Organization, 2001) superseded the previous classification of impairment, disability and handicap, which did not take account of the individual's own response to their situation. The new classification acknowledges the interaction between the individual and the personal and environmental contexts within which they live, seeking to integrate medical and social models. The terms 'body functions and structures', 'activities' and 'participation' have replaced 'impairment', 'disability' and 'handicap'.

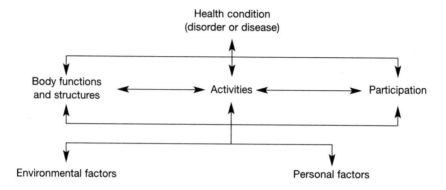

Figure 3.1 Interactions between the components of ICF-2 (WHO, 2001).

The WHO model is useful for examining the interplay between various factors and the consequent ability of older people to be able to participate in both necessary and chosen occupations. The College of Occupational Therapists are promoting the use of this classification as a framework for practice through their policy document, *From Interface to Integration* (COT, 2001).

The following sections of this chapter consider the consequences of disease and disability and the environmental and personal factors that contribute to the ability to undertake occupations and maintain independence.

Needs resulting from the consequences of age, disability and illness

In 1992, Thornton and Mountain examined the records of referrals of people to a community alarm scheme, nine out of ten people being aged 65 years and over. Data were extracted from computerized records. Only six of 395 client records surveyed gave no medical reasons for referral. When the consequences of age, disease and disability given on the referrals were analysed, this gave a far better indication of needs for community care than medical diagnosis alone, as illustrated by Table 3.2.

Table 3.2 Consequences of age, disease and disability*

	No. of times cited	% of clients
Falls	102	33
Dizziness, blackouts	74	24
Deafness	73	24
Poor mobility	65	21
Frailty	45	15
Poor vision	45	15
Paralysis	35	11
Other problems	20	6
Housebound	18	6
Chairbound	18	6
Speech problems	17	6
Limb amputation	16	5
Need to use medical equipment	16	5
Nervous, anxious etc	14	5
Condition may require urgent attention	9	3
Memory loss	6	2
Confusion	6	2
Incontinence	4	1

* Based on data from 312 client records.
Source: Cited in *Referrals to a Social Services Alarm Scheme* (Thornton and Mountain, 1992, p. 14)

Visual impairment

Approximately 80 per cent of people over the age of 60 have visual impairment. There are a number of reasons for reduced vision in the older population. These include the effects of cataracts, macular degeneration, glaucoma and diabetic retinopathy (Henwood, 1999). Cataracts cause clouding of the lens over the eye and loss of vision. They are readily treatable through surgery. Macular degeneration reduces central vision. Glaucoma leads to optic nerve damage and can lead to blindness. Diabetic retinopathy is bleeding into the eye due to poorly managed diabetes. A survey by Wormald et al. (1992) found that there was significant undetected eye disease in the population, with a significant proportion of consequent disability being treatable. The authors suggested that the introduction of the assessment of all older people aged 75 years and over could help to pick up a proportion of undetected problems. Poor vision significantly compromises quality of life and ability to undertake activities of daily living. Sensory impairment is a common risk factor for falls (Swift, 2001). If the person is living in a poorly lit environment or one beset with environmental hazards, risk is significantly increased. Landes and Popay (1993) investigated the health and social care needs of older people with vision problems living in four health districts in north-west England. They found that the extent of disability experienced by individuals could be related to a wide range of environmental, social and personal factors; for example, restricted mobility was one of the prime reasons for not having had a recent eye test.

Hearing impairment

Hearing problems are also common among older people. Between 30 and 60 per cent of all older people have hearing loss (Laing and Hall, quoted in Henwood, 1998). This can lead to communication problems, loss of self-esteem and increased vulnerability. Even minor hearing loss can lead to a preventable degree of cognitive impairment (DoH, 1999b). Some hearing problems, for example ears blocked with wax, can be alleviated through detection and treatment. Additionally, hearing aids should be provided to older people assessed as requiring them, and properly maintained.

Twenty-two per cent of older people over 60 years experience both visual and hearing impairment (DoH, 2001a). As well as being problematic in their own right, a combination of diminished hearing and sight has wide-ranging consequences for the individual's safety and ability to continue to live independently.

Poor dental care

Good oral health care has a direct bearing upon the diet the older person is able to tolerate, and their general health, happiness and independence (Fiske et al., 2000); for example, those with poor dental care may not feel able to eat in company or socialize. Studies of institutionalized older people have highlighted the deleterious consequences of poor dental health, including eating problems, weight loss, dehydration and debility. Guidelines produced by the British Society for Disability and Oral Health (Fiske et al., 2000) stated that all health care practitioners should receive training to promote oral health care. While this is primarily directed at nurses, it is evident that occupational therapists should be alert to the consequences of poor dental care for the older people they work with.

Increasing physical limitations

Progression of the ageing process is signalled by restricted involvement in long-standing occupations on the part of those who are fit and well, as described in the previous chapter. Older people who appeared quite sprightly talked about physical limitations in terms of what they now found difficult, for example not being able to hang washing on the line, catching buses, carrying shopping and cleaning windows.

During interviews with older people (Mountain and Moore, 1995; Mountain, 1998a) physical limitations were frequently described as 'wear and tear' and 'aches and pains' rather than being attributed to specific health problems. Occasionally arthritis would be cited as the causal factor, but most often older people accepted that their increasing limitations were a consequence of their age rather than any disease or condition. Individuals were most likely to describe what they were prevented from doing; for example, problems with mobility limited capability to go shopping or use buses.

> I do like to get out. If I could walk, I'd be happy. But I can't walk so far, I can get on a bus and I can go into town but then when I've been to town and I've had to walk about a bit I can only go on so long.

> It is fair to say that it all goes back to when your eyes go and you get arthritis, all the things you used to do have to be slightly altered, it's health every time.

Noticeably, for more disabled individuals, the effects of physical ageing were more pervasive and they talked about difficulties in carrying out fundamental activities of daily living like bathing or dressing.

> When I was young I was very athletic and went swimming and riding a bike, hiking and now it takes me all my time to hike up the bedroom steps. But I'm not going to complain because this is it. It's all part of growing older.

Falls

Hip fractures in older people, particularly in women, are a frequent occurrence. From a review of the literature McIntyre (1999) confirmed that the factors associated with falling are many and varied. They include illnesses like hypotension, neurological conditions, cerebrovascular accident and Ménière's disease. The existence of chronic disabling conditions like osteoarthritis, cognitive decline and limited mobility are also associated with increased incidence of falling. The risk factors for falls and subsequent fracture identified by Swift (2001) are as follows:

- easily detected balance, mobility or gait impairment;
- if the person is taking a cocktail of medication;
- visual impairment;
- stroke or history of stroke, Parkinson's disease or degenerative lower-limb joint disease;
- postural hypotension.

It is not surprising that increasing age is strongly related to increased falls. Another set of causal factors are those external to the person, for example environmental hazards, and the undertaking of what would be considered to be risky occupations for that individual. An audit of the reasons for attendance at one day hospital found that nearly 30 per cent of all admissions were as a result of a fall (McIntyre, 1999). Given that the consequences of falling can be serious for older people, with a high rate of mortality and morbidity, these could be viewed as the lucky ones! Outcome can be attributed to the nature of the fracture itself, combined with the overall fitness of the person who has sustained the fracture, often as the result of a fall (Stewart and McMillan, 1998).

> Directly I came here I fell and I've never been right since. That's why I am in a wheelchair.

It has also been long recognized that fractures have long-standing social as well as physical consequences, demanding enhanced collaboration between different medical specialities both before and following the operation, with the chances of *social deterioration* doubling over the age of 75 years (Glyn Thomas and Stevens, 1974). Research quoted by McKee (1998) demonstrated that in the short term after a fall, 40 per cent of older people undertake less activity. Anxiety and depression may accompany this lowered rate of activity. In the longer term only about half of those who have fallen regain their previous levels of mobility and their levels of independence before the fall. The significance of other causal factors in explaining poor outcomes after falls was explored by McKee (1998), who hypothesized that the way people who have fallen explain the event to themselves and others affects their ability to cope with the event. Falls are especially significant as, irrespective of the cause, they always signify a loss of control. The extent of concern about the consequences of falling is such that the NHSE funded the Chartered Society of Physiotherapy and the College of Occupational Therapists to undertake a falls audit. The aim was to investigate the extent to which the guidelines for the collaborative management of elderly people who have fallen were being implemented. Simpson et al. (1998) reported the agreed guidelines and the audit process. The guidelines are referred to again in Chapter 8.

Fear of falling

Fear of falling in itself can be problematic for older people, leading to decreased independence and isolation.

> I've got osteoporosis, so that stops me from doing a lot of the things I would like to do because I'm frightened of falling and fracturing a bone, which could disable me for life.

Not surprisingly, fear of falling is prevalent in older people who have already fallen; this is called the post-fall syndrome. A study of the quality of life and perceived health of 197 older women aged 75–84 years in Australia (Salkeld et al., 2000) illustrated this. The results of the study found that 80 per cent of the 203 interviewees would have preferred death to what they perceived to be a reduction in their quality of life if they were to sustain a hip fracture resulting in admission to a nursing home. The relationship between reduced quality of life and admission to nursing home was located in perceived loss of independence, dignity and possessions. The interpretation of the results of this study were questioned by Ameratunga and Brown (2000), who suggested that the opinions stated by the women could change over time following fracture as they learn to adapt and cope. They did, however, acknowledge the importance of the findings of Salkeld et al. thus:

> ... the study has important implications for individual patient care and preventive interventions relating to falls and hip fracture. It affirms the need for rehabilitation programmes to focus not only on enhancing patients' mobility and functional activities but also to optimize their ability to live independently and participate in social and other aspects of community life. (Ameratunga and Brown, 2000, p. 345)

Incontinence

Incontinence is the second most common reason for admission to residential care (DoH, 2001a). However, it remains a 'taboo' subject, leading to under-diagnosis and treatment (Gilchrist, 1999). Estimates suggest that 6–8 per cent of older people living in the community are affected by incontinence. The majority are in residential care, with up to 85 per cent being women. Risk factors include weakened pelvic-floor muscles due to childbirth in women, and the consequences of an enlarged prostate gland in men. However, if recognized early and treated, incontinence need not be an inevitable consequence of growing older.

Interplay between extrinsic factors and factors intrinsic to the individual

The previous section on the effects of ageing shows that it is impossible to discuss disability and frailty without raising the part that the environment plays in facilitating or limiting engagement and independence. Moreover, as Chapter 2 described, the consequences of not being able to participate can in themselves have a deleterious effect upon health.

Wilcock (1998) identified three 'occupational stressors' which can militate against health, namely occupational imbalance, occupational deprivation and occupational alienation. Imbalance occurs when an individual experiences too much of the same activity. Deprivation is concerned with lack of opportunities to carry out occupations due to limited opportunity and choice (exemplified by the limited availability of occupations in some residential care settings for older people). If a person is unable to meet their occupational needs because of societal factors and the demands that arise from external sources, they may experience occupational alienation. Additionally, Wilcock postulated that we all have to make large occupational adaptations due to factors like technological advances and changing lifestyles. She suggested that occupational dysfunction can stem from a range of social, political and ecological sources, and not purely from illness. Changing physical abilities together with external factors and circumstances will therefore shape the nature of occupational adaptations made by people as they become older.

Environmental factors

The interpretation of housing and environment is complex; for example, housing embraces factors far beyond the fabric of the building within which a person resides, to their garden and the immediate neighbourhood.

As a person becomes less independent, environmental factors are increasingly important for maintenance of well-being. Increasing age brings reduced adaptability to the environment; for example, the old more keenly experience temperature changes. Additionally the person becomes more reliant upon external cues. Comparatively early research demonstrated the increasing difficulty in coping with the environment experienced by people as they became more frail and disabled. Problems arising from the structural environment combined with social support and coping strategies were particularly important (Lawton and Simon, 1968, quoted in Cvitkovitch and Wister, 2001). Other research has found that transport, housing and use of health and social care services are strongly interrelated and affect quality of life (Joseph and Fuller, 1991, quoted in Cvitkovitch and Wister, 2001).

Knipscheer et al. (2000) looked at the relationship between the environment of an older person and incidence of depressive symptoms, applying the model of environmental docility developed by Lawton (1975). The model of environmental docility postulated the existence of relationships between the person, their environment, their subjective and objective achievements, their behaviour and their consequent mental state. Older people with decreased ability in activities of daily living will need to adapt their behaviour to meet the demands of their environment, with implications for their mental well-being. (This theory has strong synergy with the occupation for health model developed by Wilcock.) Analysis of the data from an existing longitudinal study of ageing in Amsterdam by Knipscheer et al. (2000), using the Lawton model, found that several environmental factors increased depressive symptoms. These included living in an urban environment with its crime, traffic and complex housing, not being able to undertake heavy household tasks, having a poor sense of achievement, and few contacts in the neighbourhood, particularly when combined with poor functional ability. The main issue drawn from this study is the importance of independence, combined with feeling able to influence one's environment

Housing

For the purposes of this book, housing is interpreted as being the home where the older person resides. Chapters 1 and 2 reiterated the importance of good housing for maintenance of quality of life. Housing is central to community care, and can also dictate needs for community care, in that a person's direct environment can assist or limit independence. The specific factors identified by Tinker (1995) that are related to independence are:

- design;
- conditions of the home;
- the extent of support available (either through someone coming to the existing home, or by the older person moving to housing where support is provided);
- the affordability of the current housing.

Research to explore the relationship between housing conditions and rates of mortality was conducted by analysing dates from both the English house conditions survey and national mortality data for England (Wilkinson et al., 2001). The researchers concluded that there are links between poor housing, poverty, low indoor temperatures and subsequent death. Low indoor temperatures are more likely if the house is old, has inadequate or no heating, or is occupied by people on low income. While this research was not limited to older people, it is clear that those who are ill, frail and have low incomes will be at heightened risk.

Research undertaken by Adams and Wilson (1996) confirmed the challenges of housing older people with functional mental health problems. They interviewed 41 older people with mental health problems who had been re-housed. Results of interviews demonstrated the importance of quality housing in maintenance of mental health. Good housing also conferred physical benefits. Conversely, the adverse effects of poor-quality housing on mentally frail older people were great.

Policy is now seeking to merge housing benefit paid for support services and other funding streams into a single budget to be distributed to local authorities on the basis of individual need. *Supporting People* (DSS, 1998; DETR and DoH, 2001b) was implemented from April 2003. The rationale is the provision of more flexible housing-related support services to meet the needs of vulnerable people.

Transport

Transport problems made life problematic for the older people interviewed by Mountain and Moore (1995). Some people said that they did not feel safe waiting at bus stops, and managing public transport could be difficult due to physical problems. Taxis were a way of overcoming this, with consequent financial implications.

> To go anywhere transport is very essential ... If I wish to go shopping I am unable to go as there is no one to go with me.

The more frail the older people interviewed, the more important the issues of transport became; it was one of the most cited issues by the most frail group of day-centre attenders we interviewed. Without assistance, the majority were rendered housebound as they were unable to use public services. The day-centre volunteers described transport as a 'big head-ache'.

> The main problem that we've identified as an organization is transport. Unless they get specialized transport from the door a lot of them can't go anywhere. That's why we exist and that makes transport one of our highest items of expenditure.

Cvitkovitch and Wister (2001) looked at the impact of transport needs on 174 older people living in the community in Vancouver, Canada. The sample was recruited from consumers of social care services and programmes. Results of this quantitative study suggested that targeting transport resources on those whose independence is compromised by the environment would significantly improve well-being. This relationship between transport and well-being was illustrated through the experiences of this older person who used a mobility service in Leeds city centre for the first time.

> I had a three-wheeler [scooter] and I was in Leeds the whole day. Even into the Corn Exchange, in the Schofield Centre and up in the glass lift in the wheelchair ... it was a wonderful day out.

Relationships between environment, independence and risk-taking

The living environment has a significant impact upon the independence of both older and disabled people; a well-designed environment can facilitate abilities whereas a poor setting presents difficulties and risks. A number of studies undertaken over the years have demonstrated these relationships.

In 1994, Mann et al. observed that there had been little research into the environmental problems experienced by older people. Their study involved describing the types and frequencies of problems of vulnerable older people by interviewing 127 people over the age of 60 who were receiving social or health care, and observing their home environment, room by room. The researchers found over 500 environment-related problems in the 127 homes. To analyse the data, a conceptual framework was employed. It was found that almost all environmental problems were grouped within the following formula:

Design + Maintenance + Social support $\longrightarrow$ Safety + Independence + Control

It was postulated that if design, maintenance and social support are working well, then safety, independence and comfort will be promoted. Of the three outcomes, safety must be prioritized.

Iwarsson and Isacsson (1998) also looked at the relationship between the functional limitations of older people and their home environment. Through analysis of interviews with 133 older people in Sweden aged 75–84, they demonstrated that dependence in activities of daily living correlates with housing accessibility problems, the greatest problems being experienced by those with the greatest housing barriers. They concluded that the construct of *disability* differs from *functional capacity*, as it includes an environmental aspect.

Gill et al. (1999) estimated population-based hazards from data collected on dangers in the homes of a representative sample of 1000 people aged 72 years and over. Trained nurses used a standardized checklist to rate the homes of subjects, room by room. The functional ability of the person was also noted using a valid scale. Analysis found that overall prevalence of risk factors was high, with nearly all homes having two or more hazards, and with the bathroom being the most hazardous room. It also emerged that there was no difference in risks in the homes of people with disabilities as opposed to those without, suggesting that awareness of safety was not related to personal abilities. They concluded thus:

If the epidemiological link between environmental hazards and functional decline and disability can be strengthened, then everyday functioning of older persons will need to focus on the environment as well as the individual. (Gill et al., 1999, p. 556)

The work of Agree (1999) led to the following conclusion:

Environmental factors are certainly of great importance in the appropriate and effective use of community based long-term care by disabled individuals. Environmental barriers can impede the use of many forms of assistance. (Agree, 1999, p. 441)

A further study by Gitlin et al. (2001) examined the homes of 296 older people room by room. They found an average of 13 problems with their environment in each home, with most occurring in the bathroom, kitchen and bedroom. In common with other studies the authors concluded that more work was required to examine the relationships between physical and psychological function and environmental adequacy.

The findings of this sample of studies are summarized in Figure 3.2.

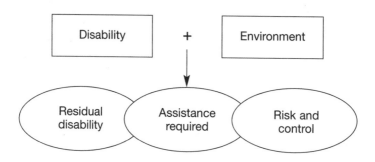

Figure 3.2 Disability, environment and risk.

These relationships between the capacity of the individual and their environment are significant for occupational therapy, and will be a reiterated theme in forthcoming chapters.

Personal circumstances

In addition to the environment, a number of issues concerned with the circumstances the individual finds him or herself in can have a significant impact upon both health status and ability to cope in the face of illness and disability. Older people can be affected by a combination of the

factors described below, in combination with the previously described setting in which they live. (Some were referred to in Chapter 2 in the section
on normal adaptations in older age, where the number and extent of
changes and losses over a given period of time were raised as being crucial in determining coping abilities.)

1. Absence of an informal care network

The nature of care networks is explored in depth in the next chapter.
What we need to consider here is the implications for the individual of
not having an available network of support, particularly when experiencing illness or increasing frailty.

The demographic profile of the older population has implications for
the availability of informal care. Those who do not have a long-term partner will not have support from partners or children. Those who married
but did not have children will also be lacking close family support.
Changes in living arrangements over the decades also bring implications.
There is a move towards one-person households. This is in comparison
with the complex family relationships that existed in the past. It is now
less likely that older people will share accommodation with other members of their family, even though, in contrast with popular belief, this was
an infrequent situation. Also, as Grundy (1995) pointed out, older people
generally prefer to maintain their own households. Given the extent of
care provided by unpaid carers, it is not surprising that those vulnerable
older people without a network of informal care are at particular risk
(Barnes D, 1997). Even when informal carers are at hand, their continued
involvement can be fragile. They can require a range of services in their
own right to sustain the caring role.

2. Living situation

It is not surprising that those older people who find themselves living
alone are at greater risk, particularly after illness or accidents.

Follow-up of older North American women living alone following discharge from hospital revealed a decline over time after return home. One
postulated reason was the poor physical conditions many of the women
lived in, with respect to their homes as well as the surrounding neighbourhoods. These findings confirmed the previously described importance of care networks and the value of appropriate equipment and
adaptations to housing (Lysack et al., 2000).

An advisory group established by the Social Services Inspectorate
(Barnes D, 1997) included an occupational therapist. They were charged
with looking at the needs of older people with mental health problems

living alone. They came to a number of conclusions, the following being of particular relevance to occupational therapy:

- The need for specialist skills, in particular those concerned with assessment, acceptance of appropriate risk and provision of protection.
- The requirement for development of training initiatives, ideally across agencies, is emphasized.
- The complexities of assessment of this group, which demand time and sensitivity if it is to be conducted properly.
- Access to advocates to help people with mental health problems get the services which best meet their needs.

3. Consequences of admission to hospital

Once an older person is admitted to hospital for whatever reason, they usually experience a decline in their independence, and go home less able than before. The fragility of hospital discharge procedures in ensuring successful return home of older people has long been recognized. A review of discharge communications (Closs, 1997) highlighted the need for improved multi-disciplinary exchange of information, particularly across the health/social care interface. A number of patient-based factors can be predictive of successful return home, for example the ability to mobilize, communication skills, lucidity, continence and extent of dependency prior to admission (Flanagan et al., 1995). The difficulties encountered by older people in the first week following hospital discharge may include lack of information, and problems with personal care and looking after their house (Mistiaen et al., 1997). Unmet needs can include information on the recovery process and help with household occupations. Relapse in the person's condition is frequently the main reason for emergency readmission to hospital, but in the case of older people this is usually accompanied by other, associated problems like living alone, carer burden and premature discharge (Williams and Fitton, 1988; Townsend et al., 1992; Gautam et al., 1996). Through analysis of data collected from three acute-based hospital units for older people, Victor et al. (2000) showed that three factors accounted for delay in discharge, namely the membership of the multi-disciplinary team, availability of a family carer and entry into institutional care. The functional status and health of the individual were less significant. Acknowledged difficulties led the Department of Health to publish guidance to assist professionals with best practice (DoH, 1989a, 1994). This knowledge, together with the need to reduce unnecessary admissions to hospital, has led to the development of a number of alternatives to hospital admission, some of which are described in Chapters 5 and 9.

4. Admission to long-term care

Depression is a common occurrence for those who have entered long-term care. The incidence of depression in nursing homes and other residential settings is widely acknowledged. It is estimated that around 40 per cent of older people in residential care are depressed (Mann et al., 1984). Having to give up one's home and independence means that the person has to relinquish many long-standing occupational routines. Despite the improvements that have been made to many care environments over recent years (Peace et al., 1997), depression may also stem from the lack of opportunities for occupation within the residential care environment.

5. Bereavement

As described in the previous chapter, the emotional distress of bereavement is great and it can be heightened by a lack of practical abilities. Widowers can be left incapable of providing a simple meal for themselves. Transportation is a common problem for bereaved women if they are unable to drive the car they possess. Women interviewed by Mountain and Moore (1995) also said that it was very difficult for them to develop a new social life and go on holidays.

> ... my oldest sister, they haven't any money. They've just both got a pension each and a little bit of savings. But they're off every day ... if they only go to Skegness or Bridlington. They're enjoying their retirement.

> There's loads of pensioners having the times of their lives going on holidays. I feel jealous when I see husbands and wives in their sixties and seventies going on holidays together.

6. The effects and consequences of illness and disability

Disability is commonly encountered in older people. Through secondary analysis of data held on a sample of 8,223 older people living in Michigan, Agree (1999) found that problems with activities of daily living increased with age, with the reporting of residual disability decreasing with greater age. The author hypothesized that the decreased impact of residual disability could be due to greater acceptance of disability or increased willingness to accept help. In accord with Figure 3.2, those living in poor or average housing reported a greater level of residual disability.

Illness in itself can have an effect upon ability to undertake occupations and maintain independence. Three examples of the many consequences of an inability to undertake occupations due to illness are described below.

A study conducted in Israel by Ziv et al. (1999) examined the problem-solving abilities and competence in carrying out instrumental activities of daily living (IADL) of 31 community-living older people receiving treatment for depression compared with 30 without depressive illness. The group was matched in all respects apart from the better educational attainment and employment records of the control group (a stated limitation of the study). The results obtained from application of six measures of IADL suggested that depression is associated with lower functioning in problem-solving and IADL. From this the authors concluded that occupational therapists should take this effect into account when planning interventions. It should also be taken into account in the case of illnesses like Parkinson's disease, where depression can often occur.

In the case of dementia, family members frequently described the fact that something was wrong with their relative in terms of observed difficulty in performing activities. Deteriorating memory was the symptom that most frequently led relatives to seek professional help, but prior to this, the confusing range of changed behaviours was a great source of anxiety (Chenoweth and Spencer, 1986).

A study undertaken in Australia by Lister (1999) explored the implications for older people of loss of ability to drive following stroke. In-depth interviews conducted with three older people confirmed the conclusions drawn in other literature that, given the importance placed on driving by society, loss of ability to drive has highly adverse implications. Problems include decreased psychological well-being (examples being loss of self-esteem and thoughts of being a burden), social well-being (isolation, loneliness and decreased participation in social events) and function (loss of spontaneity and difficulty undertaking functional tasks). The study also found that the experience of loss was variable and that participants experienced a loss of control over decisions taken to withdraw their driving licence.

7. Ethnicity

In addition to having differing cultural beliefs, health status in our society varies across different cultural groups (Cabinet Office, 2000a). Some groups are more likely to report ill health, and some conditions in certain populations are more prevalent than in the general population overall. Much of this variation can be explained by socio-economic status. However, it is also recognized that the health needs of older people from ethnic minorities can differ from that of the UK's white population. Additionally, some ethnic groups have a different attitude towards illness and disability, which will shape the attitude of the individual to their circumstances and what they perceive to be the accepted behaviour. Ironically, the access to health care by ethnic groups can be compromised.

Implications for occupational therapy

The contents of this chapter emphasize the value of the adoption of an approach that takes a range of intrinsic and extrinsic factors into account when determining the needs of older people, and the optimal responses to those needs. It also embraces a model of vulnerability in older age that takes into account medical, social and environmental factors. If this is achieved, there is no doubt that the full potential of occupational therapy will be realized for both users and their carers, and for services.

The points identified below are reiterated in the forthcoming chapters.

Adopt a holistic approach

In common with other professional groups working in the health service, there has been a tendency for health-employed occupational therapists to promote a diagnostic approach located in a medical paradigm. Conversely, those occupational therapists employed by social care agencies have been eager to set aside a medically orientated approach in favour of a social construct.

The evidence provided in this chapter underscores the importance of adopting a holistic approach towards the complex needs that older people can present with. However, to achieve this, practitioners, wherever they work, must become more focused upon the totality of needs that older people can present with, rather than being rooted in a medical or social construct.

Take account of the full spectrum of needs

The adoption of the previously described holistic approach enables the totality of needs the older person presents with to be taken into account rather than concentrating upon the problems derived from a specific diagnosis or syndrome, or a set of social circumstances. The full range of occupational therapy skills are required when assessing older people and identifying relevant interventions. Occupational therapists are trained to be able to respond to both health and social care problems, and are therefore well placed to meet a complex mix of physical and social needs that vulnerable older people can present with. This includes a consideration of environmental factors alongside the consequences of age, disability and illness, and availability of social networks. Furthermore, it is important to take time to discuss ideas and solutions with the older person as well as relying upon methods of assessment to guide decision-making.

Develop expertise

The adoption of a holistic, person-centred approach towards the needs of older people is challenging. It requires that occupational therapists continually update and refine their skill base. It also demands independence on the part of the individual practitioner rather than reliance upon the views of other professional groups. Finally, occupational therapists need to be able to work effectively with colleagues from other professions to ensure that their views are adequately conveyed and acted upon.

Be ready to respond to rapidly changing needs

The needs of older people do not remain static. They often change rapidly, in response to altered health status, increasing frailty and the challenges to managing daily life that result. This signals the importance of always listening to the concerns of older people, in combination with an approach that enables longer-term treatment and follow-up (in preference to assessment in the absence of intervention). It also indicates the importance of ensuring that vulnerable older people do not become lost to services.

Pointers for practice

- Rather than being aligned to a medical or social paradigm, occupational therapists are advised to adopt the WHO framework that crosses these constructs.

- Practitioners must ensure that they are familiar with the common causes of illness and disability in older age, as well as the consequences of ageing.

- Through observation of the older person undertaking occupations, and discussion regarding their daily lives, occupational therapists are well placed to be able to detect disorders that have not been spotted.

- Occupational therapists must be alert to the whole range of needs an older person presents with, for example the need for dental care or for hearing aids, referring on to other agencies as indicated.

- The impact of the personal, social and environmental circumstances the person lives in must be taken into account as well as the consequences of illness and disability.

CHAPTER 4

Older people and informal care

This chapter draws upon a range of policy and sociological literature to explore the informal care provided to older people by family, friends and neighbours and how service providers can help this army of carers to continue to provide support. Carers as well as the older person in receipt of care may have needs that can be successfully met by occupational therapy, with the needs of the older person and their carer frequently but not necessarily being related.

Supporting vulnerable older people in the community commands long-term support from a comprehensive network of formal (paid) and informal (unpaid) carers. In this country, the extent of informal care provision overall equates to the contributions of around 3.5 million female and 2.5 million male carers. In terms of financial worth, this amounts to between £15 billion and £24 billion each year.

However, older people as recipients of care represent only one dimension of the overall picture of informal care in this country. Chapter 2 illustrated the support offered by fit and older people in good health to their families, for example looking after grandchildren and family pets. Additionally, many older people are involved in the care of other older people, particularly if they are married.

Policy focus upon informal care

The contribution of informal carers, including family, friends and neighbours, has created tensions for the State and for professionals. Their contribution is indispensable but until relatively recently there has been little formal recognition of this vital role. The 1990 Community Care Act emphasized the rights of people to remain living in their own homes *wherever feasible and practical*. The implications of this for informal carers were wide in that it promoted the importance of their previously unrecognized contribution. However, implicit within the White Paper *Caring for People* (DoH, 1989b) was the desire to capitalize upon this unpaid labour force. Implementation of Community Care had further implications for carers. First it drew attention to the fact that carers have needs in their own right. Second it has led to a professionalizing of the role of informal carers. Similar observations have been made in other countries. A survey of the carers of people aged 70 years and over in Australia (Jorm et al., 1993) found similar patterns of caring to those in the UK. They concluded that formal care provision has to be targeted at the carers as much as at the older people they care for.

The Carers (Recognition and Services) Act of 1995 was the first formal UK policy recognition of the needs of carers. The Act, implemented in 1996, entitled carers to an assessment in their own right as long as they provide substantial amounts of care on a regular basis, and the person they are caring for is in receipt of community care. The specific requirements of this assessment are discussed in Chapter 6 on assessment. Through publication of *Caring about Carers: A National Strategy for Carers* (DoH, 1999d), the government further acknowledged the contribution of carers. The strategy is underpinned by three key approaches, namely information for carers, support for carers and care for carers. Particular attention is given to carers in employment and young carers. Within the strategy the government raises the fact that one in eight people in Britain are now carers, and that there is insufficient information available about carers from black and ethnic minorities (DoH, 1999d).

The Carers and Disabled Children Act (2000) has followed the National Strategy. This introduces a number of new entitlements for carers. Examples are that local authorities can assess carers in situations where the person they are caring for has refused to be assessed. The local authority then has to take decisions regarding whether they are able to provide services to meet assessed needs. These services are not defined within the Act but examples are given of physical assistance and training or counselling. Another aspect of the Act is the empowerment of local authorities to issue vouchers for short-term respite breaks from caring.

Networks of informal care

How does informal care fit into the overall pattern of care provision to older people? To ascertain this, we need to know who the care providers are, and the balance of formal to informal care provision. A large-scale survey of the informal care received by older people (Bond et al., 1999) confirmed that spouses and daughters were the most frequent providers of care. Also the care provided by family members was more likely to be personal or physical in nature. However, in some circumstances individuals other than those most logically identified as main caregiver were providing most of the available support. Also, those providing support might not define themselves in this role. Bond et al. (1999) suggested that the reliable identification of those individuals who provide informal care and support is a challenge to be addressed. They also drew attention to the neglected dimension of care-giving to people resident in long-term care. While the nature of caring changes when a person enters long-term care, carers do not always wish to relinquish their support.

A typology of support networks for older people (Wenger, 1992) identified five broad types of network support, dependent upon the availability of relatives, friends and neighbours, and interaction with the community and voluntary groups. Research by Herbert et al. (2000) confirmed the continuing importance of networks of care and the importance of service providers having knowledge of these networks when planning support.

The findings and conclusions drawn by Bond et al. (1999) regarding both the complexity and fragility of networks of informal care for older people were echoed in the work by Mountain (1998a). This uncovered clear discrepancies between the care described by nine older women with complex needs, the views of occupational therapists who had been involved in their treatment (and were still treating six of the nine women at the time of interview), and the care documented in the psychiatric case notes. To make clear where these differences were occurring, a method of visually displaying the care network was devised (Figure 4.1). Each of the

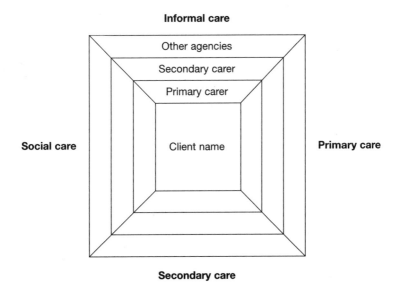

Figure 4.1 A framework within which decisions are taken about involvement in occupations.

four sides of the quadrant represents a different form of care, namely primary care, social care (including housing), secondary care and informal care. The individual is placed at the centre of the quadrant. The relationship between the form of care provided and the individual can also be attributed through the care diagram; for example, a carer closest to the centre of the quadrant represents a highly significant relationship whereas one placed further away from the centre is of lesser consequence.

Three dated care diagrams were drawn for each of the nine women. The first illustrated the care network described by the individual herself, the second the treatment and care documented in the case notes and the third the care and treatment described by the occupational therapists. The care diagrams revealed different understandings of care networks across the three data sources, even in situations where collection of data occurred within a relatively short time-scale. Not surprisingly, the care diagrams derived from interviews with each older person revealed a more complex care network than did those from the case notes or from the occupational therapists. The older people made reference to a greater number and range of care providers. Differences between the perceptions of professionals and the women regarding informal care were the greatest and occurred most frequently. All disciplines contributing to the case notes appeared to have a simplistic view of informal care and family responsibilities. One of the likely reasons for this was a transfer of information from the summary information sheet held in the case notes. The person identified on this sheet as being next of kin appeared to have been automatically translated into the most significant carer. As a consequence, for several of the women, the assumption made by professionals that family were the most important source of informal care was completely erroneous: neighbours or friends were providing the most intensive help.

This was illustrated by the experiences of Mrs KA who had cancer as well as a diagnosis of manic depressive psychosis. She had extensive needs, requiring intervention by more than one medical specialty. The case notes stated that Mrs KA's son was the main carer. Mrs KA had a very different view of this relationship in that her son had moved in to lodge with her but this was not to meet her care needs. From her viewpoint, the help received from a neighbour was of greatest significance – a fact that had not been noted in the professionally held documentation. For three other women there was no reference to informal care networks whatsoever in their case notes, even though it was a crucial aspect of their support. Professionals were clearly ignoring some important sources of informal care, and in particular that provided by the Church. In contrast to disparities in accounts of informal care, the extent of home care recorded in the case notes tended to agree with that described by the women.

This is possibly because services provided through the local authority such as home care and meals on wheels formed part of a standard package of provision to frail older people at the time, and consequently professionals would be aware of their provision.

Examination of different perceptions of the care provided to these vulnerable older women demonstrated an urgent need for improved communication between professionals involved in the treatment and care of vulnerable people. It also demonstrated the costs, both to service users and carers and to service providers, of failure on the part of professionals to listen properly to the views of the people they are trying to help. It confirmed the need for all professionals to be aware of the totality of assistance available to the people they are caring for and treating, and the existence of any gaps. The research also demonstrated an urgent need for greater coordination across health and social care agencies if policy requirements are to be met.

Caring obligations and situations

Most informal carers are family members. Daughters and daughters-in-law are the largest group of informal caregivers in the UK, particularly those aged 45 years and over (Qureshi and Walker, 1989). A proportion of these carers will be in employment. The government is considering strategies to help carers remain economically active while still maintaining their caring role (DoH, 1999d). However, concentrating upon the contribution of younger carers should not discount the caring role played by older men and women. The OPCS survey on disability (Martin et al., 1988) found that 40 per cent of the main carers of disabled people were over 65 years and 16 per cent were 75 years and older. Research by Levin et al. (1994) revealed that out of a sample of 287 people caring for older people with dementia, 57 per cent were spouse carers. Therefore there are a large number of older people who will be vulnerable due to their own health in addition to the demands of the caring role. The Department of Health (1999d) estimated that 855,000 carers provide care in excess of 50 hours per week.

Views of care provided by family members

Older people consider family and family obligations to be very important, particularly when their increasing frailty requires them to seek support. The work of Arber and Ginn (1993) identified a hierarchy of informal care situations preferred by older people. The highest preference was for care provided by the marital partner, followed by care in their own home by people from their own generation, followed by care by their children.

Mountain and Moore (1995) heard older people describe a range of family support, for example family who were close and provided support, family at a distance who also provided some degree of support, and non-supportive family or those who lived too far away. Family history and the interactions between different family members will inevitably shape the extent of support offered in later life.

> They're very important, very vital. Unfortunately we know that but they don't, so they don't all come to visit.

> I have two sons. My husband died a year and a half since and the eldest boy has been three times in 18 months. The youngest boy comes when he wants me to babysit.

Mountain and Moore uncovered some condemnation of families who do not provide support and care, but it was also clear that what was an acceptable level of family involvement varied from person to person.

> I've two very good sons. I have a son who lives in Harrogate and I go every weekend.

> Well I haven't got a family. I've got nieces and nephews. Sometimes they'll come down and other times they don't.

> I have a daughter and I just see her once a week on a Friday evening as she's a warden in sheltered housing, so she's busy working and I can't really see her during the week. I have two granddaughters. They just ring me and come down occasionally.

> As far as my son and grandson are concerned, they're not bothered about me, they're bothered about themselves. They don't come near me, not at all.

The group of older Sikh women expressed the view that their children should feel happy and fulfilled through caring for them.

> There should be give and take in families, they think of us and we think of them ... we help them in their need. They respect us, we respect them ... wherever our sons and daughters are married, we may go to their homes gladly and they may come to us happily. This is what happens in families.

> By the grace of God my children are helpful towards me. I don't have to ask for anything, they come to know of my needs without my telling them about my needs.

These interviews demonstrated the great importance they placed upon family obligations. However, given the influence of Western society upon second and subsequent generations of Sikhs, there were questions regarding the extent to which these views were idealized. Waiting for assistance from the family and the frustration this can cause for the older person was also discussed in some depth.

> They have no time. If you wish to go somewhere, they are looking after their own children ... Then the elders are left behind unthought for, the elders are kept waiting with the hope that maybe, they might or might not go, they [elders] keep sitting, looking after the house.

The interviews also illustrated how the expectations maintained by these older immigrants could be disappointed, possibly due to the fact that their children and children's children would be increasingly Westernized:

> ... both get ready and go out in the morning, even R has got a job, I feel so terrible.

> If they do not call me or if they do not take care of me then of what use is my life?

Grief resulting from bereavement could lead to a dependence upon family members for practical assistance.

> Even shopping. My son used to do my shopping. I daren't meet people.

Finch (1995) examined whether the widespread beliefs regarding family obligations are actually played out in reality. Her exploration of the views of nearly 1,000 randomly selected adults revealed that there was a consensus view that children should be the first to offer help when care was required. On the other hand there was little agreement regarding the nature of the responsibility that children have towards their elderly parents. Put more simply, it is generally agreed that adult children should do something, but there is no consensus regarding what they should do. Despite describing family obligations as unreliable in certain situations, some of the older people interviewed by Mountain and Moore indicated that it is not possible to rely upon neighbours in the same way that you can rely on family.

Views of care provided by neighbours and friends

Family care is not always available, because of changes to family structures, smaller families and geographical mobility (Qureshi and Walker, 1989). As a consequence, a substantial amount of care is provided by relatives, friends and neighbours (Twigg and Atkin, 1994).

For some of the older people interviewed by Mountain and Moore (1995), mutual care and support existed between them and their neighbours, or at least a sense that neighbours would provide support if absolutely necessary. For older people living on a particularly lawless inner-city estate it was expected that neighbours would assist each other in trying to prevent crime.

> We always tell the next door neighbour where we're going and she always tells other people.

Help provided by family members, and in some cases neighbours, included assistance with gardening, shopping and other household tasks. The extent of reliance upon informal carers for these aspects varied according to the ability of the older person to be able to pay for the help they required. If finance was not available to purchase assistance older people have to either demonstrate need according to local authority criteria or wait for people to volunteer to do tasks for them.

> I'm lucky because we get taken to Asda in the car and fetched back so we haven't any heavy carrying to do.

There was a sense of having to rely ultimately upon oneself.

> But you can't depend upon them [neighbours] all the time. I mean they're all right for a night or two but they don't want you around for years.

For some, friends were a mutual source of help and support.

> I've a good neighbour, we visit one another regularly. If she bakes she gives me something. If I bake I give her something.

However, increasing disability rendered this source of support tenuous, particularly as it was often founded upon reciprocity.

> We're all in the same boat. We can't help each other.

Research into community alarm systems for older people, where the alarm was answered by volunteers, involved interviewing friends and neighbours who had offered to act as respondents. Some stated they had not expected to deal with some of the resulting situations, particularly when the health of the older person had deteriorated over time (Thornton and Mountain, 1992).

The nature of informal caring

It has already been stated that where caring involves intimate tasks, it is usually the family who provide support (Wenger, 1992; Qureshi and Walker, 1989). Finch (1995) identified commitment, underpinned by a history of mutual care and helping, as being factors that can influence the extent and nature of care provided. The research of Clark et al. (1995) found that that the amount of care provided to an older person is greater if they are co-resident with the carer, with this also having implications for the nature of the caring role. Even though there are more admissions to residential care than moves of older people to live with their children, Healy and Yarrow (1997) described older parents living with children as an important form of supported accommodation, and identified a need for community care to support such arrangements. Through an in-depth study of 24 shared households, Healy and Yarrow (1997) found that moves of older people to live with their children had usually been instigated due to illness, with speedy decisions being taken, often without consideration of the long-term consequences. Most of the older people and their host families found the arrangement stressful, but could see no other options given the information they had available to them. Respite care to give carers a break from caring was the most frequently encountered unmet need in the study by Healy and Yarrow (1997). It should also be borne in mind that a greater amount of care overall is provided by non-resident carers who will also have respite needs.

The burden of caring and its consequences

The burden of care experienced by carers can embrace both physical and emotional demands. It can also have economic consequences. Carers of working age may have to relinquish paid employment. Additionally all carers will have to shoulder additional costs, for example heating, clothing and bedding. Even if the person is admitted to long-term care, the family may have to continue to pay. Becoming a carer also demands familiarity with the symptoms and patterns of illness in the person being cared for, and with the service system. In common with many other complex constructs, the word 'burden' is subject to many interpretations. Within a framework devised to describe carer burden, Nolan et al. (1990) also identified loss of social life and loss of the previous relationship with the cared for. Loss of the relationship is significant in the case of older people with dementia. Murphy (1986) described the feelings that the person with dementia can engender in their carer. These include anger, grief, guilt, shame and embarrassment.

Given that a good proportion of the caring role is undertaken by people who are old themselves, carers can be in poor health. Research by Levin et al. (1994) found that 40 per cent of their sample of carers coped while experiencing ill health or disability. It is therefore significant that the General Household Survey (1995) quoted within DoH (1999d) revealed that nearly 60 per cent of all carers had no visits from health or social care providers.

The tasks involved, such as lifting, can lead to carer injury. The national strategy for carers (DoH, 1999d) referred to research which demonstrated that 51 per cent of carers had suffered a physical injury such as a strained back since they began to care, and 52 per cent had been treated for a stress-related illness since becoming carers. Other studies have confirmed this finding; for example, a study by Brown and Mulley (1997) found a high incidence of back strain among informal carers of frail older people, together with unintentional injury to the older person, due to older people being put in the position of having to lift other frail older people.

The demands of caring for older people with dementia

This book has aimed to consider older people as heterogeneous human beings, irrespective of diagnostic category, with individual needs and aspirations. However, given the particular burden that caring for someone with dementia places upon the individual carer, it is appropriate to briefly consider the demands of caring for someone with dementia within the overall theme of the burden of caring.

There are a number of problem behaviours resulting from the dementia syndrome. The most problematic behaviours reported by carers during research by Reddy and Pitt (1993) were tendency to falls, disturbance at night, incontinence and attention-seeking behaviour. Mace (1990) reported that carers described difficulties such as daytime wandering, hiding things, night waking, demanding or critical behaviour, catastrophic reactions and memory disturbance, with inconsistency of observed problems stemming from uneven neurological damage.

The relationship between behavioural problems and the strain this places upon carers is well recognized. Reddy and Pitt (1993) found that the greater the severity of problems exhibited by the person with dementia, the higher the strain experienced by carers. Similarly, Greene et al. (1982) observed that carers found that the problems most difficult to tolerate were behavioural problems and the mood disturbance associated with dementia, whereas cognitive deficits were more easily managed. Sanford (1975) found that the problem mentioned most frequently by carers as being difficult to cope with (and sometimes intolerable) was sleep disturbance. Faecal incontinence was another poorly tolerated problem.

The restrictions upon lifestyle placed upon the carer of someone with dementia are enormous, with the burden of care encompassing a high level of physical and personal care needs as well as managing problematic behaviour.

The burden of spouse carers

The burden of caring has a greater impact upon spouse carers than upon other carers (George and Gwyther, 1986). The heightened demands experienced by spouse carers are not surprising, given that service providers try to preserve caring between married couples at all costs (Twigg and Atkin, 1995). The demands of caring can exacerbate existing health problems, made worse by carers not being able to take time off from caring to attend to their own health needs (Wright, 1986). Living in the same household as the person being cared for or being a close relative makes receiving adequate health and social care less likely (Parker and Lawton, 1994). This was confirmed by Mountain (1998a), who found that the marginal extent of help provided in response to the needs of this group of highly vulnerable individuals was low. The two women with partners were offered even less help from statutory care providers – another finding consistent with larger studies (Wenger, 1984; Ellis, 1993).

This spouse carer gave vent to his frustration:

> The social services were a washout. They promise you so much ... we'll get somebody to help with your cleaning, we'll get somebody to sit with her so you can go out, but nothing at all, nothing.

The women interviewed who still had partners were overly reliant upon them. Those who lived alone received more formal care overall than those who lived with others, even though their partners were also elderly. The lack of attention paid to the needs of carers was also highlighted during this research when a spouse carer of one of the older women being interviewed clearly used the opportunity provided by the presence of the interviewer to get a short period of respite for himself.

Elder abuse

The demands of the caring role can be such that it can create high levels of stress in the carer (Gilhooly, 1984), and in particular for those looking after older people with cognitive impairment. The demands placed upon carers of older people can be such that tolerance is stretched to the limit. Chronic stress can ultimately lead to breakdown of the caring situation.

The prevalence of abuse of older people is unknown. MacDonald (1997) identified the following situations where abuse of older people with dementia may occur:

- severe stress or mental illness of the carer;
- extreme provocation;
- lack of coping strategies;

- previous abusive relationship;
- punishment for past deeds;
- retaliation;
- deliberate cruelty;
- financial exploitation.

Elder abuse can occur in a range of situations including domestic and communal settings. Through a comprehensive review of the UK research, Creadie (1996) established that it is important to differentiate between different types of abuse as they will have very different explanations. Also, the characteristics of the abuser are more important than those of their victim. Therefore if the carer is unstable, has poor mental health, is older and dependent themselves or alcoholic there is a greater chance of abuse occurring. In contrast to commonly held beliefs and the conclusions drawn by authors of individual projects, the overall body of research does not support the commonly held belief that the stress of caring is the main reason for abuse.

It is estimated that one in twenty older people in the community and one in three older people in care have been abused at some time. Action on Elder Abuse, who produced these statistics, is a campaigning organization with the aim of protecting older people by driving forward policy, raising awareness, responding to cases of abuse and encouraging good practice.

In Chapter 5, where services to meet needs are described, examples of neglect and abuse on the part of paid care staff are also considered.

Measures of carer burden

Table 4.1 describes some of the frequently used measures applied to assess needs and outcomes from a carer perspective. Given new legislation that promotes the needs of carers, these and other similar measures will have increasing importance for practice. Information about all of the measures cited in Table 4.1 can be obtained from the *Outcome Measures* information pack published through the College of Occupational Therapists (Clarke et al., 2001).

Carers within the health and social care system

Some of the evidence quoted in previous sections of this chapter serves to underscore the neglect of carer needs by statutory services until relatively recently. Despite the undeniable importance of informal care for vulnerable older people, questions have been raised in the past about the extent to which health and social care practitioners, including occupational therapists, work with and assist carers (Twigg, 1992). Bamford et al.

Table 4.1 Measures appropriate for determining carer stress and burden

Instrument	Used for	Properties	Nature of questions
General Health Questionnaire (Goldberg and Williams, 1988)	Assessment of mental health	Simple self-administered questionnaire	Measures anxiety and depression in the general population
Nottingham Health Profile (Hunt et al., 1985)	Measurement of levels of self-reported distress	Simple 38-item scale	Examines the person's perceived health
Carergiver Strain Index (Robinson, 1983)	Strain in carers looking after physically impaired older people	Questionnaire with 13 statements	Can be used to measure change in levels of strain over time
Carer Satisfaction Questionnaire (Pound et al., 1993)	Assessment of carer satisfaction following stroke in their cared-for	Questionnaire	Focuses on information provided and adequacy of support
Relatives Stress Score (Greene et al., 1982)	Measure of stress experienced by carers looking after an older person with MH problems at home	Questionnaire with three subscales	Used to measure stress in relatives looking after an older person with cognitive impairment

(1998), quoted in DoH (1999d), conducted interviews with carers and identified the following needs:

- the ability to be able to maintain some form of life of their own (this could extend to social contacts and employment);
- maintenance of own health and well-being;
- having confidence in the standard and reliability of services provided to the person they care for;
- sharing responsibility with service providers, including the provision of practical and emotional support and timely assistance at times of crisis;
- having a say in the way that services are provided.

The National Strategy for Carers (DoH, 1999d) stated that carers need to be involved in service planning, and consulted individually about the services they require. In addition to the legislated assessment of social care needs by social services, health service staff should assess the health needs of carers and consider how they can help, and housing authorities may also be involved in considering accommodation needs both of carer and cared for. On first contact with services, carers should be provided with information and put in contact with organizations to assist them. (Examples of such organizations to assist carers of older people are appended.) Carers should be encouraged to feed back their experiences of services; one suggestion within the National Strategy for Carers is a comment card for carers to provide feedback about services that go into the home. Home care and occupational therapy were given as examples of services where carer perspectives might be gained in this way. The government is also promoting the value of NHS Direct to carers (DoH, 1999d). The country-wide introduction of Care Direct, whereby people can call for information about health care, social care, housing and social security, could also be a positive resource for carers. However, a recent report on older people with mental health problems noted that despite a wealth of information being available, carers still need more advice and support (Audit Commission, 2002b).

Assessment of carer needs

The assessment of carer needs is a complex process, requiring a skilled approach from practitioners. A study by Seddon and Robinson (2001) undertaken in Wales between 1997 and 1999 examined how care managers were coping with the demands of the 1995 Carers (Recognition and Services) Act, how it was being implemented through practitioners' and carers' experiences of the process. Results found that, at the time, both care managers and carers had limited knowledge of the Act and the rights it gives to carers. The authors recommended that care managers have to move beyond the limitations of the assessment and care management processes, towards a more holistic view of the caring task. To achieve this, staff training and development is required. One of the aspects that should be taken into account during the assessment process is the need for a break from caring. (The implications of carer assessment for occupational therapists is discussed in Chapter 6.)

Examples of services and interventions to meet assessed needs

One of the aims of this chapter was to discuss the needs of carers of older people and raise the contribution that occupational therapists can make within overall health and social care provision. The importance of giving an equivalent amount of attention to both the older person and their carer is emphasized through the inclusion of carer assessments and interventions throughout this book. Some of the examples of services and interventions to meet needs are now described, but the reader should also refer to forthcoming chapters.

Lifting and handling advice

Prior to providing advice on lifting and handling, health and social care practitioners are obliged to undertake assessment to meet the requirements of the 1992 Manual Handling Regulations. Therefore more information about lifting and handling needs is described in Chapter 6 on assessment. Compliance with the Manual Handling Regulations (HSE, 1992) is proving problematic. One of the consequences of the avoidance of lifting has been the more frequent prescription of hoists for use within domestic settings. There are questions about the use of hoists and other equipment for use in home settings, for example their acceptability and the limitations upon usage due to the physical environment (Tamm, 1999; Connelly, 1998). Limited evidence available following the introduction of the Regulations suggests that the needs of informal carers and the people they are caring for are complex and are not being adequately met (Cunningham, 2000). Anecdotal evidence also suggests that poor advice has led to carers lifting in situations where paid staff have refused, and unworkable solutions have been presented for application within a domestic environment. The Human Rights Act (1999) should change this as it is likely that the courts will be reluctant to grant public services immunity in negligence cases. It is therefore important to provide rehabilitation solutions and interventions through provision of equipment and training that both minimize risks to staff and to service users and carers.

Providing a break from caring

The term respite care is being superseded by the term 'provision of breaks'. Respite care is an umbrella term used to describe a whole spectrum of residential, day care and home-based services delivered to a range of users and their carers. Other terms used as alternatives to respite include regular relief, intermittent, rotating, planned, programmed or phased care schemes (Levin et al., 1994). Styles of service include residential respite care, day care, family placement schemes and home-based respite care, provided by statutory health and social services as well as the voluntary and private sector. For many people, local authorities will take the lead for arranging and funding respite services. The NHS plays a role when the person requires specialist medical or nursing care. The availability of new funding for respite care was announced within the National Strategy for Carers (DoH, 1999d). A range of professional groups are involved in the provision of respite care. Admiral nurses, who specialize in the care and treatment of people with dementia, are increasingly being employed across the country to meet the needs of both service users and their carers (Audit Commission, 2002d).

While the recent National Strategy for Carers promotes a range of services, residential provision is by far the most common form of respite available. Residential respite care is provided from a range of settings, and is most commonly the offshoot of an institutional programme. Primrose and Primrose (1992) identified three different types of residential respite provision: shared care where the person is timetabled to spend, for example, two weeks in care and four weeks at home, planned respite admissions and crisis admissions.

Day respite care can occur in hospitals, day centres or in residential facilities, with the nature of what is being provided being influenced by the provider. In theory, day care could enable carers to maintain employment, but in reality the limitations of most provision mean that this is impossible. This may change through implementation of the National Strategy for Carers (DoH, 1999d).

Users of family placement schemes tend to be less dependent and behaviourally disturbed than those attending residential or day respite services (Twigg et al., 1990). This form of innovative services is rarer in comparison with other forms of provision. A variety of home-based respite services have developed over time, largely as a result of the activity of voluntary agencies. Crossroads schemes were established in the 1970s to assist carers in their own homes, thereby providing respite. However, availability is patchy. Sitter services were initially developed for carers who need a break but refused institutional respite. Their effectiveness has been questioned as the sitter will only visit for short periods of time and there is a tendency for the carer to continue caring. As they are largely provided by voluntary services, provision across the country is not uniform, and their remit may not extend to carers of people with dementia. Sitter services may be provided at night, but this is the exception rather than the rule (Murphy, 1986). Evaluation of sitter services suggested that they could complement rather than substitute for other forms of respite service (Thornton, 1989; Levin et al., 1994). While the changing needs of carers and the person they are caring for will change over time, the number and range of providers of respite care in any one locality can make it difficult for the service system to respond flexibly and appropriately.

The prevailing theme running through the majority of definitions of short-term breaks and service interpretations is the centrality of needs of the carers. However, in the 1990s a policy shift occurred towards taking account of the needs of the user as well as that of the carer (SSI and DoH, 1993). Prevention of institutional care is the explicit aim of respite care in this country and elsewhere (Nolan and Grant, 1991; Miller, 1991). However, it can provide an opportunity for provision of therapeutic interventions to both user and carer, with the goal of improving the quality of life of both parties (Nolan and Grant, 1993). There is no doubt that the majority of carers do benefit from a break. However, the simplistic notion that informal care will be maintained if the carer is given a break from the caring role is not borne out. Moreover, the desired policy outcomes of prevention of institutional care and cost effectiveness are both ill found-ed in light of the available evidence (Mountain and Godfrey, 1995).

The General Household Survey of 1995 quoted within the National Strategy for Carers (DoH, 1999d) acknowledged that family or friends provide the most common form of break for carers. There are several rea-sons why carers might not take up respite even when it is available. These include lack of information about availability of services, lack of choice about type and timing of services, and carers' perceptions of the quality of services being offered. Take up of respite care is particularly influenced by the perceptions of the carer (Twigg and Atkin, 1994). Offers of respite are likely to be refused if carers consider that the respite service is dis-tressing and unacceptable to the person they care for. Carers can become so embroiled in the caring relationship that professional help and sup-port to help them to cope with the concept of a break from caring can be indicated (Brody et al., 1989). It may also be difficult to come to terms with different styles of respite service. This carer interviewed by Mountain (1998c) found it difficult to accept the notion of home treatment and support as a form of respite.

> Even a combination of these things [respite services] would not be as good as the respite provided by hospital. Also you'd be worried about your relatives.

The type of respite offered and accepted, and the frequency of respite, will all determine benefits experienced by carers.

Training and education for carers

In 1990, Evans reported on the development of an occupational therapy service for older people with dementia and their carers. Her paper stemmed from the question of *who is the client* with respect to the work of community staff involved with people with dementia. To explore this question, three community occupational therapists collected information over a four-week period. Details included the breakdown of the sort of work they were involved in and the contacts with patients and/or carers. Results confirmed their involvement with carers, for example providing instruction about rehabilitative techniques, discussions about respite care and giving information about services. The study also highlighted the inadequacy of statutory data collection methods for recording this type of information, and therefore the implicit agreement that it was not part of the mainstream business of occupational therapy. The value of providing training to empower carers has been underscored more recently (DoH, 1999), validating the views expressed in the 1990 paper by Evans.

Opportunities to share experiences of caring

As has already been indicated, many carers benefit from the opportunity to be able to share their experiences of caring and gain mutual support. A spectrum of resources should be available within any locality to meet needs for support and self-help. These are often run very effectively by the voluntary sector, working in partnership with other locally provided services (DoH, 1999d).

Acknowledging the end of informal caring

Informal caring may end for a number of reasons, including deterioration in the condition of the person being cared for and breakdown in the health of the carer. Recognition is now being given to the needs of carers to continue with some form of caring role, even when the person they have been caring for is admitted into a long-term residential setting (DoH, 1999d). The popular belief that there is a correlation between respite and lowered admission to institutional care fails to take into account the nature of the relationship between carer and cared for and the specific needs arising from the illness and life circumstances. Reduction in stress experienced by carers, and in particular those looking after a person with dementia, only reduces when the person is admitted to permanent residential care (Levin et al., 1994).

Implications for occupational therapy

There is a clear role for occupational therapists in assessing needs and providing advice and treatment to carers, as described in Chapters 6 and 7. However, in order to be able to respond appropriately, we first need to understand the particular needs of individual carers and their circumstances and experiences.

Understand carer needs and perspectives

Research by Mountain undertaken in the early 1990s confirmed that involvement of both users and their carers in occupational therapy assessment and treatment was transitory, with the role that occupational therapists might fulfil with respect to carer needs being under exploited (Mountain and Moore, 1996). In common with other professional groups, occupational therapists have been slow to recognize the role they have to play in supporting carers to continue with their caring role both in the community and in long-term care settings. The importance of occupational therapy involvement with carers cannot be underestimated. However, provision of assessment and interventions must be underpinned by an understanding of what it means to be a carer and the demands that this creates.

Take account of the caring context

Every family has a history, and this consciously or unconsciously shapes the reaction of members to current situations. The roles of family members will have developed and become established over time. Chapter 2 contained illustrations of caring provided by older people to other members of their families. The consequences of illness and old age can radically change patterns of established family responsibilities. It will certainly help determine attitudes towards caring. Some of the important questions for all professionals working with older people and their carers are:

- When is the line crossed from being a carer, for example of grandchildren, family pets and neighbours, to reliance upon others for daily needs?
- What are the factors that provoked that shift?
- What are the family views of that shift?
- What assistance and services do the older person and their carers require to maintain their quality of life in the community?

Understand who the carers are

The experience of caring is specific to the individual and those caring for them. This means that occupational therapists and other professionals cannot make presumptions about who is undertaking care and what is being provided. The previous sections of this chapter have illustrated how easy it is to draw erroneous conclusions, particularly if the views of the older person are not listened to properly. The totality of the network of care being received by the person has to be understood. Care networks can be very fragile, with the balance of responsibility shifting according to the contributions of individual carers within the network and the well-being of the person being cared for. If any one aspect of care is withdrawn, action has to be taken rapidly.

Understand the nature of the caring relationship

Understanding who the carers are is intertwined with the importance of understanding the contributions being made by different individuals.

This chapter has highlighted a differentiation between those with family responsibilities for providing care, and care that might be provided by neighbours and friends. However, this is not always the case, particularly for those older people with no family support. Friends and neighbours as well as family members can find themselves in caring situations that they had not originally anticipated, owing to deterioration in the condition of the older person they agreed to help.

Research on elder abuse underscores the importance of understanding the needs of the individual carers and their personal capacity to be able to maintain the caring role.

The ability of all carers to continue caring must be monitored continually, with this vigilance extending to all members of the care network.

Recognize when carers are over-burdened

Help provided to carers can be too little and too late to avoid a breakdown in the caring relationship. Caring for vulnerable older people is extremely demanding. Research has shown that provision of respite care does not usually prevent the older person entering residential care. What should be avoided is a crisis management approach to the situation, whereby the carer is overcome with stress and exhaustion before help is provided. Respite care and other forms of help should be provided to enhance the quality of life of the carer. In common with other professionals working with older people, occupational therapists have a responsibility to identify when the carer is particularly vulnerable, before a crisis is reached.

Determine carer needs and the responses required to meet them

This important area for occupational therapy practice is described in Chapter 6 on assessment and Chapter 7 on occupational therapy interventions. However, whether occupational therapy can in itself meet needs is secondary to the importance of ensuring that an identified individual or agency is responsive to needs as they arise, and is available to listen to the concerns of carers.

Pointers for practice

- Do not assume that the most significant carers are next of kin.

- Do not assume that the views of the older person and their carer will be in accord; it can be beneficial to talk with the carer and their cared-for separately, particularly if tensions are detected.

- Take into account descriptions of the whole care network from the older person's perspective, including the contributions of community resources like the Church.

- Ensure that adequate attention is paid to the health and emotional needs of carers as well as the cared-for.

- Where the carer is a spouse or is living in a co-resident household, pay particular attention to assessing their health needs in the context of the caring tasks they have to undertake.

- Have full, comprehensive information regarding the statutory and non-statutory services available to carers within your working locality.

- Be alert to changes in the well-being of the carers when visiting/treating the cared-for.

- Identify needs for respite care to meet carer needs both for health care, social and recreational activities and for employment.

- Ensure that you refer on to other agencies within the care network, particularly where necessary responses fall outside the remit of your service and your own skills and expertise.

CHAPTER 5

Services to meet needs

Given that old age is an intimate issue, which affects everyone, the provision of health and social services that would be acceptable to us in our old age ought to be a prime requirement. Older people require services to be delivered in an expert, integrated manner if optimum outcomes are to be achieved. Challenges stem from the heterogeneity of people with complex problems, the combinations of problems they present with, and the need for a range of services (including risk assessment and protection) to be delivered within available means.

There are a number of determinants that drive the nature of services. The reporting of services for older people in the media confirms that the following three intertwined factors are particularly influential:

1. Policy-makers have to balance the need for effective provision with resulting costs to the exchequer.
2. There is a long historical legacy to services for older people, the ramifications of which still impact upon what is provided today.
3. When public opinion is strong enough, it can result in changes to government policy and what is provided as a result.

It is vital that those involved in working with older people have a thorough understanding of all the factors above, as they are so influential in shaping what is ultimately provided and for whom. As a consequence this chapter is steeped in the history of service provision and the views of various stakeholders, as well as the implementation of current policy. Chapter 9 builds upon the content of this chapter by examining the occupational therapy role in various service settings.

Current context

Changing societal attitudes towards older people, described in Chapter 1, are reflected through the services provided for them. However, it must be remembered that positive attitudes to older people and ageing is a 'modern phenomenon'. Until very recently older people were neglected by successive governments, this being demonstrated through scant allocation of resources. The tendency has been for health and social care provision for older people to be set aside in favour of high-impact, resource-intensive, acute provision mainly targeted at younger people. The past failure to get services right for older people was reflected by the continued production of guidance documents and reports by the Department of Health and Social Services Inspectorate (e.g. DoH, 1997a; Barnes, 1997a; SSI and DoH, 1997a; SSI and DoH, 1997b).

Changes in the attitude of policy-makers are illustrated through the contents of a number of more recent policy documents, for example in *Modernising Social Services* (DoH, 1998b), the *National Plan* (DoH, 2000a) and the *National Service Framework for Older People* (DoH, 2001a). All articulate the need to involve people in services and provide quality provision in line with what service users and carers need.

It takes time and concerted effort for good intentions to be firmly embedded into practice. The publication of the *National Service Framework for Older People* (DoH, 2001a) was a watershed for services for older people, demonstrating a substantial, long-term commitment – something that had not been so clearly acknowledged in the past. It emphasizes the importance of integrated services and the delivery of person-centred care, with the associated need for shared information systems. The introduction of NSF Implementation groups and Local Service Implementation teams aims to ensure the translation of national policy into local action, with the requirement for a three-year implementation plan. However, it is important to recognize that there is little in the National Service Framework that is really new and, furthermore, many of the articulated standards should have already been routine practice.

Devolution of Scotland and Wales has led to different approaches towards services for older people; for example, both Scotland and Wales have published their own National Service Frameworks for older people. The Scottish Health Strategy, articulated in 2000, has resulted in a range of policy implementation documents. *Better Care for All Our Futures* (Scottish Executive, 2001) described a range of measures to promote independence and choice in older people, for consultation. While the underlying policy thrust of enabling older people to live quality lives was very similar to that emanating from London, it also included some significant differences. These included free home care for up to four weeks following discharge of older people from hospital, and free personal care. It also emphasized the need to standardize charging for services rather than allowing local variation to continue. The National Assembly for Wales has recently published its *Strategy for Older People in Wales* (Welsh

Assembly, 2003). Again the aims stated in the document reflect those of English policy, but with different approaches towards implementation, particularly in terms of funding arrangements for services for older people.

Despite an acknowledgement of limitations and subsequent attempts to improve services, the quality of health, social and community care provided for older people still often falls short of what we would wish for ourselves and for our families. The inherent difficulties of translating good intentions into actions (within resource constraints) are illustrated through the continued emergence of negative media reports and subsequent initiatives in response. In 2001 Lothian and Philp reported a bleak picture of prevailing attitudes towards older people by health care professionals, drawn from a review of the evidence. Their work confirmed that older people are both disempowered and devalued by health care, with this phenomenon not being confined to the UK. Bad practice exposed by the review included negative interactions between staff and patients, general insensitivity, little regard for privacy, and lack of information to enable the person to make informed choices. The review also found that ageism and prejudiced attitudes were prevalent among staff.

Involvement of the public, service users and carers in health and social care services has become the popular mantra of politicians, with those working in public services charged with policy implementation. User involvement is frequently mentioned. However, at the time of writing, what this means is still open to interpretation, with service providers struggling to fit this new requirement into services that were developed from a very different perspective. Until recently, opinions of those using services were not sought, and those who were seen to be complaining were viewed as being troublemakers. Furthermore, older people may need to be encouraged to challenge the system, and in particular the dominance of the medical profession.

> I was brought up to believe the doctor's word was law and therefore you don't question it. (Elderly male with hearing difficulties, Opinion Leader Research, 2001, p. 11)

Service providers must be continually vigilant if the quality of services is to be maintained. There are some signs of improvements in this area. Some of these changes can be attributed towards staff working in services making the links between existing provision and what they might expect in their own older age. This was illustrated by the attitudes of frontline practitioners working in health, housing and social care who attended seminars held at the King's Fund in 1999 and were invited to discuss their views of the current treatment, care and support of older people (Easterbrook, 1999). Attendees were very critical of some aspects of current and anticipated provision and had many suggestions for improving services. Ideas included: more adapted accommodation and greater access to rehabilitation, multi-agency one-stop shops; key workers to coordinate all aspects of treatment, care and support; and training and support for professions, particularly in the area of social and interpersonal skills.

The issues that have been raised in these introductory paragraphs are expanded in later sections in this chapter, which examines in depth the recent policy-led changes to services and the implications of subsequent initiatives.

History and legacy

The shift in political and societal attitudes that have occurred over recent years are extensive if they are considered in the context of the overall history of service provision to older people. Some of the continuing negative attitudes towards older people and the long-standing problems that pervade health and social care can be explained by the history of service provision, the nature of which has been both restrictive and paternalistic.

Murphy (1999) provided a potted history of health and social care to older people in the UK. At the turn of the last century, treatment and care of poor older people was managed by workhouses and poor-law infirmaries, in line with the poor law of 1834. An attempt in 1895 to reconsider this system failed, owing to lack of agreement within the committee. In the first half of the twentieth century, state-supported residential health and social care for older people was still being provided in this manner. 'Poor law care' was mainly run by local authorities through public assistance institutions. Given that families were expected to provide for their own, the regimes for those unfortunate enough to have to be dependent upon the state were harsh (Means, 2002). Various campaigns took place over the years to try to reform the public assistance institutions and introduce smaller residential settings.

Implementation of the Beveridge Report in 1948 introduced the National Health Service. During the same year, the 1948 National Assistance Act led to the establishment of residential care homes. Residents were allowed to keep five shillings of their pension for pocket money and contribute the rest to the local authority (Means, 2002). Since then, cost to the recipient has remained one of the main defining differences between health and social care. While health care remains free at the point of delivery, social care often has to be paid for.

The history and subsequent legacy of different elements of what continue to be the mainstays of health and social care provision for older people are explored below.

Long-stay care

Prior to recent service innovation in the form of intermediate care services, if assessment in hospital suggested that a person was not able to return home for either health or social care reasons, long-stay provision would be sought immediately.

During the 1960s there was a growing realization that long-stay hospital services for older people were frequently substandard. In 1967, Robb produced a series of emotive accounts of the deprived lives of older people living in institutionalized health care settings. She stressed the need for monitoring of standards and more resources to be spent on care of older people. However, her final remarks placed the ultimate responsibility with the staff involved in managing and delivering services. In 1972, the DHSS published minimum standards for geriatric hospitals and departments in an attempt to raise standards. A number of studies undertaken since 1972 have indicated that awareness of the need for improvements has not been readily translated into practice. In 1993, Bowie and Mountain reported observational research undertaken in 1990 on long-stay wards for older people with dementia. Observations were carried out on wards between 8am and 9pm over a three-month period. The researchers maintained diaries, providing insights into what it was like living on these wards at that time. Frequent institutional practice was observed. This included block treatment of patients, social distancing between staff and patients, depersonalization, rigid ward routines and a lack of choice or autonomy for patients. Additionally, episodes of petty tyranny, passive neglect and rough handling of patients were observed in certain settings. In contrast, episodes of patient-orientated care also occurred on some of the wards, demonstrating that provision of quality care was possible, even to the most disabled individuals and in less than ideal care settings. Another component of the same project involved an inventory of the clothing and possessions of the residents on eleven long-stay wards (Mountain and Bowie, 1992). Results found that while many patients had the basic range of clothing itemized by the inventory, some had as little as three items, with underwear being the least likely to be personally owned.

The history of provision provided through local authorities has a similar pattern. The expectations of the 1948 National Assistance Act were that homely settings for up to 30 people would be provided for those no longer able to live independently. Shortly afterwards, disputes began between health and social care providers, which continue to this day, regarding how to define those in need of hospital care as opposed to those requiring residential care only.

Aspirations of what would be provided following the 1948 Act did not match reality. A number of factors described by Means (2002) limited the

establishment of quality services. These included post-war building short-
ages, and the lack of resources to train staff who transferred to new
settings from the 'workhouses'. Therefore the conditions for older people
in residential care did not improve. This was illustrated through the work
of Townsend (1962), who presented a similar observed account to that of
Robb, detailing the impoverished existence of older people in residential
care settings.

From the 1980s onwards, the extent of private-sector residential and
nursing home provision greatly increased in the UK, funded largely
through the social security system. This enabled the majority of NHS-run
institutionalized services for vulnerable older people in the UK to close. A
small proportion of local-authority-provided social care continues. Almost
all the wards included in the study by Mountain and Bowie no longer
exist. These changes to the configuration of residential care raises questions about the deployment of staff who previously worked in older-style
settings. Additionally, it also questions whether the replacement provision
is any better, and if so in what ways. Through a review of the evidence on
elder abuse, McCreadie (1996) concluded that:

> Little is known about abuse in communal settings. It appears that psycho-
> logical abuse is the most common form of abuse and relates to many of the
> pressures of looking after people with severe disabilities. The need for
> work-based training is clearly demonstrated. (McCreadie, 1996, p. vi)

Existing evidence confirms that changes to the way in which residential
care services are provided through social care have been slow to progress,
and there are continuing questions about the quality and training of staff
working in nursing and residential care settings.

> It has taken an extraordinary long time to shake off not only the literal
> legacy of the poor law, but also the lack of vision and sense of citizen rights
> for older people associated with it. (Means, 2002, p. 12)

In 1987, Willcocks et al. conducted a survey of the lives of both staff and
residents in residential homes. They found that although the basic needs
of the residents were being taken care of, the lack of control and routines
of the home were leading to institutionalized practice. One year later, publication of the Wagner report (NISW, 1988) reiterated the need to
promote privacy, autonomy and individuality in residential care. A re-eval-
uation of residential care by the same researchers involved in the work in
1987, ten years later (Peace et al., 1997), uncovered benefits resulting from
the move from the monopoly provision by local authorities. Positive
changes included: the involvement of various stakeholders in provision,
including residents, their relatives, staff and regulators; a growing

awareness of the need to empower residents; and an overall improvement to the physical environment in which care is delivered. Aspects that were observed to be resistant to change included the continuance of a task-focused attitude towards care and a lack of training and regulation of the workforce. Barlett and Burnip (1999) confirmed the need for much greater regulation, and went on to suggest that other solutions must also be sought, for example through collaboration with other care homes, the statutory sector and with education providers. This must include the recognition of good practice where it exists.

Long-standing concerns about the quality of care provided in nursing and residential care homes have recently resulted in a policy-led response. A national long-term care charter, 'Better Care; Higher Standards' (2002), has been introduced. The aim of local charters implemented in localities from June 2000 should be to inform users and carers of what to expect from long-term care provision, through the articulation of standards and targets across health, housing and social care. Users should also be given the opportunity to feed back their views, and influence the nature of service provision. The Nuffield Institute for Health (2000) produced an analysis of the progress made by authorities in developing local charters. They recommended the need for more guidance from government. They also suggested a move away from notions of traditional social service provision, towards the inclusion of transport, employment and lifelong learning. Subsequent policy guidance was provided to health authorities and local authorities (DoH, 2001c). The Care Standards Act (2000) was an important landmark for social care provision. Two new bodies have been put in place as a result of the Act. The National Care Standards Commission is responsible for service regulation and inspection. The General Social Care Council is charged with improving standards in social care and with registering the social care workforce. It is also responsible for regulating social work training and education. Additionally, the Training Organisation for the Personal Social Services (TOPSS) is leading the development of a national training strategy and the identification of national occupational standards and a qualifications framework for social care.

Long-standing and contentious disputes between health and social care, regarding who should provide long-stay provision, continue. The requirement for local authorities and health authorities to make local arrangements for continuing care explicit was first stated in executive guidance (DoH, 1995). More recently, new guidance asked Strategic Health Authorities to ensure that joint health and social care eligibility criteria are agreed with local councils, with agreed changes in place by October 2002 (DoH, 2001d).

There is little doubt that the transfer of the majority of nursing and residential care to the private sector has increased the vulnerability of provision. The rate at which privately run care homes have been closing, largely due to changes in funding arrangements (35,000 beds lost from 1998 to 2001) is a cause for concern (SPAIN, 2001). Thus the extent of choice available to older people no longer able to live independently is diminishing. Reports by the media have shown the distressing effects of closure upon the lives of long-stay residents, necessitating a move to other accommodation when the care home they are living in closes. The transfer of provision of the majority of long-term care from health to the private and voluntary sectors also means that those requiring residential care now have to pay for it. Statistics suggest that over the next two decades 50–60 per cent of older people will be expected to pay for their own care, flying in the face of the expectation raised in the Beveridge report of *Care from cradle to grave* (Murphy, 1999). The current position is that funding for nursing and residential care is derived from a mix of public monies and personal contributions on the part of older people themselves. Approximately one-third of placements are entirely self-funded and others are expected to make a contribution, based on a means-tested assessment (Glendenning et al., 2002). Recently, the government decided that nursing care provided in residential settings for older people should be provided free, but that social care will continue to be means tested. This policy has been implemented in England and Wales, but the Scottish Parliament made the decision not to charge for social care.

Acute hospital care

Acute hospital care has remained at the hub of all services. This will now change with the recent introduction of primary care trusts, and the transfer of commissioning from health authorities to primary care. However, as with most centrally driven changes, the speed with which change will impact upon those receiving services will be much slower.

The established forms of acute provision for older people remain the following (DoH, 1999b):

- *traditional*: older people placed on either general medical wards or geriatric wards, depending upon the opinions of the referrer;
- *common admission*: sent to certain wards on the basis of assessment;
- *age-defined*: sent to wards on the basis of age;
- *integrated*: physicians with responsibility for older people within general medical wards, with access to specialist facilities as required;
- *de-specialized*: specialists in older people work on general medical wards.

In common with long-stay care, the quality of acute care for older people has frequently fallen short of what should be expected. An independent enquiry into the care of older people on acute wards in 1998 reported by the Health Advisory Service (HAS, 2000) confirmed the deficits that existed in many ward settings. These included too few staff trained in the care of older people, poor leadership, lack of attention to nutritional needs and low staff morale.

The National Service Framework (DoH, 2001a) stated that there should be a specialist older age multi-disciplinary team in every general hospital. This should include therapists of both practitioner and consultant grades. One of the roles of the team would be to disseminate best practice in care of older people across the whole organization (including accident and emergency) using a variety of methods. Identified best practice includes care protocols that take continence and nutrition into account. It also includes giving more attention to the risks as well as the benefits of hospital admission to the person. The observations of the Audit Commission (2002b) were that some beds for older people with mental health problems should be provided on every general hospital site.

Patient advice and liaison services (PALS) were legislated through the NHS Plan (DoH, 2000a), with all Trusts being required to employ PALS by 2002. They are responsible for taking the issues raised by service users and carers and bringing them to the attention of the organization, with direct access to the chief executive. They are also charged with helping staff to become more responsive to the needs of users and carers, devising appropriate training to assist with this. A further aspect of the role of PALS is ensuring appropriate user representation in planning and service delivery forums. Within the implementation document (DoH, 2002b), PALS are asked to take particular account of certain populations who may find it difficult to be heard. Older people, particularly the physically frail, those living in care homes and those with mental health problems, are specifically cited.

Day provision

Both health and social services have traditionally provided day services for older people.

Day services can provide a number of functions, for example:

- allowing staff to observe and monitor the older person and provide medical interventions as indicated;
- provision of rehabilitation;
- respite care for carers;
- provision of social and recreational activity;
- provision of rehabilitation (which may not be a feature of the facility; support and advice can be offered as distinct from rehabilitation).

There is a continuing lack of clarity regarding the role of day hospitals (as opposed to day centres) with many combinations of services falling under the rubric of day care, for example a combination of day and home support services and acute care as a day service, thus providing an alternative to hospital admission.

A series of visits by the Audit Office to day hospital facilities for older people concluded that day care was an important component of community care, assisting people to retain independence (National Audit Office, 1994). In 1994, Peter suggested that geriatric day hospitals could offer intensive assessment as well as acting as skill and resource centres for community-based services. The Audit Commission (2002b) stated that day hospital provision for older people with mental health problems should exist for assessment and short-term treatment, and day centres should concentrate upon longer-term care. However, the situation remains where even if day hospitals purport to provide active rehabilitation, in reality their remit is extremely variable. Some services can veer more towards social care than active treatment.

The evidence base to support these services is poor and conflicting. An examination of day services for older people with dementia found that the best arrangements were those where there was joint working between health and social services, with input from visiting specialists (SSI and DoH, 1997a). The most robust evidence is concerned with day hospital care for physically frail older people. The conclusions of a systematic review of the evidence concluded that day hospital services appear to be effective for older people who need rehabilitation, but there is no advantage over other forms of provision such as outpatient and domiciliary services (Forster et al., 1999). However, they may reduce use of other resources.

Community services

One of the main tenets of the Community Care Act of 1990 was that people had a *right to live at home wherever feasible and practical*. It was underpinned by two White Papers: *Working for Patients* (DoH, 1989b), concerned with reorganization of health care delivery, and the Griffiths Report on community care (DoH, 1989c). The Griffiths Report had a big impact upon the delivery of community services, particularly for older people, given that they were then, as now, the largest consumers of health and social care, with over 50 per cent of all referrals to social services being for older people. Prior to implementation of the community care reforms in 1993, social service departments were able to dispense services as they thought fit. The implementation of community care policy in 1993 brought with it an optimistic view that services for older people would be transformed.

Older people interviewed by McKenna and Hunt in 1991 were asked questions about changes anticipated in the forthcoming implementation of the Community Care Act (DoH, 1990). Areas identified for improvement by the older people included:

- travelling distances to and from hospital;
- lack of choice regarding consultant, hospital or treatment, and lack of information;
- lack of concern regarding the older person's home situation before and at discharge;
- delays in treatment.

The authors concluded thus:

> It seems evident that some elderly people are being discharged from hospital without full and proper consideration of their best interests. (McKenna and Hunt, 1991, p. 130)

Implementation of the 1990 Community Care Act has meant that social services departments are obliged carry out an assessment of needs and, if deemed to meet criteria, to provide social care in response. This process, termed care management, involves:

- determining the level of assessment;
- assessing need;
- planning care;
- implementing the care plan;
- monitoring, reviewing and reassessing needs over time (DoH, SSI and SSWG, 1991).

Community care legislation also required that social service departments identify eligibility for services, with provision of services being dependent upon the person meeting criteria set by the individual authority.

The care programme approach (CPA), introduced in 1991, is a further mandatory assessment and monitoring process targeted at people with mental health problems, including older people. This involves the assessment of health and social care needs of the person, the construction of a care plan to meet those needs, designating a key worker for each person and regular reviews of the plan (SSI and DoH, 1995). The lead for this process is taken by health agencies. The overlap between care management and care programming has been recognized by the Department of Health, who suggested that:

> The complementary principles of the health service care programme approach (CPA) and that of social services' care management should be

applied to older people according to locally agreed procedures. (Department of Health, 1997a, p. 18)

In response to assessment of needs, local authorities may provide a number of social care services, for example home care, meals on wheels, community equipment and referral for assessment of housing needs. The local authority home-help service traditionally assisted with domestic tasks around the home and shopping. In the early 1990s these services shifted to provision of personal care. Clarke et al. (1996) interviewed older people about the value of help in the home. They found that a differentiation was drawn between help with tasks around the home, which were perceived to be helping the maintenance of independence, and help with personal care, viewed as being a threat to independence. Most recently, there has been a change in the nature of home care services away from that of care, towards an enabling or rehabilitation model. However, this gives rise to questions about the continuing provision of personal care which home care has most recently been involved in. It also sets aside the views of older people who would still like to have help with housework and other associated tasks.

As with residential care, many of the social care services traditionally provided by the local authority are now provided by private contractors, either through service-level agreements with authorities or independently. This has led to some reported difficulties, for example in the interpretation of manual handling regulations by home care staff working for privately run organizations.

Community equipment services have recently received specific policy attention. A study by the Audit Commission confirmed the long-standing neglect and marginalization of community equipment services, which has led to a patchwork of haphazard and uncoordinated services across the country (Audit Commission, 2000a and 2002a). The well-reported difficulties which underpin current community equipment provision include the following:

1. idiosyncratic division of labour between health and social care providers, founded in whoever has budgetary control rather than in the needs of users of the service;
2. a further division of labour concerned with whether a piece of equipment is deemed to be provided to meet a health or social care need (this might also dictate whether the equipment has to be paid for);
3. unacceptable waiting lists for services in some areas of the country;
4. inadequate information for users and an overall reluctance to involve users in all aspects of the service.

In response the National Plan (DoH, 2000a) stated, '50% more people will benefit from community equipment services in the future.' This intention has been accompanied by financial investment for the development of integrated, appropriate services. More detail about the organization and delivery of community equipment services is provided in Chapter 8.

The established interfaces between different services

As was stated in Chapter 3, the needs of vulnerable older people often remain hidden in the community until a crisis is reached such as a breakdown in a system of informal care, a fall or a sudden illness. For other comparatively fit and older people in good health, life is manageable until an event occurs like acute illness or injury, triggering admission to hospital. Once older people have endured a period of acute hospital care, successful return home can be precarious and the ability to manage independently diminished.

Figure 5.1 shows the range of options presented by service configurations that existed prior to the promotion of a new range of services to facilitate discharge and promote independence. This illustrates a linear decision-making and placement process, with no opportunity to interrupt a prescribed sequence of events largely because the imperative to release acute beds was not supported by other options bridging hospital and home. The diagram also shows services operating separately, with minimal interface between different components.

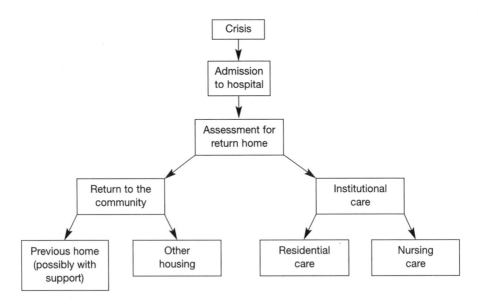

Figure 5.1 The traditional pathway of older people through the health and social care system.

In a traditional model of service delivery, once the acute phase of the illness had been managed, the older person was then either recommended for return home, possibly with support from community and day services, or for admission to institutional provision. Thus, if a person did not demonstrate ability to return home during assessment and was placed on the route towards institutional care, the chances of returning home were minimal.

Transfer of care into the community necessitates agreement between health and social care providers about the services required upon discharge, for those services to be accessible and for the necessary finance to be available to fund them (Victor et al., 2000). In the past, this process has been fraught with problems, many of which could be attributed to a lack of coordination between hospital and social services staff (Horne, 1998; Clarke et al., 1996). Different cultural standpoints and a lack of trust often led to a repetition of assessment of need once the older person had returned home (Davis et al., 1997). Additionally, needs identified in hospital might not necessarily trigger a community care assessment. Furthermore, if the older person had agreed to admission to long-term care, the likelihood of the individual being able to rescind that decision would be minimal.

Therefore the aim of acute services would be to treat the acute illness and then secure a safe discharge, and thus pass the person on to community health and social care provision or long-stay care.

Recent changes to established patterns of service delivery

Over a number of years, objections have been raised against traditional models of service delivery for older people. A study of the continuing care arrangements for older people and the commissioning of long-term care (Audit Commission, 1997) uncovered a need to rebalance care away from the traditional modes of service delivery – that of acute beds and residential care. Further to this, the National Beds Enquiry (DoH, 2000b) concluded that many older people stay in hospital longer than is necessary, and that alternatives closer to home should be sought, particularly as the majority will be less independent when they leave hospital than they were before.

A number of new understandings are accompanying the development of different forms of service for older people, the origins of which can be traced back to both policy intentions and the increasing voice of older people in our society. It is now widely acknowledged that vulnerable older people demand a high level of resource from both health and social services, and require these services to be delivered in an expert, integrated manner. This is in line with the stated aims of the government's modernization programme of improving population health, making services quick and convenient, improving consistency, breaking down service barriers and investing in staff and infrastructure (DoH, 1998a). It is also recognized that if there is a choice, older people prefer to be supported in their own home (Audit Commission, 2002b).

The new approach to service provision for older people is underpinned by a number of factors. While the majority can be traced back to policy initiatives, some of the changed foci of traditional services can be attributed to innovation on the part of NHS and social care management. The building blocks underpinning new forms of service for older people are as follows:

1. the integration of health, social care and other services for older people;
2. recognition of the value of rehabilitation services, accompanied by new services to assist rehabilitation and recuperation;
3. the involvement of older people in health and social services;
4. a needs-led, whole-systems approach to health and social care delivery, with primary and community care rather than acute care being central to the system;
5. the delivery of quality, patient-centred services.

Each of these important topics is now considered in some depth, with the resulting occupational therapy contribution to different modes of service delivery discussed in Chapter 9.

Promoting service integration

Over the last few years, successive policy initiatives have fostered the goals of integration and seamless care delivery. This is grounded in both economic and common sense. It has long been observed that older people with complex needs have changing requirements over time that should be managed flexibly by teams of health and social care professionals. Furthermore, service integration should minimize duplication and gaps.

Some local examples of integrated services for people with complex needs that span health and social care have emerged during the last 20 years (Hughes-Roberts and Redfern Jones, 1990; Ramsay and Coid, 1994). These endeavours were usually introduced as a result of the work of local innovators, and rarely generalized. However, policy-makers have only recently formally recognized the true value of service integration. New and higher profile interpretations of integration, and the mandatory introduction of new rehabilitation and care services, are shaping emerging models of practice. These incorporate health, social care and in some cases the voluntary sector. An increasing demand for skills in rehabilitation, together with the ability to deliver both health and social care interventions, mean that occupational therapy has found itself at the heart of the majority of these initiatives.

The requirement to integrate services for vulnerable people (including older people) was first articulated in an executive letter (DoH, 1997c). Following this, joint investment plans for older people (JIPs) had to be produced in partnership by health and local authorities by April 1999. Plans were accompanied by extra funding for preventive strategies and to manage winter pressures. Since 1999, all localities have been required to provide an updated plan for each forthcoming year.

The 1999 Health Act promoted new flexibilities across health and social services, so that budgets could be pooled between them. Arrangements for lead commissioning were such that either the local authority or the health authority could take the lead. Policy intentions regarding service integration and seamless care delivery for older people were mandated in the NHS Plan (DoH, 2000a) and underscored in the National Service Framework for Older People (DoH, 2001a); for example:

- a single assessment process for health and social care of older people, to be introduced by April 2002;
- integrated equipment services, to be in place by April 2004;
- a jointly appointed intermediate care coordinator to be employed in each health authority area by April 2001;
- the development of integrated falls services in all localities by April 2005;
- jointly produced protocols for the management of older people with mental health problems by 2004.

The NHS Plan (DoH, 2000a) also introduced a new service concept – care trusts. These organizations are a new level of primary care trust, responsible for all health and social care delivered to a locality. Care trust pilots commenced in April 2002.

As well as integrating across different disciplines and agencies, occupational therapists must ensure that the services provided by the profession are integrated within the same locality. This important topic for the profession is discussed fully in Chapter 9.

The policy initiative Supporting People (DoH, 2002b) (also mentioned briefly in Chapter 3) aims to improve the quality of life of vulnerable people by helping them to live in the community, promoting independent, as opposed to institutional, solutions. Implementation requires the forging of links across previously separated services, including social services, social landlords, voluntary sector agencies, local authority housing landlords,

NHS trusts and private sector housing and care provision. A new funding framework to link housing and housing-related support underpins Supporting People. Implementation commenced in April 2003.

A real issue for the integration agenda is the interpretation of the term by commissioners, managers and practitioners. Challis (1998) considered the meaning of integration within a process rather than service paradigm, suggesting that by concentrating upon tasks, the integration process can be hindered. He adopted the term *horizontal integration* to describe integration of activities occurring at the same level within the organization, with maintenance of control of certain separate processes. The merging of different processes, with the aim of reaching the final goal, is called *vertical integration*. Examples of vertical integration included care management services for people with dementia, community assessment combined with rehabilitation in the community, and linking of clinical decisions regarding admission to long-term care to care management arrangements. Success is underpinned by integration of tasks as well as organizations.

The merging of previously separated roles and responsibilities in line with the concepts of vertical integration is described within *Shifting the Balance of Power* (DoH, 2001e). This is an important document for all health and social care professions. One example of the changes required by this document is a move towards inter-professionalism in health and social care. This means that previously separated roles and responsibilities across disciplines will merge so that individuals are equipped to respond to a whole range of needs. These changes must be accompanied by pre- and post-registration training to facilitate the necessary shift in practice in line with this focus.

Maximizing the value of rehabilitation services

Given the current and anticipated rise in the numbers of older people in Western society, it is not surprising that one of the goals of policy-makers is cost-effective service provision. In the UK, as well as in other countries, this aim is being played out through initiatives to promote independence and prevent admission to long-term care. The aim of promoting independence is being accompanied by an increasing recognition of the value of rehabilitation. Through a review of the literature, Nocon and Baldwin (1998) identified the following reasons for the policy focus upon rehabilitation:

* pressures to reduce length of hospital stay in acute hospitals and provide more services in the community, meaning that people have to be rehabilitated in order to manage outside hospital settings;

- continuing care policy, which demands that health and social care agencies have explicit eligibility criteria for provision of services;
- a recognition of the importance of rehabilitation, both medical and social, in preventing residential and nursing home placements.

In 1999, the Royal Commission on Long Term Care gave its report on the future of long-term care. Metz (2000) was somewhat critical of this report, stating that there were missed opportunities to consider what older people want and to raise the potential of reducing the costs of long-term care through innovation to reduce dependency. A study of older people after fractured neck of femur confirmed that admission to residential and nursing homes was most often determined by personal and social factors (Herbert et al., 2000). The capacity of the individual to be able to benefit from rehabilitation was not usually taken into consideration, particularly if decisions are being taken at speed. Intermediate care has been promoted through government as a means of plugging this gap (DoH, 2000a, 2001a). Mountain defined the term thus:

> The term intermediate care is a *care function* concerned with the transition from dependence to independence resulting in the restoration of self care abilities. (Mountain, 1997, p. 1)

Steiner and Vaughan (1997) described intermediate care as falling between usual care systems, and possibly involving a strategic shift of services from primary to secondary care settings.

> Intermediate care may best be seen as a function, rather than a discrete set of services. That function is to facilitate transitions from medical dependence (experiencing oneself as a patient) to day-to-day independence (experiencing oneself as a person). It may also encompass the prevention of a transition in the opposite direction. The concepts of transition and restoration are central to intermediate care. (Steiner and Vaughan, 1997, p. 1)

The concept has since been translated into services, where traditional service boundaries are blurred. These are itemized in Chapter 9.

The place of intermediate care within mainstream service provision in the UK has been cemented through recent initiatives (DoH, 1997c, 2000a, 2001a, 2001g), and enhanced by the provision of government funding over a number of successive years to introduce and develop services. There are many interpretations of intermediate care services, with the thrust of the government interpretation being strongly linked to hospital discharge and the promotion of independence in older people (DoH, 2001g). The following dimensions of services are emphasized within this policy definition:

- for people who would otherwise face unnecessary prolonged stays in residential settings;
- provided on the basis of comprehensive assessment leading to a structured care plan;
- have a planned outcome of maximizing independence and enabling users to live at home;
- are time limited – no longer than six weeks;
- involve cross-professional working, with a single assessment framework, shared record keeping etc.

It is significant that the role of intermediate care in providing convalescence has been omitted from the policy definition. Additionally, intermediate care services mainly concentrate upon those older people with physical illness or frailty. There is a growing awareness that a holistic model of rehabilitation should also meet the needs of older people with mental health problems. This will require the development of specific skills on the part of care providers (Nuffield Institute for Health, 2002).

Ultimately, intermediate care for older people will become integrated into mainstream provision. Occupational therapists already make an important contribution to intermediate care services, with demand set to rise with the future development of services. The specific roles and responsibilities of occupational therapists within these services is described within Chapter 9.

Involving older people in health and social care

The White Paper *Modernising Social Services* (DoH, 1998b) required providers of social care to improve the quality of the services they provide, give choice and monitor user and carer satisfaction with services. The implementation of *Modernising Social Services* has included the mandatory requirement for all social services to undertake yearly surveys of their client base. Health policy has made similar demands; for example, the National Service Framework for Older People (DoH, 2001a) demands that all health and social care organizations have systems in place to explore the experiences of service users and their carers, including the regular use of surveys. It states that older people and their carers should be represented within every health and social care organization, with representation reflecting the cultural mix of the community being represented. Additionally the National Service Framework explicitly states that service users should have their own copies of their care plan.

Chapter 1 described how older people are becoming increasingly involved in services; for example:

1. seeking improvements to services, for example joining in the Age Concern campaigns;
2. becoming involved in local initiatives, for example the Better Government for Older People initiative;
3. representing the views of older people in service planning;
4. providing opinions of services experienced

Additionally, older people are increasingly being involved in determining the nature of the services they receive. Since February 2000, local authorities have been able to make direct payments to people they have assessed as needing social care so that they can purchase their own packages of care. Implementation has proved slow but, where it has occurred, it is most likely to be for adults with disabilities. Clark and Spatford (2001) examined the implications of applying direct payments to older people, by examining the outcomes of a nine-month pilot project undertaken in one authority. The scheme did not give older people money to buy services, but operated within the policy and practice guidance on direct payments. It enabled older people to negotiate with providers regarding when their services were to be delivered, save any unused hours for up to three months and use the service to meet the assessed needs they had identified as being most important. Results of the research found that older people who chose to employ a personal assistant received a high-quality service. However, finding someone suitable could be restricted by a lack of social networks. As the role of informal carers was not defined by the scheme, some carers used the scheme for their own direct benefit. The practice and time of care managers was challenged through the project, but they reportedly became more enthusiastic over time. In common with other projects concerned with direct payments, commitment of social services managers was crucial to success. Direct payments for older people are now being widely implemented. A recent study of the process of implementation in Wales recommended that for success, plenty of information should be available in the places frequently visited by older people. Additionally, social services care managers need to be well informed about the procedure and the support available for the older person if they choose to use direct payments.

There have been a small number of innovative projects to explore the optimum methods and potential of obtaining the views of traditionally marginalized groups of older people. Older people's satisfaction with the social services they were receiving was examined by Chesterman et al. (2001). Three outcome measures were identified: satisfaction with assessment and management of recent problems (drawn from interviews undertaken immediately after assessment), satisfaction with level of service being received (interviews six months later when the care package was established) and perceptions of their experience of social services. Analysis demonstrated the existence of relationships between satisfaction regarding service outcomes, the individual characteristics of users, their carers, available resources, the location of services and overall satisfaction with life. This research also underscored the complexity of measuring and interpreting responses to questions about satisfaction.

Barnes and Bennett (1998) reported a project undertaken in Scotland where older, frail, housebound people were encouraged to express views about the services that they were receiving. Sixty-two older people were recruited on the suggestions of home care, district nurses and social workers. All had health problems or were disabled, with 56 being users of community equipment and 60 in regular receipt of health and social services. Project workers transported individuals to group meetings to discuss their concerns. Issues discussed included home care, hospital treatment and discharge, problems of getting out, experiences of dependency, safety and security, and the accessibility of services. While this project illustrated the practical obstacles that must be overcome if frail older people are to be enabled to provide views about the services they receive, it also demonstrated the gains for services of engaging these users.

The work of Raynes (1999) involved older people living in nursing and residential care, arguably the most disregarded group of all. The project aimed to incorporate aspects of quality residential care provision identified by residents into the specification for commissioning contracts for one city council. A random sample of 50 homes was involved, resulting in 45 homes where at least one resident agreed to participate. A number of focus groups were conducted at different venues, with a maximum of 10 residents in each. All the groups agreed the following characteristics of good quality care:

1. activities in the home;
2. opportunities to get out of the home;
3. good food, choice of food and the opportunity to make a drink.

Other frequently mentioned quality issues included access to one's own bedroom, kind and knowledgeable staff and the physical comfort of the home. Half the groups raised the desirability of having equipment and adaptations available to promote self-care.

Allan (2001) provided yet another example of the benefits of encouraging the involvement of older people who traditionally have not had a voice. This work looked at the potential of consulting with people with dementia about the services they were receiving. Exploratory work with 40 practitioners and 31 older people with dementia in ten service settings demonstrated the need for a range of approaches to facilitate communication, and the requirement to consider the quality of relationship between the older person and the member of staff. It also reinforced the importance of providing staff training and support.

More recently, Raynes et al. (2001) interviewed 143 older people in focus groups and individual interviews, selected at random from 3,000 receiving home care from one city council. They were invited to say what home care services they were receiving, what they considered to be a quality service and what might be included in an ideal world. In common with other studies older people prioritized the provision of house cleaning and the provision of regular, trusted carers. They also suggested that services should be flexible, with equipment and adaptations being provided as required alongside help to enable people to get out of their homes.

Promoting a needs-led, whole-systems approach to service delivery

As Scott (1999) confirmed, treatment and care of older people cannot be fulfilled by the sole involvement of one discipline. It requires a multidisciplinary focus, and good integration between hospital and community services. Enderby and Stevenson (2000) described the range of rehabilitative services identified as being necessary to meet the extent and variability of the needs of older people living in Sheffield. These services covered the following eight domains:

1. prevention/maintenance;
2. convalescence;
3. slow-stream rehabilitation;
4. regular rehabilitation;
5. intensive rehabilitation;
6. specific treatment for acute disabling conditions;
7. medical care and rehabilitation;
8. rehabilitation for complex disabling conditions.

To maximize the effectiveness of individual services provided within a locality, they must be drawn together into a coherent pattern or *whole system* so that users are easily able to move from one element of the system to another as their needs change over time.

The Audit Commission (2002b) defined a whole system as follows:

A whole system contains a comprehensive range of services, including services which enable older people to live independent lives. It also requires a way of coordinating the services people need and guiding them through the system. (Audit Commission, 2002b)

They noted that the following aspects need to be in place for success:

1. a shared vision grounded in the needs of older people;
2. a comprehensive, flexible range of services, delivered by multi-professional teams;
3. a way of guiding people through the system, ensuring that they obtain the services they need in a timely manner.

Further work has recently been undertaken by the Audit Commission to ascertain the extent to which a whole-system approach to service delivery for older people is becoming a reality (Audit Commission, 2002c).

One of the key aspects of delivery of intermediate care services (discussed in more depth in Chapter 9) is their introduction, within a whole system, of service delivery that crosses primary and secondary health care, health and social care, and statutory and non-statutory providers. An early literature review on intermediate care determined that success required a shared vision of rehabilitation services, and for the system to be underpinned by a system of care management (Mountain, 1997). While care management is most often referred to in the context of community services, it can also be applied to other settings to produce better care and outcomes (Waterman et al., 1996). The factors improving outcome are collaboration across different agencies and services, and innovative approaches towards individual patient care and resource management. An example of how this has been applied to intermediate care services is reported in the most recent version of guidance on implementation of the single assessment process (DoH, 2002c).

The previously described integration of health and social care systems is assisting with the development of effective whole systems, where previous organizational divides are eliminated or reduced. Primary care as the first point of contact for the majority of older people has to be central to the local configuration of services.

Table 5.1 shows the components of a needs-led approach to service provision for older people. It also demonstrates the desirability of a whole-systems approach whereby the changing needs of an individual can be met over time within the same service system. It includes long-standing styles of service, for example day services (as well as specialist services) and new developments like intermediate care. Within the overall framework of services for older people, there should be subsystems to address the needs of specific user groups, for example older people with mental health problems. Accompanying these factors is an emphasis upon meeting certain quality standards. The National Service Framework for Older People (DoH, 2001a) requires the development of locally agreed protocols and care pathways to determine both arrangements at all stages and who is responsible.

Table 5.1 A needs-led approach to service provision within a whole system

Need/ problem	Trigger(s)	Interventions	By whom	Lead organizations
Frailty/ suspected risk in the community	• Request for community care • Outcome of over-75 assessment	• Assessment of home environment • Equipment provision • Housing assessment • Home care • Carer assessment • Rehabilitation at home • Day care/friendly visits	• GP/ Primary health care team • Physio/OT • Trained support staff • Care staff • Housing	• GP/primary health care team • Community and hospital occupation-al therapist • District nurse • Social worker • Home care staff
Increased frailty/risk in the community	• Request for residential care	• Admission to residential community rehabilitation • Move to Sheltered/very sheltered housing • Enhanced community support	• GP/Primary health care team • Physio/OT • Trained support staff • Care staff • Housing	• NHS acute Trusts • Social services • Private sector
Signs of mental health problems	• Outcome of over-75 assessment • Request for medical assessment • Request for community care	• Assessment of mental state • Assessment of living situation • Assessment of user/carer needs	• GP • Psychiatrist • Community mental health team • Social worker	• Care Trusts • Primary care • Social services • Secondary psychiatric services
Emergence or exacer-bation of acute condition	• Results of assessment • Crisis in the community • Breakdown of carer arrangements • Accident/ injury • Acute illness	• Day hospital attendance as an alternative to admission • Intensive treatment/support at home • Hospital admission	• Physician • Psychiatrist • Surgeon • Nurses • Therapists • Dietician • Psychologist • Social worker	• NHS acute Trusts • Care Trusts • Primary care • Social services

Table 5.1 (contd)

Need/ problem	Trigger(s)	Interventions	By whom	Lead organizations
Needs for rehabilitation, convales-cence and support fol-lowing acute condition	• Discharge from acute care • Reduced levels of independ-ence • Lives alone • Carer stress/no carer	• Intermediate care: residential or community • Day hospital/day care • Support and mon-itoring by specialist health and/or social services • Hospital aftercare services • Provision of equipment	• Therapists • Nurses • Support workers • Social worker • GP/primary health care team	• Care Trusts • NHS Trusts • Social services • Primary care • Voluntary sector
Maintenance	• Reduced levels of independ-ence • Deteriorating/ relapsing condition • Carer stress/ no carer	• Low-level monitoring • Day care • Support from specialist community services • Provision of equipment	• Therapists • Nurses • Support workers • Social worker • GP/primary health care team	• Primary care • Social services • Care Trusts • Voluntary sector • Private sector
Palliative care	• Maintenance of quality of life • Carer sup-port	• Provision of large- and small-sized equipment • Carer assessment/ teach coping strategies • Support grieving process	• Community OT • Specialist nurses • Social worker • GP/primary health care team	• Care Trusts • Social serv-ices • Primary care • NHS Trusts • Private sector

Ensuring the delivery of high-quality, patient-centred services

The earlier sections of this chapter confirm the need for action to over-come the insidious consequences of years of poor-quality service pro-vision for older people. The introduction of Clinical Governance in UK health services and Best Value in social services has been successful in that they have highlighted the need to improve the quality of services (DoH, 1998a, 1998b).

The concept of 'patient-focused care' was first introduced to the UK health system by North American management consultants in the late 1980s (Hurst, 1996). The original construct was grounded in the reduction of inefficiencies resulting from the increasing fragmentation and specialization of hospital-based services. Patient-focused care meant that services were rearranged so that the patients' needs were the basis of resource allocation – not buildings, equipment or staff requirements. Hurst described the following principles as being the distinguishing features of patient-focused care:

- the grouping of patients with similar needs;
- decentralizing services so that they are closer to patients;
- the use of multi-skilled, cross-trained staff in special care teams;
- the adoption of care protocols and integrated patient records;
- more spending on direct care and less on peripheral processes.

The concepts underpinning patient-focused care have been adopted as a core theme of the modernization agenda and now extend beyond the hospital to incorporate all aspects of health and social services (DoH, 1998a, 2000a, 2002c).

It is now recognized that adequate, ongoing training and supervision of staff is a continuing requirement for the maintenance of quality services for older people, wherever they are located. A study by Mountain et al. (1994) examined the well-being and job satisfaction of nursing staff working on long-stay wards for older confused people in one health district, through application of valid and reliable measures. Results found a high level of dissatisfaction and unhappiness among ward managers which, given their pivotal role in setting standards for the ward, should have been a matter for concern. At the time, services were being subjected to accelerated movement into the community. Mountain et al. noted that:

> Until the issues surrounding job satisfaction, stress and burnout of nurses caring for this group of patients are addressed, and until the issues surrounding management and training are explored, it is unlikely that a change of venue away from the institution will result in any radical changes in the staff experience. (Mountain et al., 1994, p. 234)

One of the aims of the training initiatives for social care staff, and the regulation of the workforce described in a previous section of this chapter, is to address the training needs of staff.

A change to the workforce to match the needs of new services is a further policy goal. The Older People Care Group Workforce Team (CGWT) is a multi-disciplinary body set up to support the delivery of innovative, integrated, user-centred services through appropriate workforce developments. One of the current priorities of the group is to support workforce planners to deliver the health and social care workforce required to provide treatment and care to older people. Achieving this goal has to take account of the shortfall of appropriately trained professionals and the potential offered by individuals who do not have a recognized health or social care qualification. The process of workforce planning has to be both dynamic and iterative to meet this challenge (Nancarrow and Mountain, 2002).

Continuing challenges for services

Whatever the intentions of service providers are, it is relatively easy to be lulled into a state of complacency whereby the beliefs of what exist do not match reality; for example, policy promotion has led to the word *quality* frequently being used to describe services. However, is this really the case and, if it is, how can quality be maintained? Furthermore, some policy objectives are proving very difficult to embed into practice, for example the implementation of workforce planning to ensure that the capacity of the workforce in terms of numbers and skills is sufficient to match needs.

Coping with increased demand for services

The factors that have led to increasing demand for health and social care services, and community services in particular, are shown in Figure 5.2.

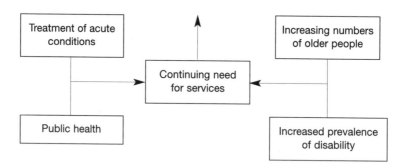

Figure 5.2 Population needs for services.

The conundrum facing government is how to deal with increasing need for services, brought about by the fact that we are living longer due to better acute care and public health. Furthermore, there is a focus upon strategies to improve health, promoted by the Green Paper, Our Healthier

Nation (DoH, 1998c). The evidence discussed in Chapters 1 and 2 confirmed that the majority of us will experience a healthy old age, particularly if we live active, fulfilling lives. Moreover, some conditions that can lead to chronicity are treatable. Inevitably, however, longevity leads to increasing demand for preventive, primary, social and secondary care services. The reality is that meeting the health and social care needs of older people is very costly for the exchequer.

> ... the costs to the NHS of providing services to this increasingly elderly population amounts to between 0.5 and 1 per cent per annum (in real terms) of the total budget of health authorities, a figure conceded by the government. (Harrison and Pollitt, 1994, p. 19)

Improving access to services

Improving access embraces two challenges: having services in place to respond to needs, and ensuring that practitioners are sufficiently skilled to be able to identify problems.

Before occupational therapists or other health and social care practitioners can assess an individual, that person has to be able to access the service system. While the aim of the government's modernization programme is service equality wherever a person lives (DoH, 2000a), questions remain about equity of access to services across the country. Moreover, older people or their carers can access few specialist services directly. Once the person becomes vulnerable they are at the mercy of the first point of contact with the service system. The next uncertainty is whether the service system is able to assess, and subsequently meet, needs. Even when an older person is already receiving health and social care services, staff can miss other problems. Banerjee (1993) examined the unmet needs of older people receiving home care. Study results found that clinical depression in older people receiving home care was not being recognized and acted upon by social service staff. A similar problem exists in primary care. Results of a questionnaire survey concerning primary care by the Alzheimer's Society (ADS, 1995) found that detection of dementia by GPs was inadequate. This was confirmed by the reports of carers. An estimated 36 per cent of people with dementia were not referred to specialist services and in 30 per cent of cases dementia was misdiagnosed as either depression or problems of old age.

Limiting age discrimination

The issues underpinning age discrimination in our society were touched upon in Chapter 1. The Foresight programme (Ageing Population Panel) (2000) stated that provision of health and social care should be age neutral.

Two forms of age discrimination are recognized by the National Service Framework for Older People (DoH, 2001a):

1. lower rates of access to services compared with other groups;
2. lesser provision of services important to older people, with occupational therapy being specifically cited.

Further to this, the National Service Framework for Older People (DoH, 2001a) devotes a chapter to 'rooting out age discrimination', centralizing the need for fair access to health and social care services, taking into account needs, not age. The document acknowledged that the aim is yet to be achieved universally. There is also recognition of the fact that some services, like joint replacement, cataract surgery and community equipment, are of heightened importance to older people.

Policy-led intentions are countered by worrying evidence about the extent to which ageist beliefs impact upon the extent and nature of the care and treatment available to older people. Despite some improvements in societal and service attitudes towards older people, questions continue to be raised about the extent of resources available to meet the needs of an ageing population.

Balancing access with service rationing

The issue of service rationing is linked to the previous section on age discrimination. This is a complex area that shifts depending upon whether a collectivist or individualist view is adopted (DoH, 1999b). The collectivist approach is to view the NHS as an instrument of the state, with the goal of improving the overall health of the population to the benefit of the state. If this is the case, then an ageist approach will prevail. The individualist approach is to consider how the individual might benefit. Therefore rationing should as far as possible be based on individualist values.

There is evidence as well as reports from the national press to support rationing of health care to older people. Through an examination of research into equity of access to cardiovascular services, Bowling (1999) postulated a number of reasons for this rationing. These included the lesser value placed upon older people by society (reflected in health policy and delivery), a belief that older people are more expensive to treat, and a lack of awareness of the evidence base to support health care interventions for older people. A survey by Age Concern England (2000) found that 77 per cent of GPs considered that age rationing occurs in the health service. Half of all Britain's 35,000 GPs expressed concern about how they might be treated in their old age. The conclusions drawn from these and other studies cast serious doubt upon the notion of older people as full citizens, given the reality of how resources are distributed across all sectors of society.

Rationing of services continues to be a feature of social care provision. Thus the goal of delivering services in response to assessed needs is compromised by eligibility criteria that ration access (Caldock and Nolan, 1994). Authorities responding to the 1999 survey of the workload of occupational therapists working for social services (Improvement and Development Agency for Local Government 2000) all operated a system for prioritization of services, with up to four levels of priority. Level 1, the most urgent group, included people with terminal illness, hospital discharges and those needing immediate help. Those in the lowest priority group included those with needs for bathing or showering equipment, and requests for small items of equipment. A recent report authored by representatives from a range of organizations concerned with older people (SPAIN, 2001) raised the deleterious consequences of the continued under-funding of social care compared with the financing of health. One effect is delayed discharge from hospital and unnecessary admission or readmission. Another is tighter rationing of services. The report identified a number of ways in which this was being enforced:

*   denying help to those with live-in carers or moderate needs for care;
*   making those with high-level needs wait for services;
*   limiting the amount, choice and quality of care received.

Case examples within the report cited a variety of situations where provision of equipment to meet assessed needs had been delayed. The report also confirmed that, at the time of writing, the number of older people receiving home care was diminishing despite the growing number of people aged 85 and over.

Balancing 'needs' with 'wants'

Discussions of rationing of social care leads into considerations of what a *need* is as opposed to a *want*. Bathing is the most frequently cited example. We can manage without a bath so in a sense we want rather than need, but most of us would agree that this is unacceptable, even in the short term. Mountain (1988a) demonstrated that while the list of care providers involved with older women with mental health problems appeared impressive, the care each person said that they actually received clearly did not reflect the extent of physical and emotional needs they described during interview. Assistance with practical, low-level interventions, for example housework and gardening, was extremely limited apart from one person who could afford to pay for private services. For those reliant upon social services provision there were difficulties in obtaining the services they really wanted, leading to frustration. This is often followed by acceptance:

> A lot of elderly people, if they can't get in the bath they'll just have a wash down, they adapt. Although they don't like it but that's the best they can do if they don't have a shower.

It was also evident that, rather than providing a creative response to expressed needs, what was being offered was dictated by the availability of a limited repertoire of provision and rigid patterns of delivery of those services. Hopefully, the previously described Direct Payments Initiative for older people will result in changes for the better.

As with other forms of social care, charges for personal services are in place. Most recently, some authorities have increased charges to try to limit serious budget deficits.

Involving the frail and old in services

While society is inviting the views of older people in good health, as described in Chapter 1, the opinions of the frail and very old are rarely sought. Viewed objectively, this paradox is puzzling, given that these are the very people who are in receipt of the service system.

Reluctance to consult on the part of service commissioners and providers can be reinforced by a reticence to voice opinions on the part of many older people receiving statutory services. Whether they are service users, carers or concerned friends and neighbours, older people in contact with services remain reluctant to complain about substandard services, or to question the decisions of professionals (Hollingbery, 1999). This reticence on the part of older people can be attributed to a number of factors. Three of the main ones are identified below.

First, consideration needs to be given to the viewpoint of those older people aged 75 years and over, who, given their age, are most likely to be receiving services. This group will have experienced health care prior to the introduction of the National Health Service, and therefore, not surprisingly, are likely to have a different attitude to health care to that of younger older people (Minkler and Estes, 2000). This can lead to a grateful acceptance of any provision. Second, trying to manage the debilitating effects of illness and frailty, as either a service user or a carer, can leave little energy for advocating for quality services. Third, it is not surprising that the tendency to accept any standard of service is exacerbated in those who are highly vulnerable and as a consequence perceive (often accurately) that their future is wholly dependent upon the decisions made by service providers. An example of fear of retribution was provided through a study of ward environment for older people with severe dementia (Mountain and Bowie, 1995). Preliminary stages of the project involved videotaping older people with severe dementia resident on one ward. This necessitated obtaining informed consent by the patients' relatives. The request for consent provided an opportunity for some relatives to complain to the researchers about the extremely poor services being provided to older people resident on the ward, whereas they had previously remained silent, possibly due to fear of repercussions.

There is no doubt that compliant behaviour contributes towards the maintenance of poor-quality services, with commissioners and providers of health and social care being all too ready to believe that lack of complaints equates with adequate provision. Interviews with frail older people (Mountain and Moore, 1995) demonstrated that while they found growing older to be frustrating, complaints were considered to be futile.

> I think that's one of the things you learn to accept. The inevitable. They'll accept the circumstance even if they don't like it.

Paradoxically, those older people and their carers who do offer their opinions can be perceived to be interfering and troublesome. Thus the continuing myth of quality services can be maintained by *not* openly inviting views from service users. Encouraging older people to have a voice in the services they receive has not been assisted by proliferation of poorly constructed satisfaction questionnaires. However, it is also evident that if older people are invited to give their views in a manner that enables a full and honest response, this can be a rich source of information upon which to base service improvements (McKenna and Hunt, 1991).

There is much to learn in this area. Therefore both service commissioners and providers are urged to share good practice. The Scottish Centre for Promotion of the Older Persons' Agenda, located at Queen Margaret University College in Edinburgh, is an example of an innovative, proactive approach towards user involvement. One of the many activities of the Centre has been the development and provision of an educational programme to enable the participation of older people in services. The course comprised four modules: drama for democracy (using drama to reflect different points of view), reviewing documents to enable the older persons' voice to be heard, having a voice in formal arenas and helping older people to tell their stories.

Implications for occupational therapy

The clinical and managerial implications for occupational therapists of working in specific service settings are described in Chapter 9. However, some common principles are described here, which should be taken into account by all professional groups including occupational therapists.

Fully understand policy and what it means for older people and services

The contents of this book, and in particular this chapter, confirm how vital it is for occupational therapists to have a clear understanding of the policy and legislative framework within which services for older people are developed and shaped. This need is emphasized with the move towards jointly commissioned and provided services. This requires all workers to understand both health and social care legislation and its implementation. It is also extremely valuable to understand the historical background to the development of services, as this often helps to explain the current position.

Clarify and agree the interpretation of key terms

It is all too easy to use terms that describe complex constructs without a clear understanding of what they mean. The word *modernization* is one example. It frequently appears in current national and local policy documents. As a consequence it has slipped into the daily discourse of health and social care staff. However, in common with a number of other terms that underpin complex constructs and are in common usage, for example rehabilitation and enabling, it can be used to describe a number of organizational processes as well as an ever-increasing variety of service options. If services are to operate in a user-centred manner, we all must ensure that we are clear about what we mean, and convey this clarity to other colleagues, those using the service and their carers.

View services from a user perspective

Those working with older people should consider what services they are likely to find acceptable in the future, in light of their own life experiences. It is also important to consider the changes that have occurred within our own communities, and in wider society, during our lifetime, as well as the changes that may take place in the future. This is a real challenge for all those working with older people.

Promote the value of rehabilitation services

Policy-led initiatives mean that the climate for promoting and developing occupational therapy services has never been better. We need to ensure that we are in a position to respond fully to the challenges posed by new forms of service, and demonstrate where rehabilitation can make an effective contribution.

Understand the whole-system service concept

To make the whole system work effectively, services have to work together, referring people on to the most appropriate settings in a timely and seamless manner as needs change. This requires a heightened awareness of the goals of other forms of provision within the locality and the ability to recognize when other services are necessary. It may also necessitate working to methods and standards established by the service system.

Embrace service integration

Occupational therapists are qualified to deliver both health and social care interventions. In the current climate of service integration this is a prime opportunity for occupational therapists to demonstrate their full potential. However, working across the health and social care divide creates new demands. It requires close working relationships with other professional groups and a shift away from rigid task demarcation within services concerned with the health and social care of the same group of people.

Pointers for practice

- Be aware of strategic policy and its implications for service development.
- Ensure that your department or service provides adequate information for patients and carers, in a format and language that service users will be able to understand.
- Take all expressed views of the service seriously, even if they are given by individuals deemed to be confused, ill or disturbed.
- Have information about the organization's complaints procedures available, and take time to explain the procedure to a person if indicated.
- Introduce methods of canvassing the opinions of the people using your service, and those of their carers.
- Understand the whole system of services provided for older people in your locality, determining any gaps and duplication.
- Work to maintain the quality of service provision.

CHAPTER 6

Assessing the needs of older people

Thorough and appropriate assessment of health and social care needs is an essential prerequisite to the provision of appropriate interventions in both health and social care. Assessment of the physical and mental well-being, functional abilities and occupational needs of older people is a key occupational therapy role. The nature of assessment both within and across professional groups is changing in line with implementation of current policy combined with the increasing voice of older people in society described in Chapter 1. This chapter will explore current policy-led requirements and how occupational therapists can most appropriately meet new demands, while at the same time maintaining professional standards of practice and using established expertise to best effect.

Policy context

Mountain (1997) noted the need to make the following changes to assessment and subsequent care planning as a result of the introduction of intermediate care services that span the health and social care divide:

- all disciplines should reappraise their assessment methods;
- needs identified through the assessment should be met by a care package that includes both health and social care elements from a range of providers;
- collaborative working between health care and social care should be enhanced.

In 2001 the National Service Framework for Older People (DoH, 2001a) mandated the introduction of the single assessment process, with full implementation in all localities by 2004. The rationale is that older people frequently have needs that span health and social care. In the past, this has meant that vulnerable older people have been subjected to several assessments of need conducted by different agencies within a short space of time.

Moreover, these assessments have asked many of the same questions. The single assessment has been introduced to both rationalize assessments and encourage different agencies to work together. The policy interpretation of the single assessment reinforces the person-centred approach to care by keeping the needs of the service user at the centre of the assessment. It also aims to reduce duplication in service provision and assessment, and utilize the skills of professionals in the most effective way to meet the needs of the service user (DoH, 2002c). In addition to assessing user needs, the extent and nature of help received from informal carers and statutory services should be recorded. The need to update information over time, and the importance of information systems that enable sharing of assessment information across different agencies, are emphasized.

The single assessment attempts to recognize the full spectrum of health and social care needs of older people. Therefore a range of providers are necessarily involved in its application and implementation. Guidance on the single assessment process is issued under the health services circular/local authority circular (*HSC 2002/001; LAC (2002)1*) (DoH, 2002d).

Four types of assessment are identified. In the *contact assessment*, basic personal information and the nature of the presenting problem are elicited. Trained non-professional workers may complete contact assessments. Assessment undertaken on first contact must cover the following domains, irrespective of the professional background of the individual undertaking the assessment:

1. user perspective;
2. clinical background;
3. disease prevention;
4. personal care and well-being;
5. senses;
6. mental health;
7. safety;
8. immediate environment and resources.

Trained non-professional workers may complete contact assessments.

Using the information obtained from the first contact assessment, professionals may make a judgement that a more comprehensive assessment or *overview assessment* is required, which will explore appropriate domains of the single assessment process. The overview assessment to explore the needs of those with more complex or pervasive needs can be undertaken by any one of a range of professional providers. Services are being encouraged to develop single assessment tools that fulfil their local needs (within specific guidelines). The Department of Health have now established a team to accredit tools for the overview assessment. Additionally, individuals are able to suggest instruments for this purpose to the Department of Health. A selection of those already endorsed by the Department of Health for this purpose can be found on the DoH website (see Appendix 3), with a number of examples being highlighted in the forthcoming tables in this chapter.

The overview assessment may then indicate the requirement for a *specialist assessment*. These assessments involve the exploration of a specific health or social care need by a professional with expertise in this area. Thus policy is now reinforcing the value of the assessment process that occupational therapists have expertise in undertaking.

Finally, the *comprehensive assessment* involves assessment by a range of professional providers for older people with more complex needs.

To prepare workers for their role in applying the single assessment process, the Department of Health has published specific guidelines for social workers, nurses, therapists, general practitioners, geriatricians and old age psychiatrists (see Appendix 3 for the web address).

Guidance for implementation for therapists specifically states that:

> While they may do their fair share of overview assessments, therapists will contribute greatly to specialist assessments and comprehensive assessments. They can offer a specialist contribution to the assessment of mobility, transfers, speech, language, eating, drinking and functional capacity, and the impact of the home and wider environment on assessed needs. In particular therapists are skilled in the assessment of the potential for rehabilitation and independence.

Instruments specific to occupational therapy that may be employed for this purpose are discussed in a later section of this chapter.

Delivering quality assessments

The benefits of the new policy-led approach to assessing the needs of older, vulnerable people are clearly indisputable. However, previous research has demonstrated that this will be a challenging task (Meetham and Thompson, 1992).

The assessment process is a particularly important aspect of a person's progress through the care system (Ellis, 1993). A quality assessment can foster the development of a successful partnership between the service user and professional, which in turn can lead to the achievement of best outcomes (Godfrey and Wistow, 1997; Godfrey, 1998). Alternatively, if the professional is overly powerful in the relationship, the user has little chance to retain control over their lives and express their needs.

The reasons why an occupational therapy assessment might be undertaken include for service purposes (so that outcomes might be measured) or to diagnose and quantify functional problems (Smith, 1992). A further dimension is assessment to provide information for users and their carers. Letts et al. (1994) suggested that a real challenge for occupational therapists is selecting assessments that incorporate the impact of the environment upon occupation. Smith (1992) also questioned why occupational therapists, with their holistic skill base, concentrate upon functional assessment and, further to this, how the assessment data is translated into interventions.

The development of quality assessment practice goes beyond identifying the necessary instruments. Through a review of assessment policy and implementation in health and social care, Nolan and Caldock (1996) identified a number of benchmarks for good assessment practice:

- Empower the user and carer, and ensure that they have full information about the reasons for the assessment before commencing.
- Take steps to make the user and carer are partners in the assessment process.
- Keep an open mind rather than being led by professional beliefs and value judgements.
- Check the understanding of the user and carer.
- Ensure that the assessment environment is appropriate.
- Take time to build a relationship with the person before commencing the assessment process.
- Explore emotional as well as practical needs, taking the relationship between user and carer into account.
- Listen to the views of the user and carer even if they are different from your own.
- Try and present ideas and solutions to the user and carer that they may not have previously considered.
- Avoid the assessment becoming a hurdle that has to be overcome before people get the services they need.
- Take all perspectives into account.
- Ensure that user and carer understand when the assessment is complete; try to agree objectives with them and explain how the outcomes will be reviewed.

Choosing the most appropriate assessment method

The occupational therapy assessment process can take several forms; for example:

- interviews with the older person and/or their carer using an interview guide;

- requesting specific information from the older person and/or their carer through a questionnaire applied in an interview situation;
- structured observation while watching the older person undertaking activities (Finlay, 1997);
- measurement of the functional abilities of the older person and their participation in activities of daily living and other occupations through application of assessment instruments.

All the above methods of assessment are used in current practice. However, there is a definite shift towards the application of assessment measures with proven reliability and validity. These measures and their properties are discussed in the forthcoming section of this chapter.

Determining what the assessment is for

Vulnerable older people can present with a multiplicity of problems. Selection of assessments must therefore take into account physical and socio-economic factors that may be present, as well as mental health problems. Bowling (1997) commented upon the limitations of many measures of functional ability in that they concentrate upon a narrow focus of activity and ignore financial, social and emotional needs. It is also vital to measure dimensions that might respond to intervention, for example problems with eyesight, hearing and speech, incontinence, mental health, functional abilities, extent of available support and quality of life (Bowling, 1995).

Assessment can take place in different settings, for example in acute hospital care, other forms of residential setting, day care or the person's own home. Different assessment scenarios commonly encountered by occupational therapists, and their implications, are discussed later in this chapter.

Through the process of reassessment, a number of assessment measures can be used as outcome measures. Outcome measures are a domain of evidence-based practice, referred to briefly in Chapter 10. Readers are also advised to refer to Clarke et al. (2001) for further details of outcome measures appropriate to occupational therapy practice.

Additionally, specialist assessments are available for those people with a confirmed diagnosis, for example: the Care Needs Assessment Pack for Dementia (Carenap D) (McWalter et al., 1998); the Frenchay activities index (Wade et al., 1985) and the Northwick Park activities of daily living index (Benjamin, 1976) for people with stroke; and the Parkinson's disease activities of daily living scale (Hobson et al., 2001).

Selecting standardized assessments

In common with other health and social care professionals, occupational therapists have traditionally employed their clinical skills to guide the assessment process, with the results of such assessments being in narrative. However, the value of carefully chosen assessment instruments is now recognized. The Department of Health make a differentiation between assessment *tools* and assessment *scales*. Within the guidance on the single assessment process, the Department of Health (2002c) defines an assessment tool as:

A collection of scales, questions and other information, to provide a rounded picture of an individual's needs and related circumstances.

A means of identifying, and possibly gauging the extent of, a specific health or care condition. (Single Assessment Process, September 2002, p. 2)

Therefore the use of standardized assessments or scales, to use the interpretation made by the Department of Health, is an integral part of an overall assessment process drawing upon a number of information sources.

Standardized assessment measures (or scales) have proven psychometric properties. They will produce consistently reliable results; for example, if two people independently assessed the same individual at the same times the results of their assessments would be the same or very similar. They are also readily comprehended so that there is no doubt regarding interpretation of the questions.

Some definitions of the commonly cited properties of standardized measures are given below:

Reliability: the extent to which the measure is consistent and minimizes random error (its repeatability). (Bowling, 1997, p. 391)

Validity: the extent to which the instrument is really measuring what it purports to measure. (Bowling, 1997, p. 393)

Sensitivity: ability of the actual gradations in the scale's scores to reflect these changes adequately – probability of correctly identifying affected person ('case'). (Bowling, 1997, p. 392)

Therefore development of assessment measures is a sophisticated research process. The common practice of customizing standardized measures, for example through altering wording and omitting or adding questions, invalidates the properties of the instrument. Similarly, if the measure has been developed for use with a specific population, it cannot be transferred for use to a different group without prior testing.

There are many assessment instruments on the market. Important considerations in the choice of assessments include:

• the psychometric properties of the instrument (reliability, validity and sensitivity);

- the appropriateness of the instrument for assessment of the multiplicity of problems that older people can present with;
- the usability of the instrument – can it be readily applied and analysed?
- is training required to use it?
- the acceptability of the instrument to the older person and their carer, including the extent to which it enables the assessment process to be owned by the recipient.

A wealth of assessment measures exist for application with older people. Some of the commonly encountered standardized measures that can be used for the purposes of comprehensive or overview assessment (as part of the single assessment process) are shown in Table 6.1. A few examples of those that might be appropriate for specialist assessment by occupational therapists (as part of the single assessment process) are given in Table 6.2.

Tables 6.1 and 6.2 are not exhaustive: other measures have been constructed to assess specific functional tasks, for example the dressing skills of older people (Davies et al., 1990) and function within the home environment (Letts et al., 1998).

It is also recommended that readers refer to texts by Bowling (1991 and 1995) for excellent reviews of measures.

Table 6.1 A sample of standardized measures used with older people

Instrument	What it measures	Properties	Usability	Applicability
Barthel Index (Mahoney and Barthel, 1965)*	Assesses functional ability – often used to establish the outcomes of treatment interventions	Popular globally but further studies of reliability required	Simple to apply. Different values applied to different activities for scoring. Popular with clinicians and researchers	Applied widely but does not provide in-depth information
Crichton Royal Behaviour Rating Scale (CRBRS) (Robinson, 1961)	10 items: 5 to examine functional ability and 5 to look at mental disturbance	Update by Wilkin and Jolley (1989)	Interviewer training required	For use with older people resident in care settings – ADL/IADL excluded

Table 6.1 (contd)

Instrument	What it measures	Properties	Usability	Applicability
Older Americans' Resources and Services multi-dimensional functional assessment questionnaire (OARS) (Fillenbaum, 1988)*	Assesses physical, psychological and social functioning	Good evidence of reliability, validity and sensitivity	Short version also available. Interviewer training required	Useful in surveys of older people
Camberwell Assessment of Needs for the Elderly (Reynolds et al., 2000)	24 areas of need covering psychological, physical, social functioning and role of carers	Good reliability and validity	Can be used by health and social care practitioners – detailed manual available	Can be used as an initial assessment, an outcome measure, service evaluation and research
Social care outcomes for older people (OPUS) (Netten et al., 2002)	Includes the domains of personal care, social contact, control, food, safety and finance, as well as info on levels of unmet need	Initial investigations suggest good validity and reliability but more studies are required	Applicable in all social care settings	Can be used as an initial assessment and then an outcome of social care packages for services and individual service users
Elderly Assessment Instrument (EASY-Care) (SISA, 1997)*	Combines medical and social assessment. Can be applied to individual and populations	Tested for validity and reliability for UK. Versions being developed for use throughout Europe	Simple to use. Can be self-completed or person can be assisted	For use in primary or community care settings only
General Health Questionnaire (GHQ) (Goldberg and Williams, 1998)*	For use as a screening tool for anxiety and depression	Extensively tested for validity reliability and sensitivity to change	Scale available in a number of lengths (12–60 items). Questionnaire, short and simple to use – designed for self-completion	Designed for use in primary and community settings

Table 6.1 (contd)

Instrument	What it measures	Properties	Usability	Applicability
Health of the Nation Outcome Scales for older adult users of mental health services (HoNOS 65+) (Royal College of Psychiatrists, 1998)	0–4 point measure of behaviour, mood, relation-ships, ADL, living conditions and occupation	Tested for acceptability, usability, sensitivity, reliability and validity	To be applied during interview by workers. Training strongly recommended	Used by MD teams to rate mental health services and repeated over time to obtain outcomes attributable to interventions
Philadelphia Geriatric Morale Scale (Lawton, 1975)	17 items measuring life satisfaction and self-esteem	Good results for reliability and validity	Rating by interview	Recommended for use in community settings
Short-Form 36-item health status questionnaire (SF-36) (Ware and Sherbourne, 1992)*	36 items measuring a range of domains concerned with health-related quality of life	Reliability and validity extensively examined	Questionnaire and scoring booklet available free of charge	Originally designed for use by US ins-urance sector as an outcome measure to detect changes in health status over short periods of time
Clifton Assessment Procedures for the Elderly (CAPE) (Pattie and Gilleard, 1979)	Two schedules: the Behaviour Rating Scale, and Cognitive Assessment Scale	Validity demonstrated by Pattie and Gilleard (1979). Weak reliability	Interviewer training required. Applied by an interviewer who knows the respondent well	For use with institutionally living older people

* Contains scales or elements that the DoH recommend could be used within the single assessment process.

Some of the occupational therapy specific assessment instruments that can be used with vulnerable older people, and their properties, are shown in Table 6.2.

Table 6.2 Some occupational therapy specific measures

Instrument	Properties	Applicability	Usability	Acceptability
Occupational Performance Interview (Kielhofner and Henry, 1988; Kielhofner et al., 1989)	Reliable and valid for an American population	Provides detailed information through a life history narrative	Need to study manual prior to use and be prepared to translate American terminology. A lot of data to analyse	Long interview process. Would need a number of sessions to complete
Assessment of Motor and Process Skills (AMPS) (Fisher, 2003)	Standardized internationally and cross-culturally	Measures quality of performance in personal and domestic activities of daily living	Attendance at a training course mandatory	Has been used successfully with older people
Canadian Occupational Performance Measure (COPM) (Law et al., 1994)*	Reliable and valid for a Canadian population. On-going work to validate COPM for use with other populations	Assesses problems in occupational performance and then measures changes in perception of performance over time	Training recommended. Training manual and training video available	Focus is upon physical limitations, though work is taking place to make it appropriate for people with mental health problems
Community Dependency Index (Eakin and Baird, 1995)*	Valid and reliable for community-living physically disabled and elderly people	Assesses independence in ADL relevant to community living	Measure available from the author	Measures physical limitations in community settings only
Mayers Lifestyle Questionnaire (Mayers, 1998)*	Work ongoing to make the measure valid and reliable for a range of populations	Gives a broad assessment of need in relation to independence in the community	Measure and guidelines for use available from the author	Looks at occupational needs in the context of lifestyle

Table 6.2 (contd)

Instrument	Properties	Applicability	Usability	Acceptability
Safety Assessment of Function and the Environment for Rehabilitation (SAFER) (Oliver et al., 1993)	Designed for use with a Canadian population – work ongoing to establish properties (at time of publication)	Assesses person in relation to their environment – 15 areas of concern	Manual and instruction video available	For use by OT with elderly people in the community
Comprehensive Occupational Therapy Evaluation (COTE) (Brayman and Kirby, 1982)	Valid and reliable for people with acute MH problems in the USA	Provides a structured format for reporting observations during initial assessment. Can then be used to measure change over time	Requirements not readily available. No special training specified but it would be necessary to study the measure carefully before using it	Used to study OT outcomes for older people with MH problems in hospital care

* Within the DoH list of recommended instruments for the single assessment process.

Comparing different standardized assessments

As there are so many assessment instruments on the market, it can be necessary to compare the properties of alternative measures when selecting those most appropriate for the purpose. The comparison of different measures to test properties and applicability is a complex research activity (Bowling, 1995, 1997). An example of research that has compared one occupational therapy measure with another instrument is described below.

Ward et al. (1998) pointed out that, despite its widespread use in a variety of environments, the Barthel Index (Mahoney and Barthel (1965)) (see Table 6.1) has not been validated for use in a person's own home. They undertook a study to compare the Community Dependency Index (CDI) developed by Eakin and Baird in 1995 (see Table 6.2) with the Barthel Index (BI). While the BI was developed as a measure of dependency in institutions, the CDI aims to assess independence in community settings. The study involved comparing two groups of older people discharged home after sustaining a fractured neck of femur, to examine which was the most appropriate measure of recovery of independence in ADL. Group 1 comprised 18 people; pre-injury ability in

ADL (estimated through interview) was compared with ability one year after the fracture. Sixty patients were in group 2, three-year post-fracture ability (estimated through interview) being compared with that at four years post-fracture. Additionally, the properties of the CDI were examined and the agreement between the CDI and BI one year and four years post-fracture. Results of statistical analysis found that the CDI tended to yield lower scores than the BI. Therefore if scores from the two measures are compared, it appears that the patients assessed using the CDI had a poorer outcome than those where the BI is applied. The difference between bodily recovery and adaptation to lowered ability is a further factor; the CDI is able to measure this recovery as a result of adaptation whereas this does not influence the BI. The authors concluded that for the CDI to gain the international acclaim of the BI, further research must be undertaken with large cohorts of patients to substantiate the properties of the measure.

Observational methods of assessment compared with standardized measures

Occupational therapists (in common with other professional groups) have tended to set aside scientific assessment instruments in favour of observational methods or locally developed checklists. However, as Table 6.1 and 6.2 illustrate, more systematic means have been developed to measure aspects that occupational therapists would have previously used observation and clinical reasoning to assess.

Studies of the reliability and appropriateness of observational methods compared with use of standardized assessments in the context of hospital discharge have drawn very different conclusions. Kneebone and Harrop (1996) developed a questionnaire to help the older person identify their own level of confidence prior to discharge home. This was based in the premise that professional opinion can be a less reliable indicator of discharge outcome than the views of the person themselves. However, when Frankum et al. (1995) compared functional outcomes of older people between two and four weeks following return home from acute care, with predictions made pre-discharge by occupational therapists, nurses and the patient themselves, they found occupational therapists to be the most accurate predictors. A study by Reich et al. (1998) explored clinical decision-making by occupational therapists in the context of risky discharges. Presentations of case vignettes of risky discharges to occupational therapists found that they were more likely to recommend return home in accord with the patient's wishes than admission to institutional care. This raises the question of whether practitioners would maintain these hypothetical clinical decisions in real life, taking into account the views of other professionals and the implications of any perceived risks.

Stewart (1999) compared the use of standardized and non-standardized assessments by occupational therapists working in social services. While the study was small and confined to the activity of one occupational therapist assessing older people referred for minor adaptations to their homes, it raised very relevant questions. Stewart found that use of a non-standardized questionnaire limited the ability of the occupational therapist to identify people who were on the margins of frailty and could benefit from further services.

A further observation about the value of applying rigorous assessments is that they provide measures or ratings that can then be used as a baseline to examine outcomes of interventions. This is difficult if the assessment process is wholly descriptive.

The message to be taken away from these diverse results is that a combination of assessment methods is most likely to be the most productive method of determining the needs of older people and their carers.

Assessments to examine specific occupational needs

Assessment is applied in a range of circumstances and settings. This section considers a number of frequently encountered assessment scenarios where occupational therapists are often involved, and the evidence base that underpins them. It also considers the appropriateness of continuing to devote resources to certain of these assessments.

Functional assessments

Assessments of the ability of an older person to undertake specific functional activities are frequently conducted by occupational therapists. Certain of these activities are classified as basic activities of daily living, for example assessments of dressing, transfers, bathing and toileting and general mobility. Instrumental activities of daily living (IADL) include assessments of domestic abilities, shopping, household management, use of public transport and money management. Assessments of ADL and IADL can be undertaken in a range of settings to fulfil a range of purposes. Wade et al. (1985) quoted in Eakin (1989) identified three types of ADL assessment:

1. checklists based on observation, with the results being a description of performance;
2. summed indices where the person is assessed on a number of items,

but where the items to be summated will not have equal weight in determining dependence or independence;
3. hierarchical (or valid and reliable) scales.

Some ADL and IADL assessment scales, for example OARS and the Barthel Index (see Tables 6.1 and 6.2), can be effectively used to evaluate progress over time (Law, 1992).

As discussed previously, the checklist to describe performance using observational assessment is most likely to be used by occupational therapists (Eakin, 1989; Law, 1992). Observational assessments of function undertaken in simulated domestic environments in ward or occupational therapy departments can be undertaken as part of the hospital discharge process. The expressed experiences of older people indicate that these assessments can be a cause of great anxiety for older, hospitalized people.

Mrs BP, a lady of 80 years, living alone with a diagnosis of depressive illness, described this experience when talking about experiences of occupational therapy assessment in hospital as part of the pre-discharge process:

> Well, they said you went to the kitchen to make a meal, if you passed you could go home, but if not you'd have to go and do it again, stay in hospital.

Egan et al. (1992) examined the accuracy of pre-discharge assessments of function for older people who had sustained hip fracture. A sample of 61 older people were assessed by an occupational therapist using the Barthel Index (BI) three days prior to discharge. Additional information collected about the subjects included role loss, depression, mental and physical health status and social support. Three weeks after discharge, independence was reassessed through telephone interviews based on the BI. The reliability of the interviews was demonstrated through a comparison with clinical ratings at follow-up appointment. Data analysis revealed a discrepancy between pre- and post-discharge levels of independence in activities of daily living, with greater dependence being reported. The authors suggest the reasons may have been due to differing interpretations of independence made by users and occupational therapists, with user views being more accurate predictors than those of the therapists. The authors conclude that functional assessment prior to discharge is not sufficiently reliable to determine the services that might be required upon return home.

Pre-discharge home visits

The requirement to assess the homes of older people and their ability to cope in the community prior to discharge was detailed in Department of

Health guidelines (DoH, 1989a). These guidelines stated that discharge procedures should:

> ... secure therapy assessments prior to discharge to ensure facilities at home are appropriate to the needs of the patient. (DoH, 1989a, p.1)

The requirement for assessment prior to return home was reinforced in the *Hospital Discharge Workbook* (DoH, 1994). The workbook identified hospital-based therapists as being key stakeholders in discharge from hospital and transfer to community services. Significantly, it promoted hospital discharge as embracing a sequence of events including pre-admission screening, the admission process itself, preparations for discharge, discharge home and post-discharge care. Therefore pre-discharge home visits are only one aspect of this sequence. Despite the rationale for the steps detailed in the workbook, the evidence base promoting the importance of fulfilling all aspects of the discharge process, and the substantial policy shifts that have occurred at national level; local practice continues to support the notion of one-off visits. Moreover, with the current speed of throughput on acute medical wards for older people the reality is that in many cases staff have little time to establish a rapport with the patient before the visit.

The pre-discharge assessment entails persons being accompanied home, usually by hospital staff, and observed in their own environment undertaking a variety of activities as requested. Both formal and informal carers may be invited to be present. The member of staff leading the visit will document observed ability to undertake the selected tasks, and balance the needs of relatives and carers with the desire of the person to return home (Bore, 1994). This necessitates taking risk factors and the capacity of community services into account. Other sources of information include the views of capacity to cope, once back home, from the patient and their carers (while the person is still in hospital) using either standardized or non-standardized methods of interview. Also, allowances have to be made for the anxiety experienced by the patient during a relatively brief observational assessment of their ability to perform a number of everyday functional activities within their own, familiar environment. The combination of the hospital management of the process together with anxieties about return home means that the older person in hospital, already at a disadvantage due to their admission to hospital, often perceives the visit to be a test that has to be overcome. The ultimate decision about their future therefore lies in the hands of the professionals (Godfrey and Moore, 1996). When interviewed about their experiences of assessment for return home, older people with mental health problems expressed their fear of both the process and its consequences (Mountain, 1998a). The situation did not allow for clarification and reassurance and left the person with no control over the process.

During the visit, equipment is frequently provided on a 'one-off' basis due to a judgement made at the time. The consequence is that the likelihood of the decision being the most appropriate one is reduced and the person is less likely to accept what has been prescribed (Clarke et al., 1996). It is well known that older people in hospital retain little of what is said to them and therefore it is important to provide written information. However, it is extremely rare for any written information to be given to the patient and their carer, either before or after the visit.

The consequent interpretation of the individual's ability to cope during a snapshot of functional activity is translated into a report for the multidisciplinary team, and in particular for the responsible medical officers. The report usually provides indicators of the extent of risk the person poses to themselves and to others if they are discharged to their prior living arrangements. Local service organizations will then dictate the provider responsible for undertaking the interventions deemed to be immediately necessary; that is, whether the responsibility remains with health, is transferred to social services or is shared.

Comparatively little is known of the effectiveness of the common practice of undertaking pre-discharge home visits in isolation from the other recommended steps in the discharge process. The extent of most of the existing research into outcomes of practice in this area is either smallscale or has been drawn out of studies that have been designed to investigate wider questions regarding the whole hospital discharge sequence (Clark et al., 1996). A systematic review by Tullis and Nicol (1999) looked at the evidence to support functional assessment of older people with dementia. Results confirmed a lack of evidence in the occupational therapy literature to support or refute the undertaking of pre-discharge home visits, attributable to a lack of available quality research. A systematic review of the effectiveness of pre-discharge visits conducted by Patterson and Mulley (1999) concluded that the effectiveness of pre-discharge visits is unproven. As with hospital-based assessment, the existing evidence base points towards the fact that assessment of an older person and their living circumstances only provides a 'snapshot in time' judgement to be made of abilities at the point of discharge and in the short term. They do not necessarily predict capacity to cope long term (Neill and Williams, 1992; Egan et al., 1992; Clark et al., 1997). Thus the focus of the visit is safety at discharge rather than longer-term safety and enhancement of independence (Clark M et al., 1996). Unfortunately, the extent of resources directed to this role can be such that there can be little time left for any other form of activity by occupational therapists working with older people in acute care. The greater benefits that can be gained when both functional assessment and home visits are followed by a plan of treatment are discussed in the next chapter.

Assessments of need for community care provided through local authorities

Assessing needs for community care is an integral component of the care management process, introduced in 1993 as a result of implementation of the 1990 Community Care Act. Prior to implementation of the 1990 Community Care reforms, local arrangements were in place for assessment of need for equipment, provided through social services. Since 1993, assessed needs have had to meet eligibility criteria as determined by the department in order for services to be received. (The rationing process that has resulted is discussed in Chapter 5.) Those in need of services have to pass two obstacles: first the community care assessment itself and second the determination of eligibility compared with assessed needs. Even if they are not centrally involved in mainstream community care assessment, assessments by occupational therapists can determine whether or not a person is eligible for equipment subsidized by social services, and financial assistance with housing adaptations.

In the future, the single assessment process described earlier in this chapter will replace local authority community care assessments for older people. However, some system to ration services will still need to be in place.

The relationship between housing and community care was also raised in the previous chapters. Assessment of housing needs is an essential component of community care. It has also been observed that assessment is the key to effective use of housing resources (Heywood and Smart, 1996). Mackintosh and Leather (1994) noted that assessment of need for housing adaptations was usually carried out by an occupational therapist. However, the legal framework for assessment of housing services is complex, with occupational therapists being required to work within the existing system (Mountain, 2000). Furthermore, the assessment of need for housing has to be placed in the context of the previously discussed eligibility criteria being operated by the authority.

Once again, the prudence of relying totally on checklists and observations when assessing needs for housing and housing adaptations has been questioned. Iwarsson (1999) developed a valid and reliable measure of housing need. The resulting instrument, named the Housing Enabler, assesses three components: the functional limitations of the individual, the physical environmental barriers and the accessibility (calculated through a combination of scores of functional limitation and environmental barriers). Research by Franklin (1998) demonstrated the need for a more holistic approach towards assessment of housing need. Results of analysis of 80 semi-structured interviews about housing need with a wide range of professionals including occupational therapists, together with observation of assessment methods, confirmed that housing need was being dictated by long-standing policies and procedures. However, there was an awareness of a need to change to a person-centred approach that acknowledged the centrality of housing in a person's life. Future implementation of Supporting People (DETR and DoH, 2001b), referred to in other chapters, will reinforce the links between lifestyle and housing.

Assessment of needs for community equipment is another area where occupational therapists continue to play a leading role. As with assessment for housing adaptations, occupational therapists assessing for equipment must ensure that they are fully acquainted with their responsibilities within case law (Dimond, 1997).

Assessments of the needs of carers

Assessment of carer needs has not been part of the established role of occupational therapists. However, this is now changing in line with the statutory requirements briefly referred to in the previous chapter.

The Carers (Recognition and Services) Act of 1995 came into force on 1 April 1996. This entitles carers to an assessment of their needs, provided that the person they care for is undergoing a comprehensive assessment of their needs. In accord with the 1995 Act, the care manager assessor is required to look at:

- the carer's views of the situation;
- the nature of the relationship between the carer and cared for;
- the tasks undertaken by the carer;
- the impact of caring upon the carer's physical and emotional well-being;
- the willingness and ability of the carer to continue caring, taking into account other responsibilities and coping strategies.

The carer has to be providing substantial amounts of care on a regular basis. While this Act did not confer any rights to services for carers, the subsequent Carers and Disabled Children Act (2000) enables the provision of services to carers. Implementation of the Act will be the responsibility of both health and social care staff as services become integrated (Seddon and Robinson, 2001).

The carer's willingness to continue caring should not be taken for granted. Seddon and Robinson (2001) recommended that assessment of the needs of carers should be guided by a framework that includes full assessment of the carer's practical and emotional needs and the incorporation of a system for monitoring and review.

Assessment should be followed by interventions, otherwise the value of the assessment is lost. The interventions that can be offered to carers by occupational therapists are discussed in Chapter 7.

Assessments for admission to long-term care

A study by Tennant (NRR, 2001) examined the thresholds of eligibility for different types of care by devising a method of objectively measuring need for different care packages to support current assessment procedures. To achieve this, a set of valid and reliable measures was identified. Different assessment packs were formulated comprising no more than three assessments per pack. A total of 618 people admitted to hospital were recruited to the study. Their average age was 80.4 years. High levels of impairment and disability were evident. However, receipt of services was low: 45 per cent received no services at the time of admission, 24 per cent one service and 31 per cent two or more services. Patients were randomized to receive different assessment packs. The study found that while measures of impairment and disability were able to discriminate between those returning home and those admitted to long-term care, no single measure of health status is able to do so. The results were used to develop an index of continuing care need.

> If admission to long-term care is a possibility, a full multi-disciplinary assessment should take place to identify opportunities for rehabilitation and reduce inappropriate admissions. (DoH, 2001, p. 33)

Assessments of lifting and handling needs

The Manual Handling Operations Regulations (HSE, 1992) created a hierarchy of measures for reducing risk to employees when manually handling others, obliging employers to ensure the health and safety of their staff and, specifically, to avoid problems of back strain through unsafe lifting and handling. The regulations state that, wherever possible, manual handling should be avoided, and where it is not possible a risk assessment should be conducted to reduce identified risk to the lowest level. There is also a requirement to keep any assessments under review. The regulations were implemented on 1 January 1993, creating a new role of 'lifting and handling advisor' in many health and social care settings. The remit of lifting and handling advisors is to educate and train staff in safe methods of lifting and handling, and ensure that the recommendations of the regulations are adhered to. However, despite a plethora of available training and events to promote safe procedures, for example the Interprofessional Curriculum Framework for Health Care Advisors (COT, 1997), those responsible for advising and implementing safe practice are continuing to experience difficulty translating policy recommendations into actions. Central to the problem is the dissonance between the requirements of the Manual Handling Operations Regulations, which are largely concerned with safe lifting and handling by staff, and the rehabilitation and care needs of the person being lifted and their carer (CSP, COT and RCN, 1997). Guidance has since been issued which encourages health staff to take real-life situations and tasks into account. However, the focus remains upon the protection of paid staff (HSE, 1992), with health and safety legislation offering no protection to carers. The need for guidance is enhanced for social services departments who are also obliged to respond to the request by carers for an assessment of their needs if the person they care for is being assessed. The situation is made more complex by the shift of social services departments from direct providers to commissioners of care services. This has led to many social services departments contracting with external agencies to provide services like home care, sometimes leading to very different interpretations of the regulations across agencies involved in the social care of the same person. Despite an urgent need for guidance on interpretation of the regulations by social care agencies, to date it is not available. Through a rigorous review of the legislation, Mandelstam (2001) raised the point that the regulations do acknowledge that in practice a completely risk-free service is not possible.

Assessment to assist with diagnosis

Assessment of occupational performance undertaken by occupational therapists can uncover problems that may not have come to light during assessments undertaken by other professionals. One example is the role of occupational therapists in memory clinics, raised in Chapter 9. Chapter 3 described the complex mix of medical, social and environmental factors that can lead to older people experiencing difficulties. The value of the occupational therapy assessment lies in the ability to take all these factors into account. Decreased occupational performance can be attributed to a number of factors, for example:

- physical ill health;
- physical frailty leading to decreased ability to undertake occupations;
- a positive choice taken by the person to decrease their levels of activity (evidenced during studies of older people in good health);
- a consequence of external life influences like social isolation or entering residential care;
- poor skills, for example a consequence of bereavement of a life partner;
- depression arising from external events like bereavement, a life-threatening illness or poor relationships;
- depression with no apparent cause;
- alcoholism;

- other forms of mental ill health;
- the onset of dementia.

Mountain (2001b) suggested that the following approach contributes towards diagnosis:

1. Look for signs of decreased occupation that cannot be attributed to physical limitations or illness.
2. Look beyond the problems presented on referral, to consider the totality of the person's lifestyle.
3. Allow the older person plenty of time to talk.
4. Talk with others the person identifies as being significant to them.

It may also require the application of standardized assessments discussed in earlier sections of this chapter.

Implications for occupational therapy

One of the debates within the profession is whether assessment and specifically assessment of function is a core skill of occupational therapy (Phillips and Renton, 1995). From an examination of the debates within the literature, the authors deduced that the assessment role of occupational therapists cannot be isolated from other aspects of their work. There are also important questions for occupational therapists working with older people about whether the profession should concentrate on assessments that provide quality information about occupational needs, rather than applying generic measures. Additionally, there are dangers in concentrating upon functional ability alone. Some of these views may be reconciled by the previously described introduction of the single assessment process.

Determine the reasons for assessment

It is crucial to understand the rationales for assessment. Is the assessment being undertaken from the perspective of the older person, their carer, or in anticipation of provision of services (assessment for admission to long-term care, for example)? The sole aim of certain assessments is to provide information about risk for the multi-disciplinary team. The occupational therapist must be aware of the implications for their own professional practice, and for users and carers of participating in these forms of assessment. The evidence cited in this chapter strongly indicates that pre-discharge assessments – frequently undertaken with older people by occupational therapists – are not effective in themselves and only give an indication of safety at discharge. Longer-term follow-up is required to help vulnerable older people to cope in the longer term.

Select and apply appropriate assessment methods

Historically, occupational therapists have been more likely to rely upon their clinical reasoning, combined with the application of 'home grown' checklists and measures, rather than selecting instruments with proven psychometric properties. Using valid and reliable measures is recommended in that they provide an accurate measure, independent of who is the assessor. They can also provide baseline data for outcome measurement. The downside is that they reduce actions, abilities and perceptions into concrete, easily understood statements so that the assessor is in no doubt as to their meaning. Such statements rarely take account of subtle difference in abilities of individuals or the complexity of the situations occupational therapists are often required to assess. It is therefore recommended that occupational therapists employ a combination of assessments, using standardized instruments as well as interview and observation. It is also important to allow the older person plenty of time to talk freely.

Ensure the quality of the process

While it is important to consider the content of the assessment, the manner in which the assessment is conducted is of equal if not greater significance. It is all too easy to forget the significance of the process for the user and their carer when it is part of everyday professional practice. The reality is that older, vulnerable people do perceive themselves to be at a disadvantage, particularly in situations like hospital discharge, where the professional view of decisions about return home can be seen as being paramount, with the assessment being a test which the user can either pass or fail.

Understand the limitations of 'one-off' assessment

The rationale behind the assessment encounter and the quality of the process can be dictated by whoever has made the referral for assessment and for what reasons. Given the occupational needs which older people can present with, it is questionable whether a one-off assessment encounter can be sufficient for needs to be determined. Mountain (1998) found that when occupational therapists accepted referrals for rapid assessment, there was little opportunity for therapist and patient to get to know each other and form a partnership to explore the recommendations that might lead to best outcomes. Those older people who had been referred for occupational therapy assessment only were fearful of both the process and its consequences. The situation did not allow for clarification and reassurance and left the person with no control over the process. Moreover, occupational therapists were more than ready to hand the problem back to medical staff once they had carried out the prescribed work, with treatment opportunities therefore being missed.

Appreciate the complexity of assessment

The previously described assessment scenarios are complex. It can be difficult to determine when assessment ceases and interventions begin, as assessment and treatment can blur. Furthermore the clear focus upon health promotion and prevention means that screening assessments are becoming more common. Chapters 7 and 8 raise situations where occupational therapy may take a more prominent role in the future through the delivery of a combination of assessment and interventions in response to assessed need.

Understand the legal implications of assessment

Integration of health and social care, and the increasing shift of occupational therapy services to community settings, mean that all occupational therapists must understand their legislated responsibilities. Social services occupational therapists are experienced at working within a legislative framework. This expertise must extend across the entire profession at both service delivery and management levels.

Pointers for practice

- Use professional judgements to determine the appropriateness of undertaking the assessment.

- Meet the requirements of the single assessment process.

- Use a range of reliable and valid measures to assess functional abilities and risk, combined with interview and observation.

- Do not alter existing standardized measures in any way as this will alter their properties.

- Remain aware of the anxieties such assessments can generate.

- Allow plenty of time to talk with the older person and their carer.

- Determine from the older person what they want and need to be able to do.

- Consider the implications for the older person of undertaking short-term, one-off assessment.

- Give the older person and their carers feedback from the assessment process as a priority and check their perceptions against the results.

- Determine the extent of informal care available and the sustainability of that care.

- Reassess on a regular basis to take account of shifting needs and changes in the informal care network.

- In the majority of cases, ensure that appropriate interventions follow assessment, by undertaking treatment yourself or ensuring that the person is referred on to a named colleague within the system of care for older people.

CHAPTER 7

Occupational therapy interventions

One of the aims of this book is to stimulate reflective practice, located in the needs of older people and their carers. This means that a prescriptive approach towards service provision and interventions cannot be appropriate. It underrates the experiences and feelings of the person who has been referred to occupational therapy, and does not reflect either the complexity of the user/therapist relationship or the relationships between the older person, their physical and social environment and their involvement in meaningful occupations. It also fails to acknowledge the complex service context within which decisions about interventions are made. Figure 7.1 depicts some of the factors that have been shown to have an influence upon the clinical decisions taken by occupational therapists (Mountain, 1998a).

Figure 7.1 illustrates the true complexity underpinning decisions about interventions. Nine contributory factors are identified, with each of these being complex constructs in themselves. The implications are that occupational therapy interventions cannot be viewed in isolation. This understanding provides the backdrop for the material in this and the forthcoming chapters.

This chapter will examine the following:

1. the professional and policy contexts within which decisions about interventions are made;
2. specific occupational therapy interventions (see Figure 7.2, p.165);
3. the underlying dynamics of the occupational therapy process.

The professional context

Discussion continues within the profession about the core aims of occupational therapy and the nature of professional practice. The passion fuelling this ongoing debate was demonstrated through the letters in the

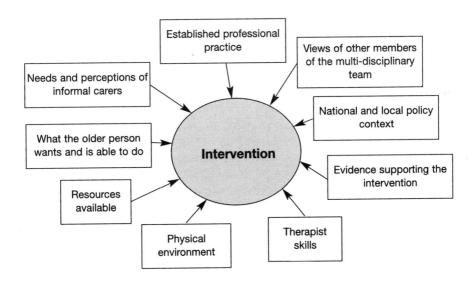

Figure 7.1 Factors influencing the nature of interventions provided by occupational therapists. Source: from research by Mountain (1998a).

British Journal of Occupational Therapy during 2002 regarding the relative significance and clinical relevance of occupational science as opposed to theories of occupational performance. It is important to understand the origins of these different viewpoints within the occupational therapy profession, and how and why they influence practice. As Chapter 2 illustrates, these perspectives need not be in conflict, as both can help us to further our understanding of the nature of occupation.

The importance of occupation underpinned the development of the profession of occupational therapy, the primary concern of the pioneers being a lack of participation in activities rather than diagnosis, disability or loss (Kielhofner and Nicol, 1989). There was an emphasis upon holism rather than the reductionism that is frequently associated with a medical paradigm.

> Occupational therapy has a great deal to learn from its history. The profession was founded on the visionary idea that human beings need, and are nurtured by, their activity as by food and drink, and that every human being possesses potential that can be achieved through engagement in occupation. (Yerxa, 1992, p. 82)

Wilcock (2001, 2002) has eloquently described the history of the profession. Her work showed how the needs of the economy during and following the war years led to the development of remedial approaches where links were made between activity and the therapeutic needs of the patient. This also led to a clearer association with medicine but unfortunately also stimulated a reductionist approach. This was reinforced by the poor image of craft and other activities within certain care settings, as opposed to the kudos that could be obtained from functionally based assessment and other interventions perceived to be of value by other professional groups. The predominance of this approach continued for several decades.

Towards the end of the twentieth century, academics outside the occupational therapy profession, as well as occupational therapists, started to observe the importance of taking into account the total lifestyle of the individual rather than just functional ability. In 1996, Challis wrote a persuasive opinion article that raised the wider role of occupational therapists with older people with mental health problems. He illustrated his point with a description of the range of occupational therapy interventions possible within residential care settings, for example providing continuity between old and new lifestyles, overseeing group work and activities, and working with carers including advice on equipment and adaptations. Steiner (2001) suggested that ability to undertake functional tasks does not necessarily reflect what the older person considers to be important to them. Focusing on ability to undertake a prescribed number of activities of daily living only reflects one dimension of an individual's lifestyle. It can also be postulated that involvement in functional abilities alone can also limit the complexities that can arise when therapy becomes a collaborative venture between user and therapist rather than a professionally led process.

Interpretations of rehabilitation

Delivery of rehabilitation is one of the cornerstones of occupational therapy practice. Rehabilitation is a complex construct, embracing a range of understandings; for example, the term is used to describe a range of service settings as well as specific interventions. This complexity was clearly illustrated during a seminar on rehabilitation with professionals held at the King's Fund in 1996:

> ... while it was clear that everyone knew what he or she meant by rehabilitation, their interpretation was not necessarily shared by others. Meanings differ according to what is involved, who benefits, who provides opportunities for rehabilitation and where. (Robinson and Batstone, 1996)

The recent, enhanced interest in rehabilitation has served to increase this complexity. Mountain (2001) noted that different interpretations are being adopted by health and social services, namely medical and social rehabilitation. The benefits of the social model are considered to be a focus upon both the views of service users and the needs for changes to society and the environment to accommodate disability. On the other hand, the medical model is said to concentrate upon curing or improving a condition through medical interventions and rehabilitation.

There are problems for occupational therapists in strictly adhering to one or other of these approaches:

1. The demography of those referred to social-services-provided occupational therapy shows that over 50 per cent of all referrals are for older people who often require assessment of health as well as social needs.
2. The practice of occupational therapy reflects a mixture of clinical and social dimensions.
3. As described in Chapter 5, the policy shift towards integrated services and the whole-systems approach towards the provision of rehabilitation services within a locality questions the appropriateness of polarized views of medical and social rehabilitation. Nocon and Baldwin (1998) examined these debates and concluded that it was more important to acknowledge the various components of rehabilitation, and the needs that are required to be addressed, rather than attributing styles of working to one model or the other.

It should be noted that other interpretations of rehabilitation have developed, grounded in the needs of specific client groups. This is evident in services for people with dementia, where the importance of activity in enhancing quality of life, as well as aspects like maintenance of dignity, relationships and psychological well-being, are promoted (Perrin, 1997). This requires us to consider the overall quality of life of an individual in the context of what they need to do and would like to be able to do, instead of concentrating upon a paradigm of rehabilitation that prioritizes interventions to improve functional ability or continued independence. The concept of personhood has also been described in relation to people with dementia. This was promoted through the work of the Bradford Dementia Group (Kitwood 1997; Benson, 2000). Personhood enables us to have a positive view of people with dementia, with a focus upon the whole person, drawing upon their strengths as well as taking into account declining abilities in some areas.

A final, important distinction should be made between rehabilitation provided by a range of health and social care professionals, and that provided through occupational therapy. As described in Chapter 2, Golledge (1998) articulated the importance of differentiating between occupation (or purposeful activity) and the use of activity for purely functional purposes, such as the use of remedial games. By underpinning rehabilitative interventions with occupation rather than activity, occupational therapists can promote a truly user-focused model of rehabilitation that is meaningful to the individual, taking into account their past and present lives, the environment within which they live and their cultural background. Therefore, throughout this chapter, the use of purposeful activity in interventions is emphasized.

Policy context

The previous chapters in this book have constantly referred to policy, demonstrating how policy and practice are inextricably linked. The policy climate for occupational therapy has never been better. Recent health and social care policy has promoted the value of rehabilitation and prevention services in helping older people to maintain health and independence (see Chapter 5). The importance of rehabilitative and preventive strategies to divert or allay admission to long-term care was an important strand of the findings of the Royal Commission on Long Term Care (1999). The report recommended that:

> Further research on the cost effectiveness of rehabilitation should be treated as a priority, but this should not prevent the development of a national strategy led by Government to be emphasized in the performance framework for the NHS and Social Services. (Royal Commission on Long Term Care, 1999, p. xxi)

Subsequent health and social care policy has emphasized the need for rehabilitation services. Most recently, the thrust has been for the development of intermediate care services, described in Chapters 5 and 9.

Interventions with individual service users and their carers

Figure 7.2 shows the intervention areas that occupational therapists working with older people might suggest or try with the older people they are working with. Categories of intervention 1–6 are reviewed in this chapter. Categories 7–9 are secondary or preventive in nature and are reviewed in Chapter 8.

Specific interventions with users

The simplicity of Figure 7.2 implies that categories of interventions are kept separate. The reality is that providing interventions in response to assessed needs is a dynamic process. Therefore one intervention might fulfil a number of goals. Also, preventive interventions might be included.

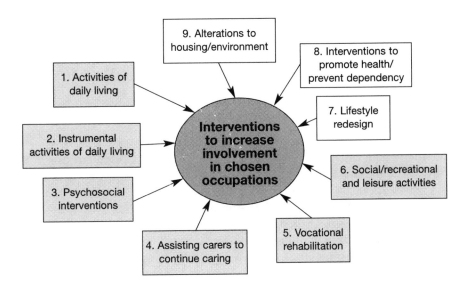

Figure 7.2 Range of occupational therapy interventions in response to assessed need.

The perceptions of the older person may indicate the need for a different approach to that suggested by the occupational therapist. Additionally, psychosocial approaches might be embedded within the entire repertoire of interventions.

Interventions in response to needs in activities of daily living

Assessments of activities of daily living (ADL) and instrumental activities of daily living (IADL) were mentioned in Chapter 6. The process of pre-discharge home visits undertaken to determine ADL and IADL abilities within the person's home were also considered. It was also stated that existing evidence strongly suggests that pre-discharge home visits undertaken to assess the safety of hospital discharge can be a negative experience for both service user and carer (Mountain and Pighills, 2003).

Maintaining coping abilities in the longer term following hospital discharge indicates a need for further interventions with older people in their own homes. Retrospective data on 139 post-discharge home visits to people aged 65 years and over carried out by eight occupational therapists working for the same hospital were analysed (Hassall, 1993). Interviews were also conducted with the occupational therapists concerned. Seventy-seven of the home visits were undertaken within one week of discharge from hospital. A variety of reasons were given for these visits, including assessment of risk upon discharge, late delivery of equipment and to see if the person was settled at home. The number of home visits carried out by individual members of staff varied from 2 to 43. The visits were not used for treatment, with the prime activities being assessment for equipment, its provision and education about usage. The study recommended better coordination of discharge arrangements and that discharge from occupational therapy should only occur when treatment is fully completed. The views of Hassall (1993) were supported by research that examined the cost and clinical effectiveness of nurse-practitioner-led patient-centred discharge planning and follow-up for frail hospitalized older people deemed to be at risk after discharge (Naylor et al., 1999). Results of this randomized controlled trial demonstrated that the intervention group stayed out of hospital significantly longer than the control group. This was attributed to a clinical intervention that was responsive to the combined effects of illness and social conditions (Naylor et al., 1999).

The rationale underpinning the wide-scale continuance of ADL and IADL assessment in the absence of interventions to meet identified needs is now being questioned by changes to long-standing patterns of service delivery (DoH, 2000a) and the promotion of new forms of rehabilitation service for older people (DoH, 2001a, 2001g). The raised profile of rehabilitation is requiring therapists to become involved as providers of rehabilitation and not merely assessors (Audit Commission, 2000b). The limitations of ending the process at the assessment stage, rather than providing interventions, are evident. Therefore if a need does emerge through functional assessment, the occupational therapist should be obliged to provide interventions as indicated, or refer the person on to an appropriate agency.

Treatment opportunities can include:

- helping the person to adapt to disability by teaching new routines to manage activities of daily living;
- providing equipment to compensate for loss of occupational performance or to facilitate participation in neglected occupations (see Chapter 8);
- adapting the environment or clothing to assist with the safe management of ADL and IADL;
- upgrading or downgrading activities to enable continued participation;
- exploring how mobility around the home, in the immediate home environment, and in the community can be maintained and possibly improved; interventions to improve mobility in older people can help to maintain independence, reduce the likelihood of falls (and their consequences) and limit admission to long-term care;
- suggesting other means of undertaking the activity, for example alternative ways of managing transport needs and shopping;

- providing equipment to help the carer assist the user with activities of daily living, for example transfers, bathing and toileting.

The central premise underpinning provision of interventions following assessment in this area is that it must be guided by what the person needs to be able to do within their environment (see Chapter 2, Figure 2.1), with occupational performance being a result of the interaction between the person, their environment and their perceptions of the context within which they live. Furthermore, it may not be necessary for the older person to be able to undertake all aspects of activities of daily living if support and assistance are in place. It may be that they wish to retain energy to enable continued engagement in other, more valued activities.

Involvement in social and leisure occupations

The limitation of an approach that concentrates upon ability to perform functional tasks has been referred to many times already. Additionally, the views of older people provided in Chapter 2 clearly demonstrated that maintaining a quality lifestyle in older age extends beyond the ability to undertake necessary tasks. It includes involvement in leisure and social activities that are meaningful to the individual. We are not the same: some of us are sociable and like to spend time with other people, whereas others prefer to be alone. As Chapter 1 described, some people still like to discover new pursuits in older age whereas others wish to continue with long-standing interests. Chapter 2 also referred to the consequences of activity deprivation.

The evidence base regarding the provision of social and leisure activities is a difficult area to locate in the absence of a description of the context within which these services are delivered. Certain rehabilitation service settings, described in Chapter 9, have concentrated upon functional abilities, setting aside the social and leisure needs of their users. In contrast, other services like day care have tended to provide a programme of group-based social activities, which may or may not be targeted at specific user groups. Existing evidence also confirms that the use of leisure and social/recreational activities has more often been used with older people with mental health rather than those with physical health problems, most likely because of the mismatch between the problems presented by mental ill health and the aims of a functional approach.

A systematic review of the effectiveness of activity programmes with older people with dementia (Law et al., 1999) involved 19 research studies into a range of interventions, including walking, conversation, self-care, social and leisure activities, assessment of motor and process skills (AMPS), individualized activities of daily living programmes, mental stimulation and music. Results of the review found that, overall, some activity programmes were beneficial. However, the evidence was weak, with more robust, larger-scale research being required. Results derived from four, more rigorous studies within the review found positive treatment effects. These support the use of activity programmes in improving well-being, communication, mental status and emotional state.

A more holistic, individualized approach is demonstrated through the lifestyle redesign programme for health promotion and prevention, described in Chapter 9, where diagnosis and service setting does not predominate. As it is difficult to disentangle social and leisure interventions from the services that provide them, the research in this area is largely given in Chapter 8. This in itself should lead occupational therapists working with older people to question the origin of some of the long-standing approaches to older people who find themselves in a specific set of circumstances.

Responding to individual occupational needs

If the full range of needs of an older person is taken into account, it is unlikely that they will solely concentrate on one occupational domain. This moves the debate on from polarized views of functional versus social activities. The occupational therapist must form a partnership with the older person and their carer so that interventions to improve or maintain performance are meaningful and fulfil the areas identified by the older person as being significant. The importance of this relationship was demonstrated through research reported by Levin and Gitlin (1992). This qualitative research involved analysis of therapists' reports of interventions undertaken with older people with chronic health conditions in their own homes, where a client-centred approach was adopted. The research revealed that the development of trust could take between two and three visits before the older person would be ready to identify meaningful interventions. Time is required before older people are willing to share their real concerns, particularly in intimate areas like continence, with views often being expressed in indirect ways. Levin and Gitlin also noted the requirement for therapists to relinquish some control in order to enable this process of collaboration and negotiation to occur.

A tool to foster this collaborative approach between user and therapist, the Community Adaptive Planning Assessment was devised by Spence and Davidson (1998). The rationale underpinning its development was the requirement to:

- make interventions relevant to the life of the individual older person;
- link future planning to past life experiences;

- take account of the occupational performance of the older person, the context within which occupation occurs and the meaning of occupations for the individual.

The appropriateness of this instrument for a UK population would have to be investigated and, at the time of writing, the authors had not demonstrated its psychometric properties. The important issue here is the thinking that underpinned the development of the measure.

A comparison of protocol-based interventions as opposed to adaptation-based interventions was conducted with older people admitted to a rehabilitation unit in America with the aim of return home or to a supported living environment (Spence et al., 1998). This used the Community Adaptive Planning Assessment. The protocols comprised interventions determined through therapist interviews with older people. The goals of interventions were increased stamina and performance of activities of daily living and instrumental activities of daily living. Emotional issues were not addressed by the occupational therapists as this was perceived to be the role of social workers. The adaptation-based intervention involved a client-centred evaluation followed by collaborative work with the older person to determine their goals, with a focus upon flexibility. The findings of the study supported the use of an approach that combined functional and emotional strategies to improve occupational performance together with a client- and family-centred approach. The research also demonstrated how seemingly simple interventions can be perceived in very different ways by the older person, their family and other service providers.

Occupation for people with dementia

Severity of illness is one of the most important considerations when looking at what might be achieved with people with dementia. A review of the literature in this area revealed a whole range of interventions, with appropriateness being determined by the extent of cognitive impairment (Mountain, in press). A comparatively early study considered that occupation for people with dementia in the form of social and recreational activities can present opportunities for social interaction that might not otherwise exist (Jenkins et al., 1977). Examples of occupation-based interventions for people with dementia include use of memory books, personalized therapeutic recreation and self-management training.

Nevertheless, rehabilitation of older people with severe dementia continues to challenge occupational therapists and others working with people with this illness.

The need for education for care staff was underscored by research undertaken in a day-care setting for people with Alzheimer's disease in

North America (Hasselkus, 1992). Participant observation on the part of the author (an occupational therapist) occurred over a four-week period. The research also included interviews with the three staff and a document analysis. Results found that the main aim of the setting was to prevent the attendees harming themselves. To achieve this, emphasis was placed upon a calming environment and making sure that any trouble was caught early. Only when safety was ensured were other aims like enjoyment and individualized care met. It was also noted that the main emphasis of care was engagement in group activities. Hasselkus suggested that for individuals in the middle-to-late stages of illness, the focus of activity programmes should be provision of respite to carers and provision of activities that are meaningful to the individual.

A UK occupational therapist, Tessa Perrin, has done much to develop thinking regarding occupation for people with dementia. Her research was based upon the following observation:

> There can be few in the health care system more occupationally deprived than persons with dementia, particularly those persons who, owing to the advanced nature of their condition, have found their way into institutional care of one sort or another. (Perrin, 1996, p. 12)

Perrin's hypothesis is located in the value of occupation in dementia and the need for a person-centred approach that takes into account the residual faculties of the individual. An example would be that cognitive approaches like quizzes and reality orientation are redundant in people with severe dementia. Perrin and May (2000) extended this thesis. They emphasized the requirement to monitor the impact of any activity upon the well-being of people with dementia, and in particular those activities that demand cognition. The notion of undertaking playful activities with people with severe dementia is promoted. This may extend to activities of childhood: Perrin and May cite the use of dolls and beach balls. This approach is skilled, and occupational therapists considering its application are strongly advised to refer to the work of Perrin and May. Some of the differences between this approach and the infantilizing, block treatment of older people in some care settings raised in Chapter 5 can be located in the individual, person-centred approach and the monitoring of the impact of the activities.

Occupation with older people with functional mental health problems

Provision of occupational therapy interventions with older people with depression presents specific challenges. This is not assisted by the currently under-researched relationship between occupation and depression in older age. The extent to which depression is caused by lack of opportunities for occupation, or alternatively that lack of occupation is a symptom of the depressive illness itself, remains questionable. Fine (2000) conducted an examination of the existing evidence base regarding the effectiveness of leisure activities for older people with depression. Leisure activities embraced dance, hobbies and games. A literature review identified six studies that examined the effects of leisure activities for this population. A further two studies looked at the relationship between leisure activities and self-esteem. Fine discussed the limitations of all the studies and in particular the failure to distinguish between the previously discussed cause and effect, and whether the activities in themselves or the increased social opportunities they presented led to improvement.

Psychosocial interventions and approaches

The notion that psychosocial occupational therapy is confined to occupational therapists working in mental health is unhelpful as it implies an approach confined to services established for specific populations. The reality is that for many older people, a holistic approach is required that draws upon a range of skills including the ability to respond to emotional needs. Some of the research illustrated in the previous chapters acknowledges the emotional needs that will accompany chronic health conditions, as do examples of preventive occupational therapy strategies described in the forthcoming chapter.

Psychosocial interventions can be used to describe a number of approaches, for example:

- Counselling – the individual is encouraged to talk through their problems and discover solutions with the guidance of a therapist. Even though occupational therapists do not complete pre-registration training with counselling qualifications, the ability to be able to listen carefully and respond appropriately must be an essential prerequisite to working with older people. For further information on techniques, readers are encouraged to refer to any one of a range of texts, for example Scrutton (1999).
- Cognitive behavioural therapy – this is one of the most commonly used therapies, and complements occupational therapy very successfully. It acts on the assumption that the beliefs an individual has about themselves and the world directly influences their feelings and behaviour. The aim is to help the person to help him or herself. It involves the identification of a focus, selection of a strategy to tackle it and monitoring of the outcome. An example easily recalled from interaction with older people, is a reluctance to travel. The key is to allow the older person to identify how this is limiting their quality of life and explore how they are preventing themselves from achieving what they wish to do. This is followed by the identification of means of overcoming the

difficulty. In the case of travel difficulties, the solution may be a graded approach to going out. For further details see Sheldon (1995).

- Activities used to stimulate a therapeutic relationship with the therapist and/or the promotion of a therapeutic experience, for example art, drama, pottery and creative writing. These approaches are the same as for the general adult population, as described by Finlay (1997).

Rehabilitation for work

It is becoming clear that the cessation of working life when the individual reaches a pre-defined age is no longer going to be the case, with working life being extended beyond the 65 years, as described in Chapter 1. Additionally, new perspectives of older people and the contribution they can continue to make to society are leading to an expectation of continuation of work in an unpaid capacity. Therefore policy presents new challenges for occupational therapists, who as acknowledged experts in the provision of vocational rehabilitation now need to translate their existing skill base to meet the needs of older workers (Mountain et al., 2001).

In a forward-thinking paper on vocational rehabilitation and the older worker, Kemp and Kleinplatz (1985) predicted the need to maintain older people in the workforce. They identified a number of special needs for rehabilitation that older workers might have. These included taking into account the aspects of the physiological aspects of the ageing process such as deterioration of the senses and lowered stamina. They also highlighted the greater side effects of medication due to altered metabolic rate, and the greater impact of disability upon older people. As discussed in Chapter 2, the authors noted that older people do not usually experience lowered intellectual abilities or decreased interpersonal skills, and are more likely to be stable, reliable workers in comparison with younger people.

Kemp and Kleinplatz (1985) identified the following as being important components of vocational rehabilitation with older people:

1. emphasizing the need for a range of abilities;
2. early intervention to prevent loss of confidence and allay the lowering of physical abilities;
3. maintaining an understanding of the physiological changes that occur in older age;
4. determining the length of time required to prepare the person for return to work.

Involvement of occupational therapists with the needs of an ageing workforce is certain to be a dominant feature of future practice.

The needs of older workers might include the following:

1. Assessment of work abilities. This is a complex area and for older people might include assessments of the following:
   - ability to continue working, including physical stamina, cognitive abilities and emotional coping strategies;
   - the nature of the person's existing skill base and the extent to which it matches the demands of the market;
   - ability to benefit from vocational training.
2. Counselling and support, for example to help determine when working life should realistically cease (in the absence of a pre-determined retirement age) and to support re-entry into the workplace.
3. Provision of community equipment and information communication technologies to facilitate involvement in work, as a home worker or in an established workplace setting.
4. Ergonomic assessment of the workplace and provision of necessary adjustments in line with the requirements of the Disability Discrimination Act (1995).

Therapeutic modalities

Over the years a number of approaches have been devised for use with older people. Reminiscence therapy, validation therapy and reality orientation therapies in particular are popular therapeutic modalities for people with dementia. However, this does not preclude their use with other groups of older people.

Reminiscence therapy

Spector et al. (1998a) conducted a Cochrane review to examine the effectiveness of reminiscence therapy for people with dementia. For the purposes of the review, they identified reminiscence therapy as:

> Vocal or silent recall of events in a person's life, either alone, or with another person or group of people. It typically involves group meetings, at least once a week, in which participants are encouraged to talk about past events, often assisted by aids such as photos, music, objects and videos of the past. (Spector et al., 1998a, p. 1)

Since the wide-scale introduction of reminiscence therapy in the 1970s, a whole industry devoted to the production of materials to facilitate such groups has developed.

Despite searching a comprehensive number of electronic information sources, as well as hand-searching journals, Spector et al. found that only two studies of reminiscence therapy met criteria for inclusion in the review. The quality of the available research made it impossible to combine study results, and the authors observed that conclusions could not be reached regarding effectiveness. Existing evidence suggested that there may be some beneficial aspects, but more research is required. The results of the review did not produce any definitive guidelines for the use of reminiscence therapy, but highlighted the following tentative implications for practice from the existing evidence base:

- For reminiscence therapy to be successful, perhaps it should be part of a continuous, ongoing programme or incorporated into the daily routine.
- Assessment for inclusion should include psychological as well as cognitive factors.
- There are some indications that reminiscence therapy can be more successful in the early stages of dementia.

It is also worthwhile considering the nature of the materials used for the purposes of reminiscence. A wide variety of 'off the shelf' products can be purchased. However, it is often the home-made prompts, tailored to the lifestyles of the older people who are participating, that can be most successful in triggering memories.

Life review

Life review or story work describes an approach that enables an individual person to talk about their life experiences including family, friends, working life, and leisure and social interests. Relevant aspects of the individual's life history are recorded to benefit the person in their current situation. Life review has a number of applications. It can be an extremely valuable way of enabling staff caring for older people with dementia to understand the people they are caring for and to respond in a person-centred way (Audit Commission, 2002b). In these situations, it might include the assembling of life story books.

Life review can also be used as a basis for assessment and subsequent occupational therapy interventions. The Occupational Performance Interview (Kielhofner et al., 1989) involves asking the person to provide a narrative of their life, identifying triggers when their circumstances changed. Life review can, in these situations, lead to painful recollections.

More fundamentally, life review can assist the older person to link their past to their future, drawing upon their experiences and strengths to enable better coping with prevailing circumstances.

Reality orientation

Spector et al. (1998b) also undertook a Cochrane review of reality orientation. This was identified as:

> A technique to improve the quality of life of confused elderly people ... it operates through the presentation of orientation information (e.g. time, place and person related) which is thought to provide the person with a greater understanding of their surroundings, possibly resulting in an improved sense of control and self esteem. (Spector et al., 1998b, p. 1)

Spector et al. noted that reality orientation was first devised to rehabilitate disturbed war veterans, and its application to the treatment and care of confused older people in the 1960s was the first attempt at psychological treatment for dementia. It can be continuous, over 24 hours, with staff providing continual cues or in a classroom format where a group meet together to undertake reality orientation activities. A search of electronic databases and hand searches of journals identified 43 publications. Application of quality criteria led to eight randomized controlled trials for inclusion in the systematic review. The results of six of these were combined using meta-analysis. Results showed that reality orientation is beneficial; however, it is difficult to identify the aspects that provide most benefit, for example amount and quality of input. The implications for practice deduced from the review were the following:

- The classroom style of reality orientation can lead to cognitive and behavioural improvements in the short term. However, there is no evidence of long-term benefit.
- Improvement over time might be sustained through classroom reality orientation being backed up by an ongoing programme.
- The main danger of reality orientation is rigid, inappropriate application.

The final point noted by Spector et al. was borne out by earlier work on the quality of ward environments by Bowie et al. (1992). They observed that the existence of reality orientation, either as a form of therapy or in the guise of environmental cues, was a common feature of such settings. A valid and reliable measure was devised to determine the number, quality and accuracy of physical reality orientation cues present on a ward – date boards, weather boards, clocks, room signs, colour coding and patient notice boards. A second aspect of the measure involved questioning the person in charge of the ward about reality orientation as a treatment, and the extent to which it was used. Subsequent application of this measure to a survey of 28 such wards found that half the wards surveyed attained poor-quality scores for this measure, for example inaccurate or absent cues (Mountain and Bowie, 1995).

A study by Metitieri et al. (2001) evaluated the outcomes of classroom reality orientation in delaying the progression of dementia, through studying patients over a 30-month period. A treatment group comprising 46 patients who received between eight and 40 weeks of reality orientation training was compared with a control group of 28 patients who received just four weeks of training. Results suggested that continuing use of reality orientation may slow down cognitive decline, with the people in the treatment group remaining in the community significantly longer than the controls.

Validation therapy

A third approach used with older people with dementia is that of validation therapy. It is defined as:

> A therapy for communicating with old people who are diagnosed as having Alzheimer's disease and related dementia. (Neal and Briggs, 1999, p. 1)

It validates the communication of the person, and is often seen to be an opposite approach to reality orientation in that it seeks to correct any erroneous understanding and ground the person in the 'here and now'.

Neal and Briggs traced the origin of validation therapy to one worker, Naomi Feil, between 1963 and 1980. She stated that this form of communication is underpinned by a number of beliefs and values. These include the uniqueness of the individual, that there will always be an underlying reason for behaviour and that this behaviour will be a combination of physical, psychological and social changes that occur during the individual's lifespan. There are 14 techniques underpinning validation therapy. Neal and Briggs conducted a systematic review to examine the evidence to support validation therapy as defined by the framework identified by Feil. A search of the evidence base identified three studies, two of which were combined using meta-analysis. It was not possible to draw definitive conclusions about benefit due to lack of evidence. The authors noted that observational studies have noted benefit, particularly with respect to an improvement in the attitudes of those providing care.

Sensory stimulation

Snoezelen was first developed as a treatment modality for people with learning disabilities and has since been used with other client groups with multiple and severe impairments. The starting point for the development of Snoezelen therapy was that institutional environments offer limited stimulation. Snoezelen involves the use of equipment that stimulates the senses in an attractive, non-demanding manner. This creates a relaxing environment that can be enjoyed and explored by the individual. Given the degree of distress and agitation that can be experienced by people with severe dementia, it is not surprising that occupational therapists and other health care workers have been attracted by the goals that Snoezelen espouses. However, enthusiasm must be tempered by awareness of the marketing techniques accompanying the sale of the equipment. The evidence base underpinning the use of this therapy is currently under-developed. Van Diepen et al. (2002) reported a pilot study to examine the effects of Snoezelen for people with dementia, compared with reminiscence therapy. They noted that only four studies examining the effectiveness of Snoezelen and including ten or more patients had been published. The methodological challenges of this form of research are well described by van Diepen et al. Results suggested that both forms of intervention can have short-term effects like reduction of agitation, leading to a more relaxed state in some people and increased stimulation for others. Most recently a Cochrane review to examine the effectiveness of Snoezelen for dementia concluded that the evidence base is as yet insufficient to be able to draw definitive conclusions regarding benefit (Chung et al., 2003).

Working with carers of older people

The demands placed upon informal carers of older people and their subsequent needs were described in Chapter 4. There is now a realization that interventions with carers can be a productive use of therapy time, but this development is relatively recent. During a seminar for study participants to discuss the results of research into the activity of occupational therapists (Mountain and Moore, 1996) the following discussion points were raised with respect to interventions with carers:

> It depends upon what area of work was being carried out and the extent of carer contact that entails. In community psychiatry of old age, occupational therapists will communicate with carers as they are present in the treatment environment.

> There is currently a lot of support for working with carers. Health Trusts are now putting more emphasis upon carer involvement and the extent of involvement can be a quality measure.

> Carer involvement should be promoted due to the cost implications of maintaining a person in the community. (Mountain and Moore, 1996, p. 24)

Occupational therapy intervention with carers can take several forms, for example:

1. provision of information and advice;
2. teaching coping and rehabilitative strategies so that the carer is able to manage the needs of the person they are caring for more effectively;
3. counselling and support;
4. assessment for, and provision of, any assistive devices and adaptations.

Mitchell (2000) provided an example of the role of occupational therapists with the carers of older people with dementia. This described the initiation and evaluation of a four-week stress management programme for carers in the health education room of a local hospital. Carers were expected to transport themselves to the group, with care for the person they cared for being made available. The outcomes for individuals attending the group were estimated using an established measure (Hodgson et al., 1998). The tentative results of this small-scale study were that carer awareness was improved and there was a decrease in some of the aspects of burden they experienced. However, whether this effect had any long-standing benefit is not known.

Working with carers mirrors the complexity of working with users. It is not a simple matter of assessing and prescribing interventions. Some of the many issues that occupational therapists must take account of when working with carers are given below:

1. *Separating the needs* of the carer as distinct from those of the older person. All too often, reports and other documentation discuss users and carers as if they are inextricably linked. The reality may be completely different. Interviewing carers separately from users can be invaluable in illuminating different needs and perspectives.
2. *Identifying carer needs*. Following the implementation of the Carers and Disabled Children Act (2000) carers may now request an assessment of their own needs. Even if a carer is not requesting a formal assessment, occupational therapists should consider the carer's needs for work, social contact, help around the home and leisure.
3. *Being realistic* about the help available to the carer. The Carers and Disabled Children Act (2000) only requires local authorities to provide help in response to assessed carer needs if the resources are available to do so. Given the financial constraints upon local authorities, responses to carer needs are not likely to be a high priority. Occupational therapists should therefore ensure that they are fully aware of all statutory and non-statutory resources available to carers in their locality. They must also resist building false expectations.
4. *The dynamics of the relationship* between the older person and their carer. As Chapter 4 described, the history of the relationship and the demands being placed upon it will create stresses. This does not always

mean that the carer wants to relinquish their caring responsibilities. In some circumstances, carers will want to continue caring whatever the personal cost, and will be reluctant to accept help, particularly respite (Mountain and Godfrey, 1995). In other situations, the carer will be on the point of withdrawing their help. It is therefore essential to explore the nature of the relationship if the resulting assistance is to be both appropriate and timely.

Approaches

The previous section of this chapter has explored some of the specific interventions that might be undertaken with older people, the undertaking of which has to be underpinned by decisions about what will most appropriately meet needs.

Table 7.1 gives examples of both the extent of information required to enable the most appropriate treatment decisions and some of the approaches (but not specific strategies) that may be indicated. It must be emphasized that the contents of Table 7.1 do not represent an exhaustive or prescriptive list. It seeks to illustrate the variety of occupational therapy interventions that might be indicated given the individual needs of older people.

Table 7.1 Examples of interventions with users

Presenting problems	Information required through assessment	Possible treatment approaches
Physical limitations/ frailty/ disability	• Tasks that are considered essential • Long-standing routines • Extent of statutory care provision • Extent of informal care available and its perceived adequacy/ acceptability/ sustainability • Leisure and social needs • Risk factors • Awareness/acceptance of risk • Perceived appropriateness of existing housing	• Teach new strategies to cope with daily occupations • Provide assistive technology and teach usage • Advise on safety and preventive measures to reduce risk • Adapt long-standing interests or explore new pastimes • Work with carers so they are able to participate in the rehabilitative process if appropriate • Suggest interventions to improve stamina and coordination if indicated • Explore environmental needs and suggest alternative use of space • Housing adaptations if indicated

Table 7.1 Examples of interventions with users (contd)

Presenting problems	Information required through assessment	Possible treatment approaches
Accident/ injury	• Cause of the incident • Any history of previous accidents • The attitudes of the person to the incident; perceived difficulties short and longer term • The outcomes of the incident • Whether the person is still working, paid or unpaid • Any care being received from statutory agencies • Extent of informal care available and its perceived adequacy/ acceptability/ sustainability • Attitudes of carers towards the incident • Perceived appropriateness of existing housing	• Undertake a risk assessment of the home environment if that was the site of the accident • Suggest reasonable adjustments to the workplace (if appropriate) • Advise on safety and preventive measures to reduce risk • Help the person to accept any long-term consequences of the incident • Suggest interventions to improve stamina and coordination if indicated • Work with carers so they are able to participate in the rehabilitative process if appropriate
Physical illness	• Attitudes towards illness and mortality • Effects of illness upon physical functioning in short and longer term • Extent of help available and for what • Current and future needs for additional support • Perceived appropriateness of housing • Involvement of other professionals/care providers	• Give lifestyle advice taking illness into account • Teach strategies to cope with daily tasks • Provide assistive technology and adaptations if indicated • Adopt a flexible approach to take account of health changes day to day and over time, grading occupations as indicated • Explore leisure interests that can be achieved within physical abilities • Advise on safety and preventive measures to reduce risk • Work with carers so they are able to participate in the rehabilitative process if appropriate
Terminal illness	• Extent of awareness of the prognosis	• Provide equipment to enable the person to stay at home should they wish to (and carers are able to cope)

Table 7.1 (contd)

Presenting problems	Information required through assessment	Possible treatment approaches
Terminal illness (contd)	• Effects of illness upon abilities to carry out occupations • Carer awareness and capacity to continue caring • Extent of overall care network • Input from other professionals	• Maximize independence • Enable continuation in leisure and social interests for as long as possible through gradation of activity and adaptive strategies • Provide counselling to discuss distress and spiritual needs to both user and carer • Work closely with other professionals involved with the older person and their carers
Changes in life circumstances, e.g. bereavement, moving home, entering residential care	• Emotional and practical implications of life changes • Any life-skills deficits • Extent of help available • Willingness to accept available help • Attitudes towards staying put in existing housing • Friendship and care networks • Leisure and social interests • Opportunities to engage in chosen occupations • Satisfaction with existing residency and surrounding environment	• Allow time to express feelings and adjust to new circumstances • Teach new life skills or revisit neglected skills if indicated • Explore new opportunities for leisure occupations and accompany/support as necessary • Work with carers so they are able to participate in the rehabilitative process
Social isolation/ alienation	• Extent of existing care network and availability of carers • Reasons for isolation and its duration • Previous lifestyle and interests • Any interplay between isolation and ability to undertake occupations • The lifestyle the person would like to have and what is feasible	• Take time to explore the dynamics of the situation before offering solutions • Offer new opportunities for socialization if indicated but resist developing a social relationship • Assess occupational function and suggest strategies/interventions as indicated • Taking full account of the dynamics under a staged approach towards the introduction of new occupations, e.g. by initially supporting new social situations

Table 7.1 Examples of interventions with users (contd)

Presenting problems	Information required through assessment	Possible treatment approaches
Social isolation/ alienation (contd)	• Social outlets in the locality	• Work with carers so they are able to participate in the rehabilitative process
Functional mental health problems, e.g. anxiety/ depression	• Duration of mental health problems • Any other accompanying problems, e.g. alcohol abuse, physical illness • Lifestyle/interests • Current use of time • Extent of help available and its perceived adequacy/acceptability • The extent of occupational function and engagement and the possible reasons for any observed and reported difficulties • Other professionals involved and perceptions of their contributions • Perceived needs for support	• Spend time talking with the person about their current circumstances and past lifestyle • Devise small strategies to improve activity levels (but be prepared for setbacks) • Communicate with other health and social care agencies and refer on for advice and specialist help as indicated • Explore needs for longer-term support • Work with carers so they are able to participate in the rehabilitative process
Signs of cognitive impairment/ early dementia	• Difficulties experienced undertaking both necessary and chosen occupations through talking to the person and their carers as well as observing engagement in occupations • The existence of concurrent problems like anxiety and depression • Participation in activities that pose a risk to self or others, e.g. driving • Any statutory care provision	• Teach strategies to enable continued independence • Provide assistive technology to promote safety and independence • Provide emotional and practical support in making necessary adjustments like having to relinquish certain occupations • Monitor the coping abilities and safety of the older person by repeat visits or through the reports of visits by other workers

Table 7.1 (contd)

Presenting problems	Information required through assessment	Possible treatment approaches
Signs of cognitive impairment/ early dementia (contd)	• Extent of informal care and its sustainability • Current suitability of existing housing and living arrangements	
Mid-/late-stage dementia	• The lifestyle of the person prior to their illness • Their life history • Care networks and the most significant people in the network • Desire and ability to remain in the community • Current and future needs for residential care	• Listen carefully and observe what the person is trying to communicate • Maintain quality of life through appropriate occupation • Provide assistive technology to promote safety and independence • Support carers to continue caring (this pertains to paid as well as informal carers) • Engage with services that will assist the person to remain in the community if this is both possible and appropriate • Continue to involve carers even when a move to residential care is the outcome
Home situation poses risk	• Observe possible hazards in the home • Observe abilities in self-care tasks • Determine the older person's views of the risks they are taking and the options available if risk is admitted • Consider the risk the person poses to both themselves and others through observation and discussion with carers • Explore extent of easily accessible help from both formal and informal sources • Determine attitudes to staying put or moving	• Offer solutions to improve safety • Suggest extra social care provision if available and indicated • Suggest day-care options which provide an alternative to home during the day • Offer advice and support to carers

The next table (Table 7.2) identifies the approaches that might be appropriate to undertake with the carers of older people, following on from the evidence of the needs of carers provided in Chapter 4. Once again, the contents do not represent the full range of strategies that might be followed. The main issue demonstrated throughout Table 7.2 is the requirement to both disentangle the needs of carers from those of the older people they are looking after and introduce a separate repertoire of responses.

Table 7.2 Examples of occupational therapy approaches with carers

Presenting problems: cared-for person	Presenting issues: carer	Information required through carer assessment	Possible interventions
All older people	• Relation to the older person • Quality of relationship with older person and attitude towards them • Physical and emotional health of carer • Time to attend to own needs • Financial demands of caring • Other caring and work commitments • Perceived capacity to continue caring in the short and long term • Residency of both carer and older person	• Perceptions of caring obligations • Resilience of carer • Impact of caring upon quality of life • Awareness of services to help carers • Importance of carer within the overall care network • Ability of the carer to be able to respond to the needs of the older person • Extent and nature of care being provided • Support being provided by statutory services and its adequacy • Support provided from other sources – involvement in voluntary/charitable sector • Willingness to continue caring • Acceptability of respite care should it be indicated	• Give the carer time to talk about their views of role as a carer • Teach enabling strategies to use with older person if indicated • Provide information about appropriate services in the locality • Liaise with other workers about support services/respite
Effects of ageing, frailty and disability	As for all older people	As for all older people, plus • Mobility limitations experienced by older person	As for all older people, plus • Provide equipment and/or

Table 7.2 (contd)

Presenting problems: cared-for person	Presenting issues: carer	Information required through carer assessment	Possible interventions
Effects of ageing, frailty and disability (contd)		• Lifting required to be undertaken by carer • Physical effects of lifting upon the carer	adaptations and teach usage • Advise on safety and preventive measures to reduce risk to older person and self
Accident/ injury/ sudden illness of cared-for	As for all older people, plus • Possible radical increase in caring demands or new caring demands (if the older person had previously been independent) • Perceived capacity to continue caring in both the short and longer term	As for all older people, plus • Attitudes to changes that have occurred in the older person • Awareness/familiarity with the caring role • Lifestyle changes for carer • Mobility limitations experienced by older person • Lifting required to be undertaken by carer • Physical effects of lifting upon the carer	As for all older people, plus • Alert other agencies to the needs of the older person and carer • Provide equipment and/or adaptations and teach usage or refer on for expert advice • Advise on safety and preventive measures to reduce risk to older person and self
Mental health problems of cared-for	As for all older people, plus • Attitudes towards mental ill health	As for all older people, plus • Actual or perceived changes in abilities/ independence of the older person • Perceptions of current and future needs for additional support	As for all older people, plus • Advise on strategies to promote continued independence • Provide information about mental health support services for carer as well as cared-for

Table 7.2 demonstrates the depth of information required from carers of all older people in order to be able to respond appropriately to their needs.

Implications for occupational therapists

Throughout this book, the need for both a sensitive and expert approach towards the needs of individual older people and their carers is emphasized. A number of considerations need to be taken account of if interventions are to be productive.

Establish a relationship with the older person

The importance of establishing a client-centred relationship with the person is indisputable. Interviews with older people revealed that those who had been prescribed occupational therapy without their knowledge and involvement felt at best uninvolved and at worst on trial (Mountain, 1998a):

> They do it with everybody.

> I thought she was from the welfare.

> I just received the letter or phone call from them.

In contrast, those who were given information and allowed some degree of decision-making felt more in control and were consequently more receptive.

> My charge nurse said she would get someone to follow me up when I came out, if that would suit me because I was in quite a long time and it was time I was going home. So I said 'Yes that would be fine' and so she said 'I've got A to come out to you, would you like a word with her on the phone?'

Interviews with older people also demonstrated that the consequences of poor referral methods could be ameliorated if the occupational therapist subsequently took time to develop a relationship with the individual.

Older women with mental health problems interviewed by Mountain (1998a) described the benefits of occupational therapy thus:

> It shows that they are trying to help you, you're not just left to carry on.

> I don't think that it's changed my life as such, but it's helped me to know there's someone helping me.

> When you come out of hospital you start getting panicky again because of all the things you cut yourself off from and to know that you've got this link is very good.

Resist the use of professional jargon

We all frequently use occupational therapy jargon without either conveying what is meant to other professions or being sure that we have the same understanding as our fellow occupational therapists. Examples uncovered by Mountain (1998a) were the differing interpretations placed upon the terms home visits and domestic assessments. If we cannot agree, then it is highly unlikely that service users and their carers will understand what is being conveyed to them. A key component of good communication is ensuring that the older person and their carer understand fully what is being said to them.

Get underneath compliance

Many of us tend to be overtly compliant in our interactions with professionals. In the case of older people, a desire to cooperate with authority figures can be exacerbated. A number of reasons can be postulated for this. These include the legacy of a generation who experienced a shortage of services and goods, the helplessness that is often engendered by care services, and fear of professionals' power, particularly when making decisions about return home following hospital admission. A fear of repercussion as perceived by older people and their carers can lead to a reluctance to clearly state needs and give views of appropriateness of suggested interventions.

It is significant that this compliance is not usually sustainable when the person is able to make choices about what they are and are not going to do. A study of community alarm systems for older people (Thornton and Mountain, 1992) found that those with pendant alarms would be selective about the situations in which they would wear the device, even though non-use was disapproved of by professionals. Indications for use were situations where they felt unwell or unsteady, or when they were engaged in, what was for them, hazardous occupations, for example using the bathroom or walking in the garden.

Research has found that overt compliance with occupational therapy can be followed by disregard for what has been advised (Mountain, 1998a). Talking to older people can reveal logical reasons for this. One lady attending a day hospital at the time of interview explained that she was not going to apply the instruction she had received from the occupational therapist in use of a washing machine as she was already receiving help with her laundry:

> I didn't bother because, well, I thought I get it done every Wednesday.

A man attending the same day hospital talked enthusiastically about the cookery sessions he was receiving and then went on to explain why he was going to continue to eat sandwiches at home:

> Well, I tell you why I don't cook at home and then you'll understand. I get my groceries on Wednesday, 7 o'clock. I start breaking into them on Saturday morning. The simple reason is I come here [day hospital] on

Thursday during the day. Friday I go to day centre and Saturday, Sunday, Monday I don't go anywhere so I make sandwiches. Saturday, Sunday, Monday, three days ... so I don't need to cook do I?

Clearly what was required was a frank discussion about this person's needs and how they might change upon discharge from the day hospital.

Another reason for non-compliance with occupational therapy can be fear of undertaking the activity itself. The same study found that older people might agree to a treatment goal for the future, but would then refuse when the event was imminent. This lady talked about her reaction to planned trips into the community:

Well, H has been once or twice ... and I've just said 'Oh I don't think I can manage it today'.

Ensure that communication is enhanced

The previous section on compliance underscores the importance of enhanced communication with the older person and their carer. Helping the person to express their true needs and feelings is a skill that must be fostered by all health and social care professionals. This incorporates meeting needs for information in clear lay language as previously described. It also embraces the nature of communication that occurs between older person and/or their carer and occupational therapist.

One of the common denominators extending across various specific therapies for older people, and in particular for those with dementia, is that their application demands that staff both talk to and listen carefully to the older person. Therefore it follows that evidence of benefit could be linked with this enhanced communication.

Help the person and their carers to manage dependency appropriately

In contrast to the value placed upon older people by other cultures, in Western society the management of people who are dependent is frequently viewed as being similar to that of young children. Thus, the person whose needs have become childlike, for example those needing help with toileting and feeding, are afforded the social status of child (Hockey and James, 1993). As the process of dependency increases, this denying of adulthood deepens. Hockey and James discussed double incontinence in older people, which is often an indication of forthcoming death but is often managed by staff in a manner that infantilizes the older person.

The differentiation needs to be made between managing functional needs and promoting needs for occupation on the part of the individual. For some older people, the use of play equipment and pursuance of occupations usually associated with children will be inappropriate. In contrast, some occupational therapists working with older people with severe dementia have promoted the notion of undertaking playful activities with severely impaired individuals (Perrin and May, 2000).

Take into account the attitudes of the older person

A study reported some time ago in the occupational therapy literature examined the attitudes of people with stroke and whether this is related to their abilities to undertake activities of daily living (Strudwicke et al., 1991). The study tested the theory that patients with positive attitudes towards their rehabilitation would perform better. Twenty-nine stroke patients aged between 40 and 78 years participated. A number of valid and reliable measures to assess physical capability, psychological state and ability in activities of daily living were applied, 2 weeks and 24 weeks after stroke. Additionally, participants were asked to keep a diary. Results demonstrated the complexity of the process of recovery. Results suggested that attitudes were the best predictors of achievement. Irrespective of physical impairment, a realistic attitude towards the stroke, treatment and exercise leads to greater progress over six months compared to those with an unrealistic attitude. The authors also noted that it is unwise to rely upon a person's initial reports of their condition and abilities, emphasizing the need for counselling to discuss the problems in depth.

Furthermore, evidence demonstrates that the quality of life experienced by an individual will inevitably be shaped by, but not be absolutely reliant upon, their level of disability and dependence. Studies of people with disabilities have shown that obtaining assistance with one aspect of life can enable a person to use their energies to undertake activities of their choice (Craddock 1996a, 1996b). Therefore the individual may exercise choice about when it is more productive for them to be dependent upon others, if that choice exists.

Deliver a holistic occupation-based model of rehabilitation

Occupational therapists working with vulnerable older people have largely concentrated upon helping a person to undertake necessary functional activities, thereby limiting their reliance upon others. Avoidance of dependency and, in some cases, consequent admission to hospital and long-term care make this a laudable use of resources. However, there are questions about the acceptability of an exclusive concentration upon this approach, given that this is only one aspect of the occupations a human being needs to engage in to experience satisfaction with their life. This is an important debate for the profession and for the wider health and social care community. The challenges of delivering truly holistic rehabilitation are discussed further in Chapter 11.

Keep abreast of new developments

Additionally, occupational therapists need to be mindful of new developments in rehabilitation research and practice, which are enabling the inclusion of groups not previously considered to be capable of using rehabilitation successfully. It is important to adopt an open mind regarding what might be achieved, taking into account the new avenues that technology, medication and alternative forms of provision are opening up.

Be responsive to rapidly changing needs

Finally, as the previous chapters have demonstrated, the needs of older people do not remain static but change over time. Therefore services and practitioners have to be both sensitive and responsive to these shifts. One way in which occupational therapists can meet changing needs is by grading occupations to match the abilities of the older person and their carer. The established approach is gradually to increase the complexity or demands of the activity as improvement occurs. This is redundant in many older people as abilities can rapidly fluctuate. Instead the occupational therapist has to employ a high level of skill to match the abilities of the older person at each encounter. This can necessitate making speedy changes to planned treatment strategies.

Pointers for practice

- Provide clear information in verbal and written formats for the person and their carer.

- Set aside time to develop a relationship with the older person and their carers.

- Assess the needs of the older person and their carers separately and identify individual interventions in response to assessed needs.

- Take into account the entire spectrum of the presenting needs rather than being confined to a medical or social paradigm.

- Devise the programme of interventions in partnership with the older person and their carers, ensuring that rehabilitation is underpinned by purposeful interventions.

- Incorporate the needs of the carer into the treatment plan by offering support and advice, teaching rehabilitative skills if appropriate and recommending respite care before a situation reaches crisis.

- Work with the entire care network of the older person, being alert to changes in the needs of the person and changes to their care network.

- Be prepared to accept that the person may want to take a measured amount of risk, balancing this with the views of carers.

- Be aware of the reasons for compliance and non-compliance.

- Be prepared to be flexible and respond to changing needs within the programme of interventions.

- Be prepared to engage with the person and their carers on a long-term basis if needs indicate that this would be beneficial and if resources allow. If not ensure that all necessary services are in place before withdrawing.

- Work closely with other members of the multi-disciplinary team.

- Measure the outcomes of interventions.

Chapter 8

Occupational-therapy-led strategies to help people to stay put

The contribution that occupational therapists can make in helping older people to sustain their quality of life and continue living in the community cannot be underestimated. Chapter 7 examined the nature of occupational therapy interventions with older people and their carers. This chapter will consider occupational therapy strategies to help people stay put in the community and retain their health and independence.

Policy context

Maintaining the health of older people has been neglected in the past, with services only responding when the person became ill and infirm. However, this has now changed, with this area of work commanding increased levels of interest from policy-makers and those charged with implementing policy.

The promotion of health commanded global attention before UK policy-makers specifically turned their attention towards this aspect. The Ottawa Charter for Health Promotion (WHO et al., 1986) was developed by representatives from 212 countries. The importance of occupation and its interplay with health is stressed within the Charter. It states that all health professionals must:

- build healthy public policy;
- create supportive environments;
- strengthen community action;
- develop personal skills;
- realign health services towards the pursuit of health.

A key government document, *The Health of the Nation* (DoH, 1992), was a watershed in the UK in that it was the first time that policy goals had been concerned with preventing rather than managing illness and disability. The goals articulated within a subsequent White Paper,

Our Healthier Nation (DoH, 1998c) (informed by the Ottowa Charter) were to increase the length of people's lives and the number of years spent free from illness, and to reduce health inequalities within society.

Prevention was specifically raised in the *Modernising Social Services* White Paper (DoH, 1998b). This referred to maintaining the independence of all older people, in addition to focusing on the needs of individuals on the margins of institutional care. Policy implementation encouraged local authorities to introduce such services. Grants were made available over a three-year period. The aim was to encourage local authorities to identify risk factors for older people and develop social care strategies to prevent or delay loss of independence.

Diminishing capacities mean that older people usually have to make lifestyle adjustments, as discussed in Chapter 2. However, there is no doubt it should still be possible to live a meaningful, enjoyable life in later years. The promotion of a healthy lifestyle, including good diet and physical exercise, necessary to achieve these goals has been translated into standards for services and for practice within the National Service Frameworks. The importance of a healthy lifestyle in preventing the consequences of major causes of morbidity and mortality in older people, namely stroke and falls, is described in the National Service Framework for Older People (DoH, 2001a). The National Service Framework for Older People Standard Eight requires:

> The promotion of health and active life in older age ... through a coordinated programme of action led by the NHS with support from councils. (NSF, Chapter 1)

By March 2004, health and social care providers were required to institute a programme to promote healthy ageing and prevent disease in older people.

Other community-based community initiatives include Health Improvement Programmes (HIMPs) introduced as a result of the Health Act (1999). These programmes require health and local authorities to work together to improve the health of the community. Working together to promote a healthy community is being reinforced through the development of Local Strategic Partnerships. These are consortia of key sectors and agencies within a locality, with the remit of fostering better communities, including regeneration of the environment.

Strategies to help people to stay put

Occupational therapy interventions concerned with prevention of accidents and disability, health promotion and retention of independence can be categorized into five main domains, shown in Table 8.1. These domains have been identified to try and make sense of what is a complex area and are therefore an over-simplification of the true picture. Each of the identified domains are not mutually exclusive; for example, the use of technology clearly overlaps with housing. Another example is the blurring that can occur between community equipment and technological applications, leading to increasing use of the umbrella term 'assistive technology'. The appropriateness of interventions are also highly dependent upon the characteristics of the individual older person at *any one time*. A fit and well older person may benefit from health promotion as well as preventive strategies. The continuing challenges of home maintenance may also signal the need for housing interventions. Sudden illness or increasing frailty will require a different repertoire of responses.

Each of these domains and its relevance to current and future occupational therapy provision is now explored in some depth.

Table 8.1 Occupational therapy interventions to help people to remain independent in the community

Domain	Aim	Implementation
Health promotion	• Promotion of health and well-being	1. Physical exercise 2. Nutrition 3. Lifestyle 4. Appropriate, well-maintained housing
Preventive strategies	• Prevention of ill health • Prevention of accidents	1. Social care interventions 2. Preventive home visits 3. Identification of environmental hazards 4. Screening for risk factors
Provision of community equipment	• Promotion of independence • Reduction of the effects of disability • Facilitation of hospital discharge • Limiting use of other forms of assistance	Provision of equipment: 1. Following hospital discharge 2. To combat the effects of limitations due to old age 3. To assist carers 4. To prevent accidents and encourage continuing independence
Housing improvement/ modification	• Giving people choice about staying put • Promotion of well-being • Prevention of accidents	1. Home maintenance 2. Preventive home modification 3. Housing adaptations

Table 8.1 (contd)

Domain	Aim	Implementation
Technology for care, independence and rehabilitation	• Giving people choice about staying put • Home safety and limitation of risk • Enabling control over the environment • Promotion of quality of life • Improving access to home-based rehabilitation	1. Surveillance 2. Environmental controls 3. Systems to alert help 4. Information and communication technologies (ICT) for quality of life 5. Engineering and ICT for rehabilitation

Health promotion

Wilcock (quoted within COT, 2001) set the ICF-2 (described in Chapter 3) in the context of the Ottawa Charter for Health Promotion. This offers a wider application of occupational therapy in the context of the health of populations and of individuals, and places occupation within the public health agenda.

Physical exercise

Metz (2000) observed that maintaining physical fitness is the most important thing a person can do to remain healthy. Using available research evidence, he drew attention to the benefit of a healthy lifestyle, for example diet and exercise and the added value of moderate exercise for older people in improving balance, reducing risk of falls and maintaining muscle size. A sample of the evidence that exists is provided below.

Venable et al. (2000) explored the relationships between the undertaking of regular physical exercise, volition as defined by the model of human occupation (Kielhofner, 1995) and the functional ability of a group of older people in good health. The specific questions posed were the following:

1. Is there any relationship between participation in exercise and abilities in activities of daily living?
2. Is there a relationship between exercise and perceived psychosocial functioning?

This study was small scale, involving 48 older people living in the com-munity who voluntarily participated in group exercise at a range of venues; therefore the results were inconclusive. The benefits of exercise were evident, but whether there was a causal relationship between exer-cise and independence levels was less clear. The authors point out that increased confidence can be the reason.

An evidence-based review to examine whether exercise can reduce falls and falls-related injury in older people was undertaken by Provence et al. (1995). Results of a meta-analysis concluded that falls can be reduced through exercise. The range of exercise techniques considered by the review included endurance, flexibility, balance, Tai Chi and resistance for between 10 and 36 weeks.

The value of exercise in the prevention of falls was endorsed by a sys-tematic review of the evidence on prevention of falls and subsequent injury in older people (Effective Health Care, 1996).

Research reported by Robertson et al. (2001) demonstrated the ben-efits of individually tailored home exercise programmes in reducing falls in older people. It was also shown to be cost effective.

Diet and nutrition

Occupational therapists have not generally been involved with diet and nutrition. However, given the deleterious consequences of poor oral health raised in Chapter 3 there are questions regarding whether this should remain the case. Assessment of abilities to prepare food and drinks, particularly where the abilities of the older person to cope fol-lowing hospital discharge are being questioned, is a long-established occupational therapy role. We need to reconsider this skill base and whether it can be transferred successfully in a cost-effective manner to populations of comparatively older people in good health, with the aim of maintaining health and well-being.

Lifestyle redesign

Jackson et al. (2001) described lifestyle redesign as:

> ... a process of occupational analysis whereby clients acquire knowledge about the characteristics of occupation and an understanding of the impact on their lives, and then apply these skills to develop a healthy routine of occupations. (Jackson et al., 2001, p. 11)

The study of elderly people in good health (Jackson et al., 1998) was concerned with the effectiveness of preventive occupational therapy for older people, interventions being based upon application of occupational science theory and research. This research is so important for occupational therapy that it is worth recounting it in some detail. It was undertaken in America between 1994 and 1997. The protocol for the occupational-based interventions delivered through the study were grounded in the results of a pilot study concerned with living a meaningful existence in older age, referred to in Chapter 2. This drew attention to the interpretations placed upon occupations by older people, how decisions are made about involvement in certain occupations and how older people (in common with us all) enjoy occasional excitement and a break from routine. The study was also based in the positive results of a meta-analysis of the effectiveness of occupational therapy for older people (Carlson et al., 1996) and the development of occupational self-analysis described by Clarke in Mandel et al. (1999).

The research involved a randomized controlled trial of preventive occupational therapy to community-living older people over a nine-month period, compared with social activity groups run by individuals with no training in the field and with a third control group who received no intervention. The intervention group received information in eight areas: an introduction to the power of occupation, ageing, health, transportation, safety, social relationships, cultural awareness and finances. Finally, participants were asked to undertake their own occupational analysis, through the creation of a book of information gained during the nine months and their own experiences of the programme. This enabled them to redesign their lifestyle to promote their own health. The information was delivered through a mix of presentations, discussion, exploration and experience. Study outcomes included physical health, mental health, occupational functioning and life satisfaction. Results of the study confirmed that the well elderly programme had a significant benefit upon preventive health care. In comparison those regularly engaged in social activity experienced no extra benefit to those in the control (Clark FA et al., 1997). Moreover, benefits were maintained six months later without further intervention (Clark et al., 2001). Even though the authors stressed the benefits to the profession of replicating this study, this has not been undertaken, and information about the numbers of occupational therapists adopting this approach is not available. Completion of the study led to the production of a manual to assist practitioners to implement the interventions (Mandel et al., 1999).

Preventive strategies

Prevention can be interpreted in many ways, for example provision of assistance in the home, maintaining the physical comfort and structure of the home and maintaining social networks to reduce loneliness. It is a concept that overlaps with health promotion, drawing together several of the topics already addressed throughout this book within other chapters. A systematic review of the literature on preventive strategies for older people (Godfrey, 1999) concluded that while there was robust evidence to support prevention in the context of health and disability, this was not so for social care preventive strategies. However, the commonality of a number of factors which lead to successful development of preventive strategies are realized, for example cross-agency collaboration and involving older people in setting priorities (Lewis et al., 1999).

Preventive home visits

Preventive home visits are often described in the context of the role of health visitors. However, they can readily come within the remit of occupational therapy. Involvement of occupational therapy may well increase with the shift of emphasis to health promotion and prevention supported by a primary-care-led health service. However, the existing evidence to support their undertaking is contradictory, as illustrated by the following examples of reviews of research in this area.

A systematic review of the effects of preventive home visits to older people living in the community (van Haastregt et al., 2000) included only robust evidence from 15 randomized controlled trials. The definition used of preventive home visits was visits to older people living independently, using a comprehensive geriatric assessment format. The stated goals of these visits were to reduce or treat observable problems or prevent new ones. The outcome measures used by the selected trials varied, for example improvement in physical function, improvement in mental well-being, number of falls, mortality and admission to hospital or nursing home. The conclusions drawn from this work were that there was no clear evidence to support preventive home visits and that more research is required to determine which aspects of the visit can lead to real benefit. However, a later meta-analysis of a review of home visits for health promotion and preventive care undertaken by Elkan et al. (2001) suggested that these visits were significantly related to reduction in mortality and admissions to long-term care. The authors acknowledged that their findings differed to those of van Haastregt et al. (2000), suggesting that this was attributable to the pooling of data through meta-analysis. The authors of both studies strongly supported the need for more research to examine which aspects of such visits can lead to benefit and to explicate the extent to which the person being visited was compliant with suggestions and interventions.

The message to be taken away from this robust population-based research is that participation in further exploratory research by occupational therapists is advised, while the devotion of limited resources in the absence of evaluation may not be.

Specific aspects of preventive home visits have been explored in other studies, namely:

1. identification of environmental hazards;
2. preventive visits as part of the primary care assessment of older people aged 75 years and over;
3. screening of those perceived to be at risk of falling.

These processes together with examples of the evidence to support them are described below.

1. Identification of environmental hazards

Clemson et al. (1992) recognized the lack of research into the preventive role of occupational therapists and the lack of standardized assessment measures to assess home hazards. Twenty-two home visits to people aged 65 years and over were conducted by seven occupational therapists and rated in situ by two occupational therapy raters. Analysis of results using the Kappa coefficient of reliability showed that the reliability of the ratings of some aspects by the occupational therapists were excellent, but for 19 items on the 59-item checklist a poorer inter-rater score demonstrated the need for further guidelines for assessment. Further research by Clemson and colleagues (1999) has led to the development of a valid and reliable assessment for occupational therapists to use to objectively identify hazards which may lead to falls in the home, the aim being prevention. The Westmead Home Safety Assessment is available in both long and short forms, accompanied by a manual.

As a component of their research, McLean and Lord (1996) developed a home environment risk checklist based upon existing safety checklists for homes in Australia with modifications by occupational therapists with experience of assessing home hazards. The checklist is replicated in Table 8.2 to demonstrate the impact of cultural difference.

It can be seen from Table 8.2 that one or two items in the checklist are less appropriate to the UK. Additionally certain items are omitted that might be deemed appropriate to observe in this country, for example frayed carpets and kitchen safety. The relevance of using a mix of observation, interview and culturally appropriate assessment instruments was raised in Chapter 6.

It must also be emphasized that, while many older people live in poorly designed homes with environmental barriers and hazards, the need to maintain control over the home setting combined with well-established routines means that advice regarding safety is not always adhered to.

Table 8.2 Home hazard checklist (Source: developed by McLean and Lord (1996))

Factor	Risk indicator
Access	No rails or support on two or more steps
Lighting (lounge)	Only table or standard lamps in use
Mats	Able to be moved with the foot With curled or frayed edges Made of towelling or with inadequate rubber backing
Power-point positions	Located close to the floor
Kitchen	Polished floors No resting position near the refrigerator
Bedside light	Absent
Shower/bath	No grab rails No non-skid mat
Laundry area	Inside with two or more steps without a rail to the outside

2. Assessment of people aged 75 years and over by primary care

As part of their contract, GPs are required to offer all older people on their lists aged 75 years and over a home visit and assessment, the aim being that of prevention and the identification of unmet need. Given that guidance does not contain any specific recommendations about how the assessments should be conducted it is not surprising that the responsibility has been devolved, in many cases to other members of the primary health care team. Through analysis of 480 such assessments, Nocon (1993) found that nurses were most likely to recognize the need for referral to occupational therapy. During another phase of research, interviews with 100 older people undertaken revealed that only 47 per cent had been offered an assessment, with 25 taking up the offer. Of those assessed, 17 needed community equipment of various types but none of this group had been referred to occupational therapy. The research indicated the requirement for GPs to be better informed about occupational therapy services, but also questioned the extent of resources required to manage unmet need. An aspect not raised by Nocon, but discussed elsewhere in this book, is the importance of accurate assessment to meet needs, particularly in the case of community equipment. More recently Bath et al. (2000) promoted the value of using standardized methods to measure health and functional status of older people during the over-75 assessment. Their research promoted the application of EASY-Care (SISA, 1997) by primary care staff, referenced in Chapter 6.

A number of studies have been conducted to examine the nature and extent of the needs of older people being managed by primary care. Awareness of community occupational therapy by people over the age of 65 years on the list of one GP was examined by Goldthorpe and Lloyd (1993). An 80 per cent response rate was achieved (out of a total of 410 surveyed). Analysis of the results found that over half of respondents were unaware of the services listed in the questionnaire. Those reportedly in need of services were people with arthritis, cardiovascular disease and mental health problems. One third of respondents had an unmet need that could be met by occupational therapy. Edwards and Jones (1998) obtained similar findings. A survey of a random sample of 1405 people aged 65 years and over living in the areas covered by three health authorities uncovered unmet needs for basic and relatively inexpensive equipment. They suggested that needs for equipment could form part of the over-75 assessment in primary care.

3. Screening to try and prevent falls

Continuing concerns about the high numbers of falls by older people is expressed by the extent of Department of Health funding which has been allocated for both research and therapy audit in this area (Simpson et al., 1998). One of the conclusions drawn from a systematic review of evidence of effective strategies for preventing falls and injury in older people (Effective Health Care, 1996) was as follows:

> Home visits and surveillance to assess and where appropriate modify environmental and personal risk factors can be effective in reducing falls. This can be carried out by nurses, health visitors, occupational therapists or trained volunteers. (Effective Health Care, 1996, p. 2)

A Cochrane review on interventions to reduce the incidence of falls in older people (Gillespie et al., 2000) concluded that service commissioners should consider the health care screening of all older people perceived to be at risk. This should be followed by interventions to reduce the risk posed by the older person themselves and the risk factors presented by their environment. However, this sets aside who decides upon the level of risk that would indicate the need for a visit, and the balance between the cost of the visits with benefit as described in the previously cited reviews by van Haastregt et al. (2000) and Elkan et al. (2001). Furthermore the evidence from other studies cited in this book (Ballinger and Payne, 2000; Thornton and Mountain, 1992) found that older people have to consider themselves to be at risk and in agreement with the practitioner regarding the approach to be taken. The review also suggested that the evidence to support other interventions such as exercise alone or health education programmes is inadequate.

Supporting independence with assistive technology

Community equipment can be instrumental in assisting people to live independent lives (Winchcombe, 1998; Audit Commission, 2000a, 2002a). The term includes devices that are relatively cheap and readily available, like tap turners and toilet seats, to more expensive items like environmental controls, stair lifts and hoists. More recently, the interpretation has widened to that of assistive technology. This has been defined as:

> Any item, piece of equipment, product or system, whether acquired commercially, off the shelf, modified or customized, that is used to increase, maintain or improve functional capabilities of individuals with cognitive, physical or communication difficulties. (Astrid: A Guide To Using Technology With Dementia Care, Marshall, 2000)

Therefore in addition to community equipment, assistive technology embraces housing adaptations such as grab rails and ramps. It also includes technological solutions to promote independence and facilitate safety. Occupational therapists remain the professional group who are instrumental in assessment for, and provision of, community equipment and housing adaptations.

A briefing prepared by NCCHTA (2000) determined two levels of provision of equipment and adaptations – that to try and ensure safe discharge, and that provided for preventive purposes or to promote independence. The paper also acknowledged knowledge gaps.

> It is not currently known whether facilitating early discharge through minimal equipment provision is enabling or disabling in the long term.

> The cost of minor adaptations and equipment is under £100. However, the output volume and relative cost implications of inappropriate or delayed provision is high. (NCCHTA, 2000, p. 1)

In a review of ICT applications, Curry (2001) identified a number of applications that can contribute towards the maintenance of independence and promotion of social inclusion such as falls alarms, motion sensors, emergency alarms, lifestyle monitoring, on-line assistance and video conferencing.

The ageing population, combined with the possibilities that technology presents, is leading to considerations of technological applications for older people. Metz (2000) acknowledged the benefits that can result from technological developments of assistive technology but also observed the high prices and under-developed designs. In 1998, an expert working group was convened to examine the challenges and opportunities the ageing population in Europe presents for technology (Etan, 1998). They suggested that the challenges were prevention, the introduction of new forms of domestic and health care and the application of appropriate technologies and technological adaptations. The National Strategy for Carers (DoH, 1999d) gives examples of technology that might give assistance to carers to continue caring. Most of the exemplars given are concerned with promoting safety of the cared for.

Assistive technology can perform a number of functions. These include the following:

- helping to prevent accidents: it is known that provision of equipment is key in preventing accidents and maintaining dignity and independence (Aminazadeh et al., 2000);
- enabling independence and quality of life: timely provision of assistive technologies can contribute towards decisions about house moves or entry into residential care.
- ameliorating the effects of illness and disability, particularly following a period of time in hospital.
- assisting to care, as detailed in the National Strategy for Carers (DoH, 1999d).
- facilitating involvement in work and leisure activity, and promoting social roles.

The delivery of appropriate assistive technology embraces the following aspects, each of which incorporates a number of processes:

1. supply;
2. provision;
3. utilization;
4. return, maintenance and recycling;
5. user involvement and feedback;
6. evidence of effectiveness.

The functions and organization of the different aspects that come under the rubric of assistive technology, namely community equipment, housing adaptations and modifications and technology to promote independence, are considered below.

Community equipment following hospital discharge

There is a long-standing evidence base to support the benefits of equipment provision following discharge, provided that education and follow-up regarding usage are adequate. There is also a requirement to take changing needs into account.

An early study by Thornely et al. (1977) looked at the use of equipment by 150 people six months to two years following discharge from one acute hospital. The reported utilization rates were 56 per cent for bath seats, 67 per cent for toilet aids and 73 per cent for grab rails. Reasons for non-use included poor instruction, poorly fitting equipment and lack of confidence. A study conducted in Sweden came to similar conclusions. Parker and Thorslund (1991) reported a study of the use of equipment by 57 people aged 74 years and over living in one rural community. At the time of study, all disabled people in Sweden were entitled to free access to equipment through a national, health-led, reportedly bureaucratic system, with no follow-up or recycling after issue. The study sample was drawn from the data collected for another study, with each volunteer being assessed at home by a therapist trained in research techniques. As well as assessing the functional abilities of the person, the therapist also evaluated the home and noted any adaptations made to facilitate independence. The 57 subjects had 422 items of equipment between them, with an average of seven items each. Twenty-nine per cent of issued equipment was for mobility, 20 per cent for personal hygiene, 20 per cent for communication and the remaining 11 per cent to meet a mix of other needs, for example cutlery, long-handled reachers and special scissors. In line with the distribution of equipment provided, the most common problems experienced were concerned with mobility and bathing. Seventy-five per cent of the equipment was being used. Reasons for non-use were primarily due to changes in functional abilities, demonstrating the importance of follow-up, review of the needs of the person and recycling of unused items. The study concluded that occupational therapists have an important role to play in identifying solutions to problems experienced by older people living at home. However, a greater level of involvement may necessitate advising other care providers to assess and provide equipment rather than occupational therapists being directly involved in all instances.

Neville-Jan et al. (1993) examined utilization of equipment by older people three months after hospital discharge. The study was initiated due to increasing demand upon the skills of occupational therapists, a 100 per cent increase in the demand for equipment, and observations by a community occupational therapist of the non-use of equipment and ill-fitting items. A survey questionnaire was sent to 80 people identified through hospital records as having been issued equipment for permanent use. Analysis was based upon 50 returns. Patient diagnosis was primarily stroke, arthritis and hip fracture. The non-utilization rate at the time of the survey was 36 per cent, with toilet frames and bath boards being the items of equipment most commonly not being used. (The authors observed that this might be an underestimate as non-responders may have also been non-users.) The study resulted in some local policy changes. These included limiting the issue of equipment while in hospital to that which assists with toileting, hygiene and eating. Post-discharge home visits were initiated to evaluate environmental, social and personal needs in the context of the person's daily living routines. Other equipment could be issued at this stage with at least two follow-up visits. The study also raised further questions about the adequacy of occupational therapy pre-registration training in this area.

Community equipment to combat the effects of limitations

There has been some research to examine the implications of equipment usage compared with other forms of assistance. Research by Agree (1999) found that people using a combination of personal care and equipment were three times more likely to report residual difficulty than those just using equipment. One reason could be that increasing limitations might make using equipment impossible without help. Use of equipment alone was associated with lower levels of self-reported residual disability than use of personal care alone. Agree deduced that:

> Environmental factors are certainly of great importance in the appropriate and effective use of community based long-term care by disabled individuals. Environmental barriers can impede the use of many forms of assistance. (Agree, 1999, p. 441)

Another population-based study of use of equipment as a strategy to reduce the effects of disability was conducted by Verbrugge et al. (1997). This paper raised the implications of accepting personal assistance, as opposed to using equipment. Equipment can enable a person to retain personal independence but the appearance of the item and the skill that is required to use it could be a disincentive. The conclusions drawn concurred with the study of Agree et al. (1999) in that equipment is the best strategy for reducing and resolving limitations resulting from disability.

> Equipment by itself is more efficacious than personal assistance (alone or combined with equipment). The results pertain to people with moderate to severe disabilities; they are likely to be true or more so for persons with mild disabilities. (Verbrugge et al., 1997, p. 391)

Community equipment to enable participation and social inclusion

Until recently, the potential of community equipment in assisting people to fulfil societal and social roles was set aside. However, there is now a growing awareness of the potential of community equipment in assisting with work and leisure as well as necessary functional tasks. Schweitzer et al. (1999) examined how assistive technology can contribute towards participation in leisure activities by older people at home. It involved supplying equipment to facilitate participation to 17 out of a randomly selected sample of 25 older adults. (The sample was drawn from a larger study.) Twenty devices in all were supplied and training provided in usage. Follow-up interviews were conducted with participants to explore their experiences. The study confirmed the value of providing equipment to enable participation in valued leisure occupations, and re-engagement with abandoned activities. However, a few factors were uncovered that could limit this value. These included resistance to any changes to the physical arrangement of the home or changes to routine, and a tendency to opt for 'low-tech' solutions. The study uncovered a need to customize existing devices or develop new ones in response to this need.

Providing community equipment

Providing simple items of equipment to older people in response to assessed needs involves a number of processes. According to Gitlin and Burgh (1994) these are:

1. selecting a device;
2. choosing an activity to practise using it;
3. timing of introduction of the device;
4. deciding where to instruct the person;
5. giving instruction;
6. reinforcing usage.

Selecting a device

Selection of an appropriate item can be limited by lack of information on what is available. Goldthorpe and Lloyd (1993) conducted a postal survey to 410 older people who formed the practice population of one GP. The respondents were asked about their awareness of community equipment and what their needs for equipment were. Of the 336 who responded, over 50 per cent were unaware of the services listed. These included descriptions of home adaptations, equipment to help mobility, washing and dressing, and eating and drinking, and to assist with food preparation. Over one-third stated that they had needs that might be met through this provision. There is no reason to doubt that these results still have validity.

Even if they are aware of services, many older people still find it difficult to access what they require. Some of these issues have already been raised in Chapters 5 and 6.

It has been suggested that delays in waiting for equipment causes the individual to suffer loss of dignity as their way of life is compromised (Easterbrook, 1999). This effect is increased if when the equipment is provided it is of poor design, unattractive or shows signs of wear and tear. One of the participants in the King's Fund seminars on services for older people provided an alternative view:

> I want a stylish old age – give me a Conran-designed zimmer frame.
> (Easterbrook, 1999, p. 8)

It is beyond the scope of this book to discuss evaluations of specific items of equipment for disability. However, the implications of specific evaluations are relevant within the context of service delivery and organization. On behalf of the Department of Health, the Medical Devices Agency funds three Disability Equipment Centres to undertake the Disability Equipment Evaluation Programme. The programme is concerned with undertaking research-based, comparative evaluations of equipment designed to assist people with disabilities and older people, the aim being to enable individuals and organizations to make informed choices about the purchase of equipment. The rigour of these evaluations is indisputable. What is unknown is the extent to which they are taken into account by those involved in purchasing and prescribing equipment. The Agency is now rewriting its evaluations for consumers with assistance from the consumer organization RICA (Royal Institute for Consumer Affairs), as user awareness of the equipment they need and are being offered will increase. The Foundation for Assistive Technology (FASTUK) is devoted to providing information and research about community equipment and assistive technology. One of the responsibilities of FASTUK is to review the research in this area for the Department of Health.

Instruction

The importance of giving timely, accurate instruction in the use of equipment is indisputable, evidenced through the findings of a body of research over a 25-year period. The majority of research into the usage and effectiveness of equipment has been in relation to the needs of people with arthritis, an area of high volume and demand.

Schemm and Gitlin (1998) examined how occupational therapists teach people how to use equipment to assist independence with bathing and dressing. The study involved 86 hospitalized people aged 55 years and over, receiving rehabilitation for orthopaedic conditions, CVA or lower-limb amputation, and 19 occupational therapists. Each person received an average of two to three pieces of equipment for bathing and dressing and were satisfied with the training they received in their usage. Average training received was two and a half sessions (10 minutes per session) to teach the use of equipment for dressing and one session (9 minutes) to teach use of bathing equipment. Occupational therapists perceived that those people who evaluated the equipment positively had better knowledge of its use.

Another study, undertaken in Canada, looked at the effectiveness of disability equipment prescribed for people while in-patients in a situation where hospital-based occupational therapists were not able to follow patients into the community (Finlayson and Havixbeck, 1992). This study looked at user satisfaction with the education they received on how to use the equipment, equipment usage following discharge and user opinion on the quality of the product. All those who received equipment during a four-month time-frame were asked to participate in the study. Questionnaires and interview schedules were applied to 29 people who had been issued a total of 83 pieces of equipment. While the use of these non-standardized measures compromised the study, results do concur with the previously cited, more rigorous evaluations. Each person received an average of nine minutes' instruction on four occasions, with an average of 31 minutes education in all. Seventy-five per cent of the allocated equipment was being used on follow-up. It was concluded that while service users' perceptions were that education in equipment usage was adequate, usage could be improved by home visits before discharge, and spending time obtaining the history and perceptions of the user.

A small audit of the importance of providing adequate information about equipment at the time of installation, in this case raised toilet seats (Packham, 1999), reiterated the findings from research. The audit found that users had received inadequate information at the time of installation, with the result that safety was being compromised in four out of seven cases. The results of these studies emphasize the significance of education upon the outcomes of equipment provision.

Outcomes of equipment provision

Wielandt and Strong (2000) reported the results of a review of the literature on user compliance with prescribed equipment. The findings of 31 studies were synthesized to identify the following five factors which impact upon compliance:

- *Medical related*: Diagnosis can influence compliance, for example whether the person has a deteriorating condition and whether there are other concurrent medical problems.
- *Client related*: Influencing factors, such as age, housing, individual preferences and coping mechanisms.
- *Equipment related*: The relationship between inappropriate equipment and non-usage. This could include safety and working conditions, equipment which does not fulfil the task, and appearance.
- *Assessment related*: The value of home visits for assessment, and involvement of the person and their family in assessment for equipment.
- *Training related*: The extent of instruction the user receives.

The paper concluded with the observation that there is need for comprehensive evaluation to identify the factors which increase the active engagement of users in assessment for and prescribing of equipment.

McCreadie et al. (2002) involved older people in evaluating assistive technologies. Four focus groups were held with 37 older people identified from a range of constituencies but all with some level of disability. Scenarios of functional activities were used to get participants to identify the situations that caused them the most difficulty. The problems most frequently identified were climbing stairs, getting in and out of cars, bending and reaching, getting out of bed and getting in and out of baths/showers. They also raised problems in accessing information about devices to help. All were able to suggest solutions to their difficulties. The second phase of the study involved the incorporation of suggestions from the focus groups into two design solutions, one being a stair-climbing aid and the other a cataloguing system based upon descriptions of functional problems, giving the equipment that might then meet needs. Prototypes were presented to the focus groups for testing and feedback. The authors concluded that older people are very capable of being active evaluators of assistive technology.

Organization of community equipment services

Research evidence has strongly affirmed that many difficulties stem from the manner in which equipment services are organized, managed and delivered. How provision of equipment is strategically organized can have major implications for access and outcomes. Delays in provision can lead to compromises, reduction in quality of life and dissatisfaction with the service.

The organizational context within which equipment is provided is usually complex. In the UK, equipment is supplied by statutory services to those assessed as being in need, with the private sector supplying the statutory sector. There are a number and variety of options available within this framework, fostered by the commercial enterprise that underpins the supply (Mandelstam, 1997). At the user level, the extent of financial and equipment options can prove confusing. Provision of equipment to those people assessed as being eligible as a result of their needs can be undertaken by both health and social care agencies. The nature of the equipment once dictated which agency provided. This divide was known to be problematic and led to disputes between agencies where the needs of individuals extend across health and social care (Winchcombe, 1998). However, the requirement to integrate community equipment services, mandated through the National Plan (DoH, 2000a), should in the future ensure that people do not have to wait for a service owing to organizational constraints. Service development should draw upon the evidence base regarding different aspects of equipment provision, for example the use of attractive, appropriate items, and the need for a system of recycling.

Housing adaptations

Housing adaptations are structural alterations to the home environment. According to Mandelstam (1993) this includes minor alterations like grab rails and removable ramps as well as major adaptations like house extensions, shower units and fixed ramps. Recent research to look at the effectiveness of housing adaptations in seven local authorities (Heywood, 2001) confirmed the benefits of this form of intervention for the person themselves, their carers and other family members. Minor adaptations were reportedly beneficial for nearly all those who responded. They prevented accidents and concerns over the likelihood of accidents, and helped to maintain independence. The author concluded that these represented real value for money. Major adaptations had the capacity to profoundly change people's lives for the better. Benefit was most likely to be experienced where users and their carers had been fully involved and the home respected. Problems occurred most often where the original specification was faulty. The report strongly recommended that increased spending on housing adaptations would be a worthwhile use of public funding

Smith and Widiatmoko (1998) reviewed six Australian studies and estimates based on expert opinion to try and determine the cost effectiveness of preventive home modification in reducing falls in people aged 75 years and over. An occupational therapist and a specialist provided expert opinion on falls in older people. The outcome measures they identified included the rate of falls, the number and type of injury after a fall and the subsequent treatment. The results of the study indicated the benefits to be gained from such interventions but further research is recommended.

Home improvement

It is now widely recognized that helping older people to maintain their homes and gardens not only helps to allay the fears of losing control of their environment, but also helps to reduce hazards and minimize risk-taking behaviour. Older people can also be fearful of having to move from homes they have lived in for many years, and therefore welcome interventions that can enable them to stay put. The National Strategy for Carers (DoH, 1999d) promoted the need for carers to have good information about housing options, tenancy rights, and repairs and adaptations to their home.

One of the objections raised in discussion groups with older people during a study of quality of life in retirement was the segregation of older people in society that can result.

> I'm 81. I mean, as I say, there's one 90, there's one 94 in the place where we are. But to me, I don't like to be with old people ...

Demands for assessment for housing adaptations by occupational therapists in the context of community care have led to the escalation of waiting lists, with people categorized as being a lower priority for services, sometimes having to wait for long periods. An example given by the Department of Environment (1997) is the need for minor works to property as a component of care packages which can be delayed, with one solution being a partnership scheme with a housing association. They recommended that:

> Housing and community care strategies should consider how elderly and disabled people can be helped to carry out essential repairs and adaptations (e.g. through home improvement agencies working alongside occupational therapists). (DoH/DoE, 1997, p. 10)

Klein et al. (1999) described a home adaptations and repair agency in the USA where the agency contracts with occupational therapy consultants to identify the most appropriate changes to the older person's home to enable them to continue to live independently. The remit of this service included the provision of minor repairs, the installation of minor adaptations like grab rails, and major modifications like shower rooms and stairlifts. The occupational therapy assessment involved the person, the family, their home environment and how these factors are related. Information is ascertained by getting the person to discuss their daily routine and the challenges it presents, followed up by observations of how common activities around the home are managed. Specifically, the home evaluation described by Klein et al. required details on household composition and medical information, functional deficits resulting from medical problems and information about the structure of the house. The authors emphasized the need for collaboration between the therapist, the person and their family throughout the assessment, and consideration of solutions to meet identified need. Following this, the therapist has to work in partnership with those who will undertake the work. The programme described by Klein et al. (1999) included follow-up visits by the occupational therapist to ensure that modifications were being used appropriately and safely.

Care and Repair England is a charity established in 1986 to improve the housing and living conditions of older and disabled people. The aim of the organization is to support initiatives that help people to live independently in their own homes. This is being achieved through the promotion of home improvement agencies (HIAs) to help people to repair and maintain their properties. The work of the HIAs is complicated and often requires collaboration with a wide range of professional groups including occupational therapists, architects, surveyors, environmental health officers, social workers and benefits-agency staff. They are most often provided through social landlords such as housing associations. Recognition of the potentially wider role of HIAs in helping people to stay put led to research to examine the possibilities. In 1997, Care and Repair England conducted a mapping exercise to examine how HIAs were moving into other areas of service delivery (Care and Repair England, 2001). There was a 62 per cent response rate to the survey, with 78 per cent of those responding offering more than one extra service. The most common additional services offered were handyman services, fitting of small adaptations like grab rails and hand rails, installation of home security systems and provision of advice on security, and helping people to improve the energy efficiency of their home. Other service provision included gardening and decorating services, providing community alarms and rapid response for essential repairs following hospital discharge. Seventy-three per cent of responding agencies had attracted funding to provide additional services.

The initial mapping exercise was followed by a more detailed exploration of this diversification through questionnaires to 13 HIAs. This confirmed that HIAs are well placed to respond to the housing and social care needs of older and disabled people. Three experimental projects in different UK locations were asked to comment on the actions that their clients might have taken if they had not been available. Analysis of responses revealed three categories of response: admission to residential/nursing home, having to pay for the work or increased need for support from other services. Most recently, Care and Repair England commissioned a survey to look at the ways in which housing-related initiatives are working to improve people's health (Easterbrook, 2002). This study found projects concerned with falls prevention and home safety, home maintenance, provision of information and training in home safety and energy efficiency of the home, and facilitation of hospital discharge. The 'Should I stay or should I go?' initiatives to support the development of housing options services for older people are currently being monitored by Care and Repair England, to evaluate their impact (Hambly and Adams, 2003).

Technology to promote independence

In 1998, an expert working group was convened to examine the challenges and opportunities the ageing population in Europe presents for technology (Etan, 1998). They identified the potential of technology in providing care and support to individuals in their own homes, the challenges being prevention, the introduction of new forms of domestic and health care and the application of appropriate technologies and technological adaptations. The National Strategy for Carers (DoH, 1999d) gave examples of technology that might assist carers to continue caring. Most of the exemplars given are concerned with promoting safety of the cared for, providing a slightly different slant on the use of technology to promote and maintain independence. Additionally, Internet shopping and telephone befriending schemes are raised. The range of areas for technological development include the workplace, housing, transport, communication and mobility (Etan, 1998). This rapidly developing agenda contains many challenges for occupational therapists. These include involvement in the development of systems that meet user and carer needs, evaluation of the application of technology from the perspectives of user and carer and a reconsideration of rehabilitative interventions in light of the contribution of technology.

A range of systems for monitoring a person in their own home is already available. Woolham and Frisby (2002) identified three categories of technology that can be placed in an existing property:

1. stand-alone technologies that do not link into other systems;
2. technologies based on community alarms, and which can include smoke and gas detectors;
3. SMART systems that filter information from a range of sensors linked to a computer system installed in the user's home.

Examples of these applications are provided below.

Systems to alert help

The tenet underpinning community care policy – that
enabled to live independently wherever feasible and

growth in the development of community alarm systems for older people (Thornton and Mountain, 1992). Providers of these services include local authorities, housing and the private sector. Systems have become increasingly sophisticated over the years, as technology has developed, but essentially they are reliant upon the telephone network. The communication equipment in the house is a small trigger designed to be worn by the individual. These used to be heavy pendants worn around the neck, but small, discrete items are now available. When the button on the device is pressed, it sends a radio signal to a telecommunication unit in the house (this will also have an alarm button). The unit may have a built-in telephone or sit alongside a separate telephone. The unit is then connected to a call receiver through the telephone network. Operators at a central control point communicate with the caller to assess the urgency of the call and whether or not a visit is required. The call receiver is also linked to a computerized database, which holds information about the caller, and their call record. If a visit is required, the operator has to call a respondent. Some services employ wardens for this purpose whereas others rely upon volunteers, often relatives or neighbours. In some locations the service is provided free to those who meet stated eligibility criteria. In others users pay a portion of (or all) the costs.

This technology is particularly valuable for those older people who have fallen or are at risk of falling. The role of occupational therapists in the identification of those who could benefit is evident. Following on from this, potential users can benefit from professional help to acquire the best available service to meet their needs, and information about it. Given the commercial nature of the community alarms market, this is particularly important. There are also benefits to be gained from occupational therapy involvement when a call has been made, for example to identify environmental hazards (in the research undertaken in 1992 by Thornton and Mountain, falls accounted for 26 per cent of all alarm calls in the two case study services).

In 1992 Thornton and Mountain noted that:

> The assumption that older people ought to be permanently protected against risk pervades the design, marketing and provision of community alarm provision. There is little evidence of alarm systems being used to allow older people coping alone at home greater control over their lives. (Thornton and Mountain, 1992, p. 39)

More recently, one of the major commercial companies, Tunstall Telecom, have developed falls monitors, providing an alert to respondents when the wearer falls.

Environmental controls

These systems enable a person to have control over their environment through the application of technology. Analysis of the success of environmental control systems (ECS) with frail older people has been conducted by occupational therapists in Canada, working in partnership with industry and a university (Vincent et al., 1999). Five case studies were undertaken to examine the success of ECS in increasing independence of the person and reducing the burden upon their carer. The computerized system was able to perform domestic activities activated by remote control, give verbal reminders and ensure domestic control. Five people were identified to receive the ECS in their own homes. Their impairments included arthritis, Parkinson's disease, poor eyesight and mild dementia. Three were over 75 years old. Research included a questionnaire regarding the technical performance of the equipment, and assessment of caregiver burden. Results found that while the systems reduced the dependency of the individuals, caregiver burden remained high. The stress upon carers was reduced when the system worked, but increased when it failed. It also did not reduce the burden associated with activities such as dressing, shopping, transport and budgeting.

Systems to improve quality of life

The Foresight Panel (2000) suggested that ICT could be harnessed to improve the quality of life of older people, particularly in light of the leisure opportunities it can present. Examples provided are accessible information for planning journeys and en-route journey planning, design of products, and systems to accommodate minor impairments. A conference convened by the AgeNet research network in 1998 was devoted to examining the benefits and potential of the Internet for older people. One of the papers of particular relevance to occupational therapists considered ergonomic issues relating to use of the Internet. Current research is looking at a whole range of new applications, and adaptations to existing technology. Examples include the wider potential of mobile phones to meet the needs of older people and how to facilitate transport use by older people, for example by providing advance warning of the progress and arrival of public transport.

Systems to support independence

Mynatt and Rogers (2001/2002) suggested that determining how technology can assist older people should be placed within the context of why older people have to move from their own homes to alternative living arrangements. One of the prime reasons is an inability to undertake activities of daily living. A number of possible solutions were identified by Mynatt and Rogers including systems to help people get in and out of the bath, monitoring the vital signs of the bather and improving medication adherence through prompts.

The University of Stirling, in collaboration with a number of European partners, has been developing and examining the potential of assistive technology with people with dementia. The project has led to the development of a guide to using technology in dementia care (Marshall, 2000). The Northampton project described by Woolham and Frisby (2002) had a different aim in that it explored whether technology could be used to reduce the stress experienced by carers of older people with dementia, and delay admission to residential care. The devices used were linked to community alarms, so that the alarm is activated when the older person is at risk. Table 8.3 shows the framework embedding the user of this technology, as identified by Woolham and Frisby (2002).

Table 8.3 The infrastructure system required to promote the use of technology for people with dementia (Source: Woolham and Frisby (2002))

1. Identify person with dementia	
2. Assess the needs of the person with dementia	• Describe living circumstances • Analyse the needs of the person • Identify the problems that need to be solved • Identify potential technology and alternatives and suppliers • Consider ethical issues
3. Prepare the care plan and arrange services	• Recommend technology • Complete an ethical protocol • Choose solutions and decide • Approve funding • Order equipment
4. Implement the care plan; operationalize services	• Install equipment and test • Arrange social response to alarm • User acceptance
5. Review	• Reassess person with dementia • Monitor equipment • Maintain equipment Or • Remove equipment

Readers are referred to the work of Woolham and Frisby for a clear breakdown of responsibilities within each of the processes shown in Table 8.3.

Smart homes

Smart homes represent the application of technology to housing, and as such represent a mix of environmental controls and systems for surveillance. Demonstration homes have been developed in different countries. In the Netherlands they have developed a 'Very Smart House for Older People', where control systems monitor every aspect of the house and could also monitor the medical condition of the inhabitant (Etan, 1998). In the UK, a number of agencies have been active in examining the value of smart-home technology, including the University of Stirling. The Joseph Rowntree Foundation collaborated with academics and housing providers to build two demonstration homes in York and Edinburgh in 1998–99. The success of the homes reportedly lies in the greater independence of those with sensory impairment, reduced mobility or memory loss, through the application of technology. Two examples of the features of these homes provide a flavour of how such systems can be harnessed. A door entry system can give visual alerts (for example, lights flashing on and off) and displaying a picture of the caller on the TV. The user can subsequently talk to the visitor through the TV control. The home security system will confirm whether doors and windows are locked. Infra-red sensors can monitor for intruders and provide a visual as well as audible alarm. It can also be linked to warden-call systems. Research and development is ongoing to identify further technological applications.

Use of technology for care, support and rehabilitation

These approaches are still in their relative infancy in this country, but are certain to impact upon the working lives of occupational therapists in the near future. They are raised in this chapter, as current applications overlap with the prevention agenda. However, there is little doubt that technology will soon become an integral feature of occupational therapy.

Occupational therapists working in Northern Ireland have already been involved in a technologically driven project concerned with delivery of home care (South and East Belfast Trust, undated). The use of technology to support carers' needs for information, education and support was reported by Hanson and Clarke (2000). This European project aimed to maintain the independence and quality of life of frail older people and their carers. The system involved use of the television with additional technology, a video telephone and a small camera. This enabled carers and their cared for to access support from district nurses, GPs and a welfare rights officer, as well as obtain information through the television. Despite an approach being made to 12 family carers, only three agreed to participate. Response to the equipment was explored through a case study approach. The researchers attributed the low response to invitations to participate in the project to the length of time most had been caring. Some carers felt that they did not have adequate time to devote to the project, particularly where their caring situation demanded a lot of time. Also, it was postulated that carers at an earlier stage of their caring career might have greater need for the system. The technology itself was a further factor that could have added a low response rate. Older people are willing to use technology as long as they consider it to be useful to them. Another observation worth noting is that the system raised expectations of services that could not always be met. The conclusions were that technology has potential when applied in specific circumstances in close collaboration with providers of health and social care, emphasizing the need for a service infrastructure as described by Woolham and Frisby (2002).

Implications for occupational therapy

The agenda covered in this chapter describes a range of exciting new opportunities for occupational therapists. It is evident that the profession has much to offer in the areas of health promotion and prevention. We can be instrumental in the development of local strategies to help older people retain their health and independence. We can also be at the forefront of testing new technologies, helping older people and their carers to be involved in this testing, and in the integration of technology into services and homes. However, to achieve this, we need to keep abreast of new developments and how they might be exploited, and ensure that our skill base is sufficiently developed to meet these demands.

Use opportunities to introduce new services

Implementation of health and social care policy described in Chapter 5 has led to the introduction of primary care trusts and is also fostering the integration of health and social care services. The contents of this and previous chapters have indicated where proven, unmet needs for occupational therapy exist, particularly in primary and community care settings. Health promotion and prevention are areas of work where other professions already provide a service, particularly in primary care settings. We must therefore ensure that our involvement complements rather than duplicates existing work. Wider service reorganization presents a prime opportunity both to reconsider the best use of scarce occupational therapy resources in light of this unmet need and to consider the introduction of new, responsive services.

Ensure the effectiveness of new areas of work

The evidence base cited in this chapter indicates the lack of consensus concerning some areas of involvement, for example the efficacy of preventive home visits. While the evidence base in these areas is underdeveloped, this does signal a need for caution in service developments. Given resource implications, and the extent of unmet need that exists in the community, involvement in any new area of work must be preceded by a consideration of the evidence in light of a local-needs analysis. The challenge is how to respond appropriately to ever-inflating demands, balancing the benefits of introducing preventive strategies with the increased costs that these will accrue.

Balance the demands of equipment provision with other areas of work

The provision of community equipment, described within this and previous chapters, is an important aspect of the work of occupational therapists, but it has also historically limited the ability of some practitioners (particularly those employed by social services) to use their skill base to maximum effect. Current policy interest in what has been a neglected area of service delivery is leading to a revisited focus upon the type of equipment that is acceptable to service users, and the effective organization and delivery of services. On the one hand, we must not lose sight of the fact that this equipment can be instrumental in helping some older people to remain at home. On the other we must ensure that this involvement does not detract from other aspects of work. Consequently, there is an urgent need to think of new ways whereby assessments for equipment and its allocation can be undertaken in a timely manner, possibly by delegating more routine tasks to support staff. Furthermore, provision of equipment should be woven into total packages of occupational therapy interventions rather than being a separate aspect.

Involve the older person and their family fully in provision of assistive technology

The previously described relationships between functional ability and environment described in Chapter 3 impact upon ability to be able to use assistive technology. To be beneficial, assistive technology has to be useable within the person's environment. This means that it has to fit into the available space and into the routines of the person and their family. Additionally, the extent to which the device is perceived to be required by the individual themselves will influence usage. This requires full involvement of the older person and their carers.

Work to improve the quality of community equipment provision

With the needs of users in mind, we must rise to the challenge of improving the quality of community equipment and how it is provided. Users require adequate information about what is available. The benefits of inclusive design have not yet impacted significantly upon the assistive technology market in the UK. However, the importance of well-designed items should be promoted and incorporated into purchasing decisions. The market must be encouraged to produce items that are well designed and reasonably priced. This is a prime opportunity for occupational therapists to campaign for and demand on behalf of older users, the services that they would find acceptable for themselves.

Develop the expertise necessary to deliver complex packages of interventions

Ideally, occupational therapists working with older people should be able to respond to needs in the areas of health promotion and prevention agenda, as well as providing specific rehabilitative interventions, as described in the previous chapter. Delivery of this mix of interventions is demanding, requiring a high level of expertise on the part of the individual occupational therapists. It also requires knowledge and networks that extend beyond statutory health and social care provision to services provided by education and by the voluntary sector.

Keep abreast of new technological developments

Technology is developing at a rapid rate. The introduction of technology will create new organizational and knowledge demands upon workers. Occupational therapists must work with other key agencies and individuals to ensure that the necessary infrastructure is in place (including skilled staff) to be able to use innovations successfully. To achieve this, it is important to remain well informed of new developments and their potential applications.

Help older people to accept technology

Future generations of older people will be familiar with technology. Information and communication technologies are increasingly being used by older people. However, a number still need persuading of their value. This perception is not helped by commonly held perceptions of older people as being outside the mainstream user base of technology. If technological solutions are to be adopted, occupational therapists and others working with older people must help them to become familiar with equipment, and address their concerns and questions. Research is required to determine the best systems to meet needs. The involvement of older people and their carers in the development of these applications should improve their appropriateness and therefore the extent of take-up.

Pointers for practice

- Exploit all opportunities to promote a healthy, balanced lifestyle in all older people.

- Use the opportunities presented by reorganization to introduce new, forward-thinking services.

- Develop knowledge of, and links with, agencies involved in health promotion and prevention work.

- Undertake preventive interventions if the scope of your role will allow this, for example as part of the 75+ assessment by primary care.

- Identify aspects of your current workload that might be successfully undertaken by less-qualified individuals and seek ways in which these aspects might be successfully delegated.

- View assessment for, and provision of, community equipment as part of a package of rehabilitative interventions, rather than the sole outcome.

- Measure the outcomes of assistive technology from both service and user perspectives.

- Get involved in training initiatives for less-qualified staff so that you might be released to concentrate on more complex areas of work.

- Explore the potential of technology to improve the lives of older people and their carers, ideally in partnership with users, carers, engineers and computer consultants, so that acceptability as well as technical application can be properly considered.

CHAPTER 9

Occupational therapy interventions within specific service settings

Chapters 7 and 8 considered the occupational therapy interventions that can help older people to maintain and regain their health and independence. However, occupational therapists do not work in isolation. They work within organizational frameworks and settings and with other workers. Chapter 5 described the historical and current context within which services for older people operate. This chapter will examine the occupational therapy contribution within the service context.

Research has demonstrated that the setting where an occupational therapist delivers interventions can be critical in determining the nature of the interventions undertaken and their demonstrable success (Mountain, 1998a). Figure 7.1 illustrated the range of factors that contribute towards the nature of occupational therapy interventions. They included the physical treatment environment, the resources available and the perceptions of other members of the multi-disciplinary team – all factors that come within the rubric of treatment environment.

The treatment environment directly influences the clinical or 'professional' confidence of the individual occupational therapist, with this shaping the clinical decisions taken (the importance of professional confidence is examined in more depth in Chapter 11). The clinical decisions taken by the individual therapist will have a direct impact upon the activities suggested by the occupational therapist and the resultant nature of the service experienced by service users and carers. These relationships are illustrated in Figure 9.1, with the powerful influence of the treatment environment being evident.

Working with older people is an area of high demand and high volume. Given the ever-increasing demands for the services of occupational therapists, it is crucial that occupational therapists are employed to work where they can be most effective. When thinking about resource allocation, it is necessary to consider the following:

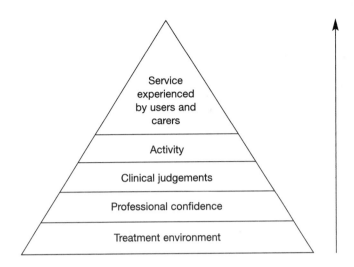

Figure 9.1 Relationship between treatment environment and service quality.

1. The services where occupational therapy has a clear, provenly effective contribution, as opposed to those where occupational therapy might not be so beneficial.
2. The nature of the treatment setting itself. A whole variety of factors make some environments sympathetic to the delivery of occupational therapy, while others present barriers.
3. The expectations of occupational therapy within specific service settings and where changes are required to maximize value.
4. How older people and their carers access occupational therapy services, including the factors that facilitate or alternatively block access.
5. The contribution of occupational therapy within the whole system of services for older people.
6. The changes in occupational therapy practice that are required to meet the demands of new services for older people.

This chapter examines all of these issues in the context of both new and established forms of service, and services for specific groups of users.

The range of inputs provided by occupational therapy is extensive. Figure 9.2 illustrates where occupational therapists may currently work with older people and their carers. Within each of the domains identified in Figure 9.2, occupational therapists adopt a range of roles and make a variety of contributions. The following sections of this chapter review the roles and contributions of occupational therapists for specific user groups and within defined and generic service settings, with reference to the evidence base that underpins them.

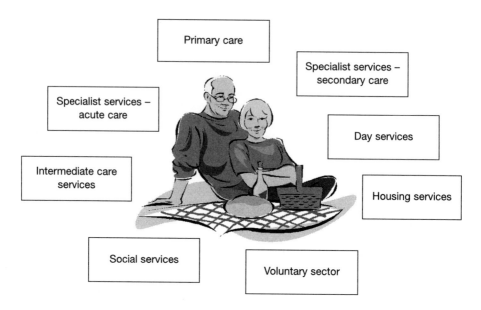

Figure 9.2 The occupational therapy contribution within the system of services for older people and their carers.

Rehabilitation services for specific user groups

Specialist rehabilitation services have developed within both acute and secondary care to meet the needs of defined user groups. While these services need not be confined to older people, the majority of people they will serve will be over the age of 50 years. This is an area of practice where more investment has been made to examine the benefits of rehabilitation. These services are provenly successful within the context of the following:

- multi-disciplinary involvement (including occupational therapy);
- the existence of many aspects to assess and treat;
- where rehabilitation occurs in several stages.

However, which aspects of treatment lead to specific benefits remains an area for further research. There is clear evidence to support the effectiveness of rehabilitation when it is part of an overall package of care, for example in stroke care, cardiac rehabilitation and comprehensive geriatric assessment (Sinclair and Dickinson, 1998). This can largely be attributed to the research investment made by charitable funders. Given that this effort has not been replicated for other conditions, there are unanswered questions regarding the transferability of this evidence base. The following section will describe these rehabilitation services and the specific occupational therapy contribution.

Services for people with stroke

Evidence demonstrates that many people who have sustained stroke can derive benefits from active rehabilitation and advice at all stages of the care pathway (Forster and Young, 2002). Additionally, robust evidence has demonstrated the benefits of well-organized rehabilitation (Stroke Unit Trialists Collaboration, 2002).

Guidelines have recommended that rehabilitation should commence as soon as possible after the stroke (Intercollegiate Working Party, 1999) and that rehabilitation should continue until maximum recovery has been achieved (DoH, 2001a). The evidence to support the development of specialist multi-disciplinary stroke services both within acute hospital care and within community settings is robust. Survival and recovery are more likely if people are admitted to a specialist stroke unit within a general hospital, served by an expert multi-disciplinary team. A stroke care co-ordinator is often identified within specialist provision. Their role is to coordinate assessment and adequate discharge arrangements including the transfer of information to community services, and ensure that community equipment and adaptations are in place (DoH, 2001a).

However, significant differences in the availability of specialist stroke services, and in institutionalization following stroke, exist across the country (Rudd et al., 2001). In some locations, provision is reportedly basic, with rehabilitation being targeted solely at discharge from hospital and with little monitoring following return home (Tyson and Turner, 2000). Interviews with people who have experienced stroke confirmed a lack of satisfaction with rehabilitation services and a desire (or unmet need) for more directed rehabilitation in the critical period, immediately post-discharge (Pound and Gompertez, 1999). This may change with the mandatory introduction of stroke units across the country (DoH, 2001a).

There is a reasonably substantial and growing body of evidence to support the benefits of occupational therapy with people with stroke. Gilbertson et al. (2000) showed that providing domiciliary occupational therapy to a group of people discharged from hospital with a diagnosis of stroke improves functional outcome in the short term, but it was unclear whether these benefits would be sustained over time. Each person identified for the enhanced service received a programme of occupational therapy, tailored to his or her specific needs. Treatment sessions therefore involved interventions to improve participation in self-care, domestic or leisure occupations, and liaison with other agencies to provide advice, services and equipment. The study concluded that rehabilitation should extend beyond discharge from hospital into the community.

The majority of the existing evidence base regarding occupational therapy has concentrated upon abilities to undertake functional activities, with the goal of increasing capacity to participate in occupations concerned with maintenance of independence. To examine the effectiveness of interventions to promote leisure occupations after stroke, Parker et al. (2001) conducted a randomized controlled trial in five sites across the UK. Surprisingly, and in contrast with the results of a previous, smaller-scale study (Drummond and Walker, 1995), there was no significant difference found in the group randomized to receive additional leisure interventions compared with those who received only interventions to improve abilities in activities of daily living. The authors recommended that, in the absence of an evidence base, therapists should not always assume their interventions are effective. Taking into account the paradigm for involvement in occupations described in Chapter 2, it could be postulated that undertaking essential tasks to maintain independence took priority for the participants over other non-essential, but more desired occupations.

Another randomized controlled trial of community occupational therapy, aimed at improving functional abilities (Walker et al., 1999), demonstrated that occupational therapy provided for up to five months at home for people not admitted to hospital following stroke significantly reduced disability and handicap.

Services for people with hip fracture

The value of a multi-disciplinary community-based approach towards the management of older people with hip fracture, incorporating early discharge, was first raised over ten years ago (Kreibich et al., 1991). This search for new styles of service was a response to the increased incidence of these injuries in older people, together with a realization that the postoperative treatment provided orthopaedic wards was not meeting the needs of this group of patients.

Well-coordinated services in hospital, combining the expertise of orthopaedics and medicine for older people, therapy services and social services, can improve outcomes (Royal College of Physicians, 1989). Stewart and McMillan (1998) provided an overview of the various services that have developed to rehabilitate older people with hip fractures. Rehabilitation is now an acknowledged crucial component of such schemes. The early hospital discharge scheme for post-operative management of people with hip fractures, followed by rehabilitation at home, is now perceived to be an optimum package of services. However, as

Stewart and McMillan pointed out in 1998, these services were only available to the minority.

Clinical guidelines produced by the Scottish Intercollegiate Guidelines (SIGN; web address in Appendix 3) have used robust evidence to guide clinical practice. The following statements are supported by strong evidence:

- Early assessment of occupational therapy needs in collaboration with other members of the multi-disciplinary team.
- Early rehabilitation to promote independent mobility and function, with an emphasis upon walking and activities of daily living.

Kirkland and Mitchell (1995) described an occupational therapy service within a fractured hip management team located in one Australian hospital, using a case study as illustration. The authors suggested that this service differed from mainstream occupational therapy provision in orthopaedics in that it involved a blanket referral to occupational therapy services, early access to information (often when the person was still in casualty), followed by details of post-surgical outcomes. Determination of abilities and lifestyle prior to the fracture was a key aspect of the information-gathering process. Information about lifestyle and living conditions, together with condition following surgery, enabled early implementation of an individualized occupational therapy treatment programme during admission. This might include a visit home to ensure that necessary equipment is in place. Contact with physiotherapy and occupational therapy was maintained for a period of time following discharge, during which time rehabilitation would be continued as indicated and equipment removed if the person regained their pre-fracture abilities.

Services for people with Parkinson's disease

Occupational therapy interventions with people with Parkinson's disease are not usually initiated until the later stages of the disease, though the integration of health and social care and development of intermediate care facilities may result in individuals accessing rehabilitation earlier. Most people with Parkinson's disease will access community rehabilitation services only until their medical condition requires admission to in-patient care. Even then, specialist services are not always available, with the majority of admissions being to general medical wards. Interventions can include support to reorganize daily routines, introduction of adaptive strategies and advice regarding the provision of specialist equipment. Deane et al. (2001) published a Cochrane review of the existing quality evidence to support the efficacy of occupational therapy for people with Parkinson's disease. The review initially identified eight studies, embracing a range of treatment strategies. These included physical exercise, social and leisure occupations, interventions with the aim of improving mobility and gait, functional activities, education sessions and relaxation sessions. Due to methodological limitations, only two of the eight studies met the criteria for inclusion in the review. Results showed that the existing evidence is not currently robust enough to support occupational therapy for people with Parkinson's disease. However, this is most likely to be due to lack of research investment rather than the ineffectiveness of interventions. The reviewers highlighted the need for standardized practice, which might in the first instance be based upon a survey of expert occupational therapists working in this area. Both charitable funders and the Department of Health have recently acknowledged the need for research investment in this area.

Services for people who fall

Swift (2001) summarized the wide-scale significance of fall prevention and treatment for services:

> Treatment and prevention of falls in older people spans primary and secondary prevention, diagnostic ascertainment and assessment, acute medical and surgical care, functional assessment and rehabilitation, continuity and organization of follow up, and for some patients, long-term supportive or institutional care. (Swift, 2001, p. 856)

Specialist services for older people who have fallen or who are at risk of falls are being developed in line with the standards set in the National Service Framework for Older People (DoH, 2001a). Risk factors can extend to unsafe housing, previous fracture and fear of falling. These services should cross health and social service provision and be available to all those older people at risk with their agreement. The remit of the service is to undertake a specialist assessment by a falls service in collaboration with health and social care.

A range of professionals including occupational therapists are involved in falls services. Interventions based upon this assessment should be agreed with the older person and their carers. One of the consequences of the assessment might be referral to intermediate care services, described in a further section of this chapter. Another option raised in the National Service Framework is for the person to go home with the occupational therapist for a risk assessment of their home. It is evident that the timeliness of this assessment and subsequent interventions is a key factor.

Guidelines for managing falls by physiotherapists and occupational therapists (Simpson et al., 1998) included the following:

- interventions to improve the older person's ability to withstand threats to their balance, including balance training, muscle strengthening and provision of aids and adaptations in a preventive capacity;
- the identification of environmental hazards and either removing them (with consent) or teaching the person about the risks and how to avoid them;
- discussions with the older person to identify how they have managed any previous falls, and agreement on strategies for managing any future incidents;
- determining the extent of fear of falling, and intervene to increase confidence and balance.

Most recently the National Service Framework for Older People (DoH, 2001a) stated that most people will need rehabilitation following a fall whether or not they are admitted to hospital, citing the guidelines for physiotherapists and occupational therapists.

Ballinger and Payne (2000) reported a qualitative study of accounts of falling in older people. Semi-structured interviews were conducted with 20 occupational and physiotherapists working in hospital settings and eight older people who had been admitted to hospital following falls and subsequent fractured hips. Interviews with the therapists revealed that they generally believed that falls were both predictable and preventable, and attributable to the characteristics of the individual person and/or their environment. In contrast the older people interviewed implied that the falls were either due to bad fortune or the fault of others, emphasizing their capabilities at the time, thus detracting from their vulnerability. Ballinger and Payne (2000) recommended that therapists need to be sensitive to the people they are treating and their beliefs if a therapeutic partnership is to be formed. This means adopting a less prescriptive approach, taking into account the implications for the older person if they agree with the therapist's interpretation of events and reasons for them.

Services for people with cardiac problems

A review of effective practice in rehabilitation (Sinclair and Dickinson, 1998) noted the benefits of active cardiac rehabilitation. Interventions span health promotion, preventive strategies and lifestyle change (discussed in the previous chapter) to provision of active rehabilitation strategies following illness. However, much of the existing emphasis is upon services for men of working age. The rehabilitation needs of women and of older people tend to have been set aside. A study to look at what motivates older people to remain physically active after a myocardial infarction (MI) indicated that providing training to improve physical activity or having experience of physical activity prior to illness were both more likely to have an impact upon subsequent lifestyle (Stanhle et al., 2000). However, the small numbers in the groups studied does indicate a need for further study to validate this finding. A qualitative study explored risk factors for cardiovascular disease in a group of people who had experienced a first MI (Murray et al., 2000). Those interviewed were between 31 and 74 years old. Findings indicated a need to provide people with an opportunity to discuss their understanding of cardiovascular risk as part of the rehabilitation programme. This needs to take into account the perceptions of users and carers.

Services for people with mental health problems

As was mentioned in Chapter 5, a system of service provision should be accessible within each locality.

The following range of services has been identified for older people with mental health problems, and their carers (Williamson et al., 1995, p. 36):

- domiciliary assessment and care where appropriate;
- support for carers;
- day care;
- respite care;
- multi-disciplinary outreach;
- acute in-patient assessment and care;
- rehabilitation;
- longer term in patient care;
- liaison/consultation;
- education and research.

In contrast with services to meet needs following physical illness, services for older people with mental health problems have received less attention, both from policy-makers and from service commissioners. There is less specificity regarding the services and interventions that should be provided and patchy evidence to support service development. A substantial number of services provide a social function and aim to provide respite for carers (discussed in Chapter 4) rather than rehabilitation.

The National Service Framework for Older People (DoH, 2001a) suggested that a comprehensive mental health system for older people should include the promotion of good mental health, early detection and diagnosis, an integrated approach to assessment, care planning and treatment, carer support and a specialist mental health service. Occupational therapy involvement could occur within any of these service elements.

An advisory group established by the Social Services Inspectorate (Barnes D, 1997) included an occupational therapist. They were charged with looking at the needs of older people with mental health problems living alone. They came to a number of conclusions, the following being of particular relevance to occupational therapy:

- The need for specialist skills, in particular those concerned with assessment, acceptance of appropriate risk and provision of protection.
- The requirement for development of training initiatives, ideally across agencies.
- The complexities of assessment of this group, which demands time and sensitivity if it is to be conducted properly.
- Access to advocates to help people get the services which best meet their needs.

The Audit Commission (2002b) recommended the provision of specialist multi-disciplinary teams for older people with mental health problems. Teams should act as the focus for the single assessment process, described in Chapter 6. The report stated that occupational therapists should be core members of these teams. Unqualified members of teams need to be trained in mental health and supported by their qualified counterparts.

Many mainstream rehabilitation services for older people exclude those with mental health problems. The development of intermediate care services provides recent evidence of this. However, the value of providing tailored rehabilitation services to older people with mental health problems is leading to a reconsideration of what might be achieved. In particular, the rehabilitative potential of people with dementia is being explored. It could be argued that many of the interventions undertaken by occupational therapists and others in this area are rehabilitative in nature, even though they were not previously interpreted as such owing to prevailing views of the treatability of dementia. Huusko et al. (2000) evaluated the impact of intensive geriatric rehabilitation for people with dementia who had sustained a hip fracture. The study was a sub-analysis of a larger four-year study of the effectiveness of rehabilitation for older people with hip fracture. All 238 participants were fully mobile prior to injury. Patients were randomized to receive intensive geriatric rehabilitation or standard care. Those in the rehabilitation group received specialist multi-disciplinary rehabilitation. This included specific rehabilitative interventions, advice, training, and provision and use of equipment to assist with daily living. In contrast with popular opinion, results found that people with hip fracture and mild or moderate dementia can often return to the community. Three months post-operatively, rate of return home for those with mild dementia were as successful as for people without a diagnosis of dementia.

Memory clinics are a specialist service for people with dementia that is gaining popularity. The increase in the number of memory clinics in the

UK has been stimulated by the licensing of a number of drugs that claim to slow down the progress of the disease (Lindesay et al., 2002). There are also benefits to be gained from providing an early diagnosis (Luce et al., 2001). Most memory clinics have developed within the remit of existing NHS service provision, with some clinics embracing the expertise of occupational therapists. Their main function is to provide an accurate diagnosis and provide the older person and their carer with advice and information. The majority of services also initiate and monitor treatment. Other identified functions undertaken by some services include education and training, screening for drug trials and other research, and undertaking medicolegal assessments.

Other services for older people

Aside from identified rehabilitation services for specific user groups, there are a number of other services where occupational therapists work with older people, and where rehabilitation can be of benefit.

Accident and emergency

Ensuring that hospital admissions are necessary and in the best interest of the older person is leading to a number of initiatives. The siting of occupational therapists within accident and emergency departments is gaining popularity. A specialist section of the College of Occupational Therapists now exists to promote this aspect of the work of occupational therapists. There is a small but growing body of research to support the investment.

Lee et al. (2001) described the introduction of a rehabilitation assessment service within an accident and emergency department in Canada. Development of the service was underpinned by a literature review. This identified recommendations about the use of functional assessments and the value of a multi-disciplinary approach towards the care of older people. The service used a systematic approach to targeting and assessing older people at risk. Three assessment tools were identified for examining physical performance, self-reports of functional ability and gait. Additionally information was collected about insight into problems, living situation (including environmental barriers), extent of informal care available, use of equipment and history of falls. A study was subsequently conducted to examine the appropriateness of providing this service in A&E and the extent to which it guided decision-making. Eighty older people who had been assessed in this way were asked to complete a checklist-style diary for six weeks following their visit to A&E and participate in a follow-up telephone interview. The difficulties inherent in asking vulnerable older people to participate in this way led to only six people completing all aspects of data collection. However, evaluation of the initial data on the 80 older people found that no single factor determined the reason for the visit, and the consequent resource requirements. A combination of factors have to be taken into account including level of functioning prior to illness, availability of support, physical ability and living situation. The authors also observed that introduction of the service had promoted collaborative team working in the department.

A report of the introduction of a similar service in the UK suggests that wider benefits might also be derived, as this quotation from a patient demonstrates:

> I learned from the occupational therapist how to pace my illness. I was trying to do too much; shopping in the morning, visiting my wife in nursing home in the afternoon. Together we worked out how I could do what I wanted without being overcome by tiredness and my chest problem. It really helped. (Quoted in James, 2002, p. 25)

Carlill et al. (2000) audited the outcomes of a pilot occupational therapy and social work service established to serve an accident and emergency department. The service was for all age groups, but the majority of referrals received were for older people. Reasons for referral to the service included concerns about mobility, function and ability to cope once home. People referred to the service were observed undertaking functional activities by the occupational therapist. Results might indicate referral back to the A&E team for admission to a setting other than acute care or discharge home. If the recommendation was to return home, equipment could be supplied to facilitate this. The person might also be visited on return home. The audit indicated the value of the service and the need for this to be provided seven days a week for extended hours. It also underscored the value of equipment loans in enabling discharge.

Close et al. (1999) examined strategies to prevent falls by older people. People aged 65 years and over presenting at the accident and emergency department of one hospital following a fall (during a specified seven-month period) were randomized into a control or intervention group. The 184 people assigned to the intervention group had a detailed medical and occupational therapy assessment. The 213 people in the control group received standard care. Individuals in the intervention group had a detailed medical assessment in the day hospital. This was used to identify the primary reason for the fall, and refer on to other services if indicated. The medical assessment was followed by one home visit by an occupational therapist. The occupational therapist conducted assessments of function using the Barthel Index and functional Independence Measure. Environmental hazards were assessed using a checklist developed by the

Health and Safety Executive. The emotional consequences of the fall were examined using the falls handicap inventory (Rai et al., 1995). Following assessment, education and advice on safety was offered, and modifications to the home carried out if indicated. The research occupational therapist also provided small items of equipment if required, with referral being made to social services occupational therapy services for larger items. Older people who had received the service were followed up by postal questionnaires every four months for a year after the fall. Results showed that that the number of subsequent falls by people in the intervention group was significantly reduced, as were the numbers of recurrent falls by individuals. Results were concurrent with previous studies in that many older people had multiple risk factors which could result in falls; but the primary cause was frequently an environmental hazard. The authors also point out that older people attending A&E departments are a high-risk group who are both accessible and receptive to intervention.

> We conclude from our findings that there is now a strong case to incorp-
> orate falls and injury prevention strategies of proven efficacy into routine
> clinical service. (Close et al., 1999, p. 96)

Day provision

Traditional patterns of resource allocation mean that occupational thera-
pists often work within day care settings. Mountain (1998a) found that the clinical activity of occupational therapists in day hospitals was influ-
enced by the many inherent problems and historical methods of service delivery that had been established over the years, compounded by the practice of placing relatively junior staff in such settings. One example was compliance with nursing staff in the delivery of a programme of social/recreational activity. This detracted from focusing upon specific needs of individuals. Another observation from the same study was the requirement, on the part of service users, to be sociable and to participate in group activities. As one reluctant day hospital attender described it:

> They'll all be having groups and noise.

However, one older person resident in hospital at the time of interview would have willingly accepted day hospital admission as an alternative:

> If I could get home every night things would be all right. I don't want to be
> a burden on my wife but I don't want to leave her – we've been married
> over 50 years.

Sainty (1990) explored the most effective way of identifying those older people attending a day hospital who might benefit from individual occupational therapy. Experimentation with different methods of identification indicated that direct referral to the occupational therapist by other disciplines led to some people being missed who might potentially benefit. Also it was noted that the reasons given for referral tended to be of a general nature. Sainty concluded that interviewing all new day hospital attendees as well as accepting referrals was the most effective and workable system.

Most recently, there have been moves to improve the focus of day provision, for example through the development of day hospitals that offer true alternatives to in-patient admission, integrated day hospital/day care services, and day hospital as a form of intermediate care service. A randomized controlled trial reported by Burch and Borland (2001) compared rehabilitation outcomes at a day hospital for older people with a day centre. Attendees were assessed on their health and functioning to provide a baseline, and then again six weeks, three months and one year later, through application of a number of valid and reliable measures. In total 105 people were included in the study. The day hospital patients were found to be significantly more impaired in their functional ability than the day centre clients at baseline. However, three months later this gap had closed. The authors deduced that both models of day provision had the capacity to offer successful rehabilitation. However, meetings with the staff involved in the trial revealed problems with offering active rehabilitation in day centre settings. Interviews exposed difficulties over discharge from day centre, lack of rehabilitation facilities in day centres and cultural difficulties with the relationship between social care staff and visiting health workers.

Occupational therapy managers are urged to look carefully at the nature of the day setting, its clarity of purpose and the specific contribution occupational therapists can make.

> ... the problems of creating a climate of change in an existing institutional setting (which day hospital represents) cannot be underestimated. (Mountain, 1997, p. 4)

The need to determine the evidence to support the continued provision of rehabilitation through day hospital services is demonstrated through the current investment being made by the department of health in a major randomized controlled trial, due to report in 2006 (Parker, 2002).

Social services

> Services such as home helps, respite care and occupational therapy are often crucial in enabling older people to remain in their own homes. (Royal Commission on Long Term Care, 1999, p. 9)

Due to the policy underpinnings discussed in Chapter 5, the main role of social services occupational therapists has been that of assessment for and provision of community equipment and assessment for housing adaptations. These services are not a rehabilitative service in themselves and have therefore been raised in Chapter 6, and also in the previous chapter on preventive strategies. However, they are an important component of the rehabilitative process and can be a key aspect of community care for many older people.

Regrettably, the imperatives to assess for (and deliver) equipment and housing adaptations have resulted in the full capacity of social-service-employed occupational therapists not being fully exploited. A study by McCloughry and Murphy (quoted in DoH, 1999e) found that the involvement of occupational therapy in home care reviews could lead to a reduction in the demands upon the service if other enabling strategies like community equipment were introduced as well. The study also found that occupational therapy involvement alongside social work in 21 referrals for long-term care led to 12 people remaining at home with occupational therapy intervention.

A randomized controlled trial by Logan et al. (1997) examined the benefits of enhanced occupational therapy provided through social services. This involved 111 people referred to one of three social service departments within one city following discharge from hospital after stroke. The group was randomized to receive either standard or enhanced social services occupational therapy. At three months those receiving the enhanced package were more independent in mobility, household tasks and leisure than the control group. However, the benefits experienced by the group diminished over time to that of reduced mobility only. Those receiving the enhanced service also had more items of equipment. It was concluded that a dedicated service improved the timeliness and efficiency of the service and were highly beneficial in the short term, but more evidence was required regarding longer-term benefits.

Residential and nursing care

Despite a policy emphasis upon services to help people stay put in their own homes if they choose to (DoH, 1990; Royal Commission on Long Term Care, 1999), for a small minority of older people, this is no longer possible due to the extent of their illness and/or disability.

The 2000 Health Survey for England (DoH, 2001g) confirmed that 65 per cent of people in residential or nursing homes have a serious locomotor disability and 54 per cent experience problems with personal care. A study of the rehabilitation networks of older people after fractured neck of femur (Herbert et al., 2000) found that admission to residential and nursing home was most often determined by personal and social factors. The capacity of the individual to be able to benefit from rehabilitation was not usually taken into consideration. Therefore there are questions regarding the extent to which incapacity increases following admission and the benefits of providing rehabilitation in these settings.

One of the factors equating with quality by residents of nursing homes in the study by Raynes (1999) was provision to enable participation in occupations. It has been estimated that 40 per cent of older people in nursing and residential care are depressed (Mann et al., 1984). Several reasons can be postulated for this, including the relinquishing of long-standing occupational routines, the loss of one's home and the occupational deprivation that can exist in such settings. Green and Acheson Cooper (2000) examined the factors that lead to maintenance of occupational performance by nursing-home residents. Qualitative interviews with the matrons of 20 homes within one postal district were conducted to investigate how they addressed the occupational needs of residents. The authors acknowledged the limitations of the study in that it was restricted to staff; residents were not involved. Analysis of the data found that, in common with other studies of care environments, the attitude of the matron was key in setting the philosophy of care. They concluded that the ad hoc involvement of an occupational therapist would not be sufficient to support the level of activity on a day-to-day basis, but could be valuable in supporting the matron and facilitating the necessary organizational changes.

A small study by Green (1995) examined the outcomes of introducing a programme of occupations into a nursing home. Observed and reported benefits on the part of staff, residents and their relatives included enjoyment, animation and relief of boredom. Green noted the willingness by some staff to become involved in the delivery of the activity programme, indicating a potential training role for occupational therapists.

This awareness of the importance of providing rehabilitation and occupation in nursing homes is gathering pace. This is demonstrated through the references and practice examples provided in an information pack produced by the King's Fund (2001). Most recently, the PPP Foundation have funded a study being undertaken to examine whether individualized occupational therapy provision in nursing homes has an impact upon the incidence of depression. The results of this research are expected in 2004.

Intermediate care

Occupational therapists have to be able to respond to needs for rehabilitation of vulnerable older people at risk of readmission to hospital or admission to long-term care. In their review of the American literature on rehabilitation of older orthopaedic patients, Flanagan et al. (1995) noted that several factors are predictive of return home. These included the ability to mobilize, communication skills, lucidity, continence and extent of dependency prior to admission. They commented that:

> It is imperative that such patients continue to receive physical and occupational therapy after discharge, either at an outpatient facility or at home. Many elderly patients who are frail ... would benefit from a relatively low intensity but lengthy in-patient rehabilitation program. Such a program may best be provided in a nursing home setting or as part of a sub-acute rehabilitation program. (Flanagan et al., 1995, p. 91)

This observation translates into the concept of intermediate care, a concept that has recently been embraced by policy-makers and translated into a range of service provision. The rapid introduction of intermediate care, together with the umbrella nature of the term, has led to some difficulties:

> The term intermediate is often used in a confusing way and is applied at different times to different service settings or roles. (Audit Commission, 2000b)

It is significant that the notion of convalescence, a key element in earlier constructs, appears to have been set aside in the policy interpretation.

The term is currently being applied to a variety of services, for example rapid-response, supported discharge and outreach from hospital, and hospital at home. These are described in full in Table 9.1.

Table 9.1 Summary of intermediate care service types, evidence and staffing (Source: adapted from NHS Executive South West Regional Office et al., 2001)

Service	Description
Rapid response	• Prevention of avoidable admissions through rapid assessment by specialized teams • Referrals from GPs, A&E, NHS Direct, Social Services • 24-hour access to short-term support
Hospital at home	• Treatment at home for a condition which would otherwise involve an acute admission • Used to avoid admission or facilitate early discharge
Residential/ hospital-based rehabilitation	• Short-term programme of intensive rehabilitation • Community hospital/residential setting • For patients who are medically stable but require rehabilitation to facilitate independence • Can be step-down (post-acute) or step-up (admission avoidance)

Table 9.1 (contd)

Service	Description
Domiciliary assessment and rehabilitation	• Specialist multi-disciplinary teams that assess need at home or post-acute discharge, and organize packages of care to meet rehabilitation needs
Supported discharge	• Short-term package of care • Enables post-acute recovery at home at an earlier stage • Sometimes provided by a community rehabilitation team
Day rehabilitation	• Short-term programme of intensive therapeutic support • Up to six weeks • Provided in local authority, private residential home, day centre or day hospital • May also provide rapid response service

Additionally, a number of organizations including the voluntary sector and independent sector are providing services. Help the Aged are currently involved in a range of intermediate care services and have funded an evaluation of their effectiveness.

It should be noted that an 'experimental approach' has been adopted towards the introduction of intermediate care services, with a sharing of good practice in the absence of an existing robust evidence base. Therefore the majority of guidance has been developed out of examination of the components of various services rather than from research and evaluation. Through an examination of services that existed at the time, Vaughan and Lathlean (1999) identified a number of key factors that can be indicative of the success of intermediate care. These are:

• leadership and support, and clinical champions;
• financial commitment;
• audit of local need;
• dedicated project management;
• time for schemes to mature;
• communication between different health professionals – team spirit;
• trust placed in staff.

It can be seen from Table 9.1 that a number of the traditional services provided for older people have been translated into intermediate care provision with the accompanying policy requirements for no more than a six-week period of rehabilitation. It has already been noted that older people with mental health problems are largely being excluded. There is an indisputable need for further, more robust evidence, particularly given the conversion of many existing services. For example, a controlled trial of hospital-at-home services (one of the services that can be intermediate care) indicated that they are an acceptable alternative to hospital admission but not significantly better in terms of quality of life experienced by the patient, their physical functioning or how acceptable they find the service to be (Richards et al., 1998).

The central involvement of occupational therapists in the delivery of intermediate care service has substantial workforce implications for the profession. In 1997, a review of the literature to support the introduction of intermediate care services recommended the following, if good outcomes are to result:

- well-founded multi-disciplinary team assessment and treatment;
- the enhancement of the role of certain staff to allow them to fufil specific roles;
- the need to centralize the user and carer at all stages of the process.

While the wide-scale introduction of services in the absence of evidence to support them is questionable, it can also provide opportunities to explore new methods of working. Intermediate care represents a number of important challenges for occupational therapy practitioners and managers, and for other health and social care professionals. It also poses a number of cautions. These are summarized in the following table.

Table 9.2 The challenges and cautions posed by intermediate care services

Challenges	Cautions
Effective, multi-disciplinary team working	Inadequate or discriminatory referral systems
Identified team leadership	Isolated services that fail to relate to others
Development of a common philosophy of treatment and care	Emphasis on physical function rather than what the older person needs and
Good working relationships with other provision within the total system of care including acute and primary care	wishes to do and their social care needs
	Neglect of the on-going training needs of qualified and unqualified staff
Regular team meetings	
	Lack of career progression
Flexible approach to work, including 'out of hours'	
	Failure to measure patient and service outcomes

Table 9.2 (contd)

Challenges

The training, guidance and continuing
development needs of support workers

Documentation and dissemination of
information about the service and the
approaches being taken to add to the
pool of knowledge

Adoption of specific roles by occupational therapists within services

Over time a number of identified roles within different service settings
have emerged.

Discharge coordination

Given the acknowledged problems of successful discharge of older people from hospital, services have been put in place to facilitate hospital
discharge and assist the person during the post-discharge period. Closs et
al. (1995) evaluated a supported early discharge scheme for older people
admitted to an orthopaedic unit, with a dedicated occupational therapist
coordinating arrangements. In this scheme, the occupational therapist
took the patient on a pre-discharge visit and subsequently discussed discharge arrangements and the services that ought to be in place. Following
discharge, the occupational therapist then followed the person up by telephone at regular intervals at 1, 4, 16 and 52 weeks to assess progress and
service take-up, with visits being undertaken by a liaison nurse if the person was considered to be at risk. An examination of the experiences of
older people, their carers, GPs and other community staff indicated that
the service met patients' goals for return home in addition to meeting the
needs of the service for speedy discharge.

Studies have demonstrated the benefits of discharge planning in terms
of reduced readmission rates, length of admission and increased satisfaction (Closs et al., 1995; O'Caithan, 1994; Shiell et al., 1993). However,
these evaluations of individual schemes tend to be reliant upon the commitment of individuals. A robust review of outcomes over a number of
studies meeting pre-determined criteria was inconclusive (Parkes and
Shepperd, 2001).

Care management

Assessment and care management were the cornerstones of the 1990 community care reforms in the UK. As stated in Chapter 5, care management involves determining the level of assessment required, assessing need, planning care, implementing the care plan, monitoring, reviewing and reassessing needs over time (DoH et al., 1991). In some social services departments, the care manager role will be taken by an occupational therapist. This role for occupational therapists is being promoted in situations where they are the most involved professional (College of Occupational Therapists, 1999) and is supported by the existing evidence base (Mountain, 2000).

McGloughry and Murphy (1998) conducted a pilot study, which clearly demonstrated that occupational therapy involvement in care management can lead to improved outcomes for older people and for services. An occupational therapist was placed in an assessment and care management team, the intention being to examine if this would divert older people from residential and nursing homes and reduce the need for home care. Results showed that occupational therapy was able to help a third of older people referred for assessment for long-term care to stay at home. Most frequent interventions were provision of minor adaptations and small items of equipment.

The concept of care management has developed over time to underpin specific services. Several examples of integrated service provision for frail older people are underpinned by the care management process. It can enable needs identified through assessment to be provided through a care package containing a mix of health and social care interventions, met by a range of providers. Despite the demands they make upon care providers, the indications are that these services are more beneficial than those involving single care providers (Challis et al., 1991, 1996). Care management services for frail older people are being extended to provide alternatives to institutional care (Challis et al., 2001).

Key working

The role of the key worker is to act as the prime point of communication regarding the treatment and care of people with complex needs. It was specifically promoted through the concept of the care programme approach (DoH, 1997a). Since the introduction of care programming, the need for good communication between different agencies and individuals has been emphasized by the policy-led promotion of care pathways that extend across health and social care. It is evident that occupational therapists are equipped to undertake the role of key worker successfully, particularly given that the profession extends across the health/social care divide. Payne et al. (2000) reported a review of the literature on transfer of patient information across health and social care (including hospital discharge). They were able to conclude that the identification of a key worker was the most effective strategy for transferring information, particularly through providing a point of contact for workers from the hospital and community. The challenges of the role were also emphasized, particularly the need to bridge the divide between health and social care. The National Service Framework (DoH, 2001a) promotes the importance of key working or care coordination, underscoring its value for people with mental health problems.

Changes to established occupational therapy input

The previous sections of this chapter have examined the occupational therapy contribution for specific user groups and within defined service settings, and the changes that are taking place, for example the development of integrated services and the promotion of a user focus. Alongside these changes, significant shifts are taking place *within* occupational therapy services for older people, creating new opportunities and challenges. The final section of this chapter looks at the nature and possible impact of some of these changes.

Integration of occupational therapy services

The long-standing employment of the same professional group by both health and social services, and the consequent overlaps and gaps across hospital and community, make occupational therapy services themselves prime targets for integration (Mountain, 2001a). The benefits of integration of occupational therapy services are indisputable, with the previous divides between the profession (particularly at the time of discharge from hospital) resulting in duplication of effort, or alternatively people failing to receive the services they need (Clarke et al., 1996). Thus occupational therapy is becoming a litmus test for other forms of service integration (Mountain, 2002).

A comparatively early project explored options for integrating occupational therapy services in one health district (Herbert and Mort, 1996). While confined to the integration of the work of one discipline across health and social care, the suggestions arising from this work offer a paradigm for wider application. The project identified three possible levels of integration: conservative, evolutionary and radical. The conservative level described work towards integration at a provider level for example

agreed standards across health and social care, retention of existing commissioning arrangements taking into account agreed standards, and
development of formal links across health and social care management
systems. This form of integration is most often described in the practice
literature. The evolutionary model put forward by Herbert and Mort
(1996) suggested the appointment of a project manager to manage the
change process. The remit of this post would be to promote the integration agenda through management of the process from an organizational
perspective. A further aspect would be to ensure that practitioners receive
the necessary training for successful implementation. Locating documented examples of this form of integration is problematic. However, it
is known that, following the recommendations of Herbert and Mort, this
approach was implemented within the health district under review, leading to integration of occupational therapy services for older people and
people with disabilities. The final, radical approach they put forward was
grounded in joint commissioning across health and social care, with the
creation of a single point of access to services. An example of this radical
form of integration can be found in Northern Ireland, where health and
social care services are already integrated. Another project to examine the
feasibility of integration of occupational therapy services, in one district of
Scotland, came to similar conclusions to Herbert and Mort, identifying
four options ranging from better joint working on key aspects to wider
integration within the health and social care framework (Cointet, 2000).

A whole-systems approach towards occupational therapy

Chapter 5 looked at the pathways taken by older people through service
systems. The nature of the whole-service system and the different elements it embraces will dictate the referral routes taken by older people
into occupational therapy, how information is passed on from referrer to
occupational therapists and the quality of that information. Additionally,
the quality and success of referral will be dependent upon the knowledge
of the referrer. Mountain (1998a) found that older people referred to
occupational therapy from acute or secondary care services were given a
variable amount of information by the referrer. Methods of referral of
older people with mental health problems to occupational therapy did at
times reveal scant regard for the views of the person concerned and their
carers. This study also highlighted the timeliness of referral. Referrals
stemming from other services like day hospital or in-patient care, as
opposed to referral from community sources, had different implications
for the individuals concerned.

The reconfiguration of health services in the UK towards a primary-
care focus and integration of health and social care offers new

opportunities for occupational therapists to improve referral patterns and shape input into services. One of the clear benefits of health and social care integration for people is that the same group of occupational therapy staff can be involved in the transfer of care from hospital to community (Mountain, 2000).

Figure 9.3 illustrates a whole-systems approach towards the rehabilitation of older people.

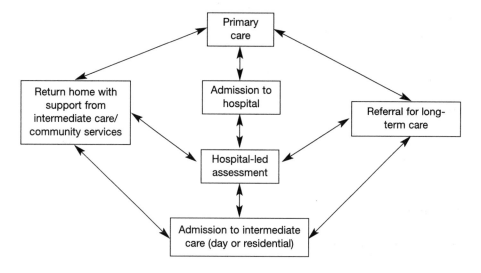

Figure 9.3 A whole-systems approach to assisting older people to return and remain at home.

A person-centred approach underpinned by a philosophy of rehabilitation would allow older people to move into and out of different health and social care services provided within their locality as their needs change over time, lessening the need for critical decisions to be taken in haste. Additionally, if occupational therapists were united in their approach, communication flow across the system would be enhanced and the development of a longer-term approach towards rehabilitation would be a real possibility.

The community practitioner in occupational therapy

In 2001 the College of Occupational Therapists produced a consultation document, *From Interface to Integration* (COT, 2001). The profession has accepted the principles it articulates. The document promotes the establishment of a community practitioner in occupational therapy; the role of this practitioner would be to provide services in the community, with specialist services continuing to be provided by therapists skilled in those areas. This new form of practitioner will be able to combine many of the roles of occupational therapists in existing health and social care settings.

How this principle of in-reach rehabilitation services might be applied to frail older people is illustrated in Figure 9.4. Assessment would be undertaken by community-based occupational therapists, in liaison with hospital staff and the range of primary, intermediate care and community facilities within the locality.

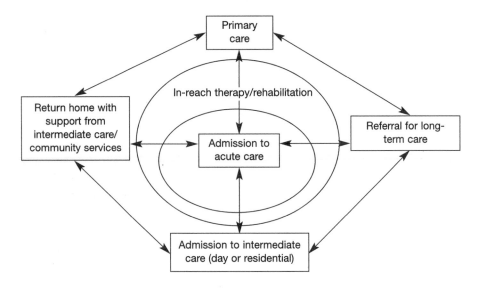

Figure 9.4 The incorporation of in-reach occupational therapy services into a whole-systems approach.

Implications for occupational therapy

Improve knowledge of policy and its implementation

If occupational therapists are to extend their role fully into the community in the manner described within the Blom Cooper report of 1989, understanding of health and social care policy, together with the implications of implementation for the profession, local services and the individual, is essential. This must be promoted through pre- and post-registration education as well as through continuing professional development.

Have clarity of purpose

Rehabilitation and the specific role of occupational therapists in delivery of interventions have to be clearly defined within specific service contexts. Clarity regarding service philosophy, objectives and those who are likely to benefit is likely to lead to improved outcomes for patients.

Develop a role in education and training

The expertise of occupational therapists can be used to train support staff to carry out rehabilitation. This is important where demand exceeds supply, and where strategic shift of services demands the delivery of rehabilitation on the part of staff previously employed to fulfil a care rather than rehabilitative role.

Deploy limited resources most effectively

Rehabilitation in primary and community care settings is leading to increased demand for occupational therapy services. In ideal circumstances, all services involved in the rehabilitation of older people would have access to qualified occupational therapy. However, as this is not possible, staff should be deployed selectively in services where occupational therapy is demonstrably effective or where indications of benefit are positive. Furthermore, all service developments should be evaluated.

Deliver the most appropriate service provision to meet needs

The need to change our views, expectations and responses is most clearly demonstrated through the increasing use of technology in care and rehabilitation. However, it must also be borne in mind that change is not always associated with new developments. There can sometimes be a return to more traditional methods and beliefs. One example is the adoption of the concept of intermediate care services in response to a previously neglected acknowledgement of the value of a period of time dedicated to rehabilitation before a person may be able to return to the community. Another, more fundamental return to core values is the resurgence in interest in the curative effects of occupation. Occupational therapists must take full advantage of the opportunities presented by changes in services and attitudes, to put in place effective services to meet the needs of the older people they serve.

Respond to the needs of a generic workforce

The accelerated development of a generic workforce is one of the consequences of the increase in community-based integrated services like intermediate care. There are insufficient numbers of trained staff to meet demand. Occupational therapists must therefore be prepared to devolve simple rehabilitative tasks to a generic workforce, thus releasing the time of trained staff to target and apply their expertise to greatest effect in situations where care needs are complex. Additionally, a generic approach can meet individual needs more appropriately, for example a person who requires basic nursing care as well as assistance with their independence skills. An essential, but frequently neglected requirement is the involvement of trained staff in the design and implementation of appropriate training programmes to generic workers.

Take medical and social factors into account

In the past, most specialist rehabilitation services were located in inpatient settings. However, over time, certain provision has moved into community settings. Services for specific user groups allow occupational therapists and other staff working in these settings to develop a body of expertise. However, these services are often delivered within a medical model of rehabilitation. This can limit the occupational therapist's ability to deliver social interventions in response to assessed needs. Conversely, working in a social model may lead to neglect of health needs. To use their skill base to full effect, occupational therapists have to balance the benefits of increasing specialization with a continued awareness of the full range of needs older people and their carers will have.

Pointers for practice

- Understand how strategic policy is being interpreted at local level and the consequences for occupational therapy services.

- Anticipate demands for occupational therapy stemming from policy initiatives.

- Determine the whole system of health and social care provision in your locality and the current and future role of occupational therapists within that system, for example deployment of staff into new primary-care-led services.

- Develop relationships with occupational therapists working with older people in other areas of the service system and identify ways of working together, even if you are employed by different organizations.

- Allocate scarce occupational therapy resources to services where the practice and research evidence indicates that a need is being met and the service is effective.

- Do not base decisions about resource allocation upon long-standing custom and practice.

- Agree clear operational definitions for services.
- Evaluate and audit service developments.
- Get involved in the training and education of other professionals and of the generic workforce.

CHAPTER 10

Using and generating evidence to support practice

The aim of this book is to draw a picture of the world of older people living in the UK at the beginning of the twenty-first century, and describe appropriate occupational therapy responses to those older people. Use of available research and practice literature has served to objectify the views expressed by the author and helped to indicate where occupational therapists should be directing efforts to increase their effectiveness.

There is little doubt that research and evidence-based practice have become a central concern of the occupational therapy profession over the last decade. This can be attributed to a number of external factors as well as a desire on behalf of occupational therapists themselves to deliver quality interventions grounded in best evidence. The professional code of conduct for occupational therapists working in the UK states that:

> Occupational therapists have a duty to ensure that wherever possible their professional practice is evidence-based and located in best practice. (College of Occupational Therapists, 2000)

The College of Occupational Therapists' research strategy was first published in 1997 and updated in 2001 (Ilott and White, 2001). The updated strategy places a greater emphasis upon both 'corporate action and personal responsibility'. It states that all members should make use of existing tools produced by the college to foster evidence-based practice, and use time allocated for audit, evidence-based practice and research as effectively as possible. Given these professional imperatives, it is appropriate to consider how evidence-based practice and research can be woven into occupational therapy practice with older people.

Policy context

Ensuring that practice is underpinned by evidence of effectiveness is now a political as well as professional imperative. All practitioners are required to use evidence to underpin their practice, so that both quality and effectiveness are assured, and the 'post code lottery' approach towards service provision is minimized (DoH, 1997b, 1998a). The introduction of National Service Frameworks from 1999 onwards, which are in themselves underpinned by evidence as far as is possible, require services to meet specified standards within given time scales, thus trying to ensure that provision of equivalent quality and effectiveness is available across the country.

The implementation of policy requires the actions shown in Figure 10.1 to be undertaken, with a number of mechanisms in place to assist with this.

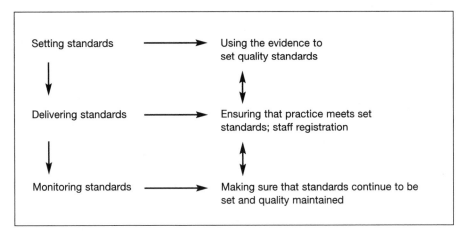

Figure 10.1 Requirements of current policy.

The 1997 White Paper *The New NHS: Modern, Dependable* (DoH, 1997b) placed some responsibility for evidence-based practice upon established professional organizations. In 1998, the White Paper *A First-Class Service* (DoH, 1998a) introduced the concept of clinical governance. This is a framework that encompasses a range of quality initiatives. The application of evidence-based practice, implementation of clinical guidelines and standards for practice and the appropriate involvement of users and carers all fall within the rubric of clinical governance (Sealey, 1999).

A number of new regulatory bodies for health and social care professions now require practitioners, as a condition of their continued registration, to engage in continuing professional development and to ensure that they keep their practice up to date. The Health Professions Council (HPC) is the regulatory body for occupational therapists.

National bodies have been put in place to encourage, and in certain situations, mandate an evidence-based approach towards treatment and care through the identification of best evidence and the development of evidence-based standards and guidelines. The National Institute for Clinical Excellence (NICE) was established as a special Health Authority for England and Wales on 1 April 1999. It is part of the NHS, with a remit to produce high-quality, evidence-based guidance for professionals, patients and the public. The work of NICE includes the development of clinical guidelines for health care practice through a number of Collaborating Centres (an interpretation of clinical guidelines is provided in a further section within this chapter). It also involves the commissioning of health technology appraisals, so that the evidence for specific interventions can be drawn together. NICE also has the remit to develop and encourage clinical audit. Over time, implementation of the advice produced by NICE should limit inequities in access to health care and interventions. One example pertaining to older people is the appraisal of anti-dementia drugs, which has led to a requirement to prescribe if the medical practitioner considers that it will be of benefit. Prior to this, purchase of the drug was left to the discretion of health authorities, resulting in inequitable availability across the country.

The Social Care Institute for Excellence (SCIE) was established on 1 October 2001. The aim of SCIE is to provide independent advice to users of social care, their carers, social care practitioners and service managers. The work of SCIE includes reviews of research evidence. It also aims to harness the experiences of those who deliver social care (termed knowledge-based practice (Fisher, 1998)), and disseminate this knowledge. SCIE wishes to encourage the active involvement of all those involved in social care and disseminate the knowledge base widely. A number of local initiatives independent of SCIE exist to promote a culture of evidence-based social care and research utilization by social care staff, for example Making Research Count and the Centre for Evidence-based Social Care based at the University of Exeter.

Given the moves to integrate health and social care, it is important that occupational therapists take account of the work of NICE and SCIE. Practitioners and managers are being supported in the implementation of an evidence-based approach through a number of national knowledge management initiatives, for example the National Electronic Library for Health and the Electronic Library for Social Care.

Clinical effectiveness

Clinical effectiveness has been defined as:

> The extent to which specific clinical interventions, when deployed in the field for a particular patient or population, do what they are intended to do,

i.e. maintain and improve health and secure the greatest possible health gain from available resources. (NHSE, 1996)

The NHSE enlarged on this definition by identifying the need to demonstrate benefit in terms of efficacy and cost effectiveness.

Sealey (1998) identified a number of activities that are associated with clinical effectiveness:

- evidence-based practice;
- critical appraisal skills;
- standards, clinical guidelines and care pathways;
- clinical audit;
- cost effectiveness and efficiency;

Some of these processes are briefly reviewed below in the context of services and interventions with older people. However, reference to Sealey and other texts is recommended for more detail.

Evidence-based practice

Evidence-based practice is the use of best evidence in making decisions about the care of individual patients (Sacket et al., 1997). The evidence base can also be employed during decision-making about services, and it underpins the standards required by all the National Service Frameworks in line with the policy requirements described in Figure 10.2.

Evidence-based practice involves:

1. finding out what is known already;
2. synthesizing the evidence;
3. incorporating the evidence into decision-making;
4. identifying evidence gaps.

Promoting a culture of evidence-based practice in the workplace requires a number of strategies to be put into place. The following activities can help to embed such a culture:

- identifying gaps in clinical knowledge and using information resources to search for evidence;
- participating in guideline development;
- developing local standards for practice:
- undertaking regular audits;
- introducing or joining journal clubs;
- seeking the views of service users and their carers.

Practising in an evidence-based manner does not mean undertaking primary research. The College of Occupational Therapists recommends that all practitioners should be active consumers of research, but only a small proportion of the profession should be actively engaged in research.

The links between different elements of evidence-based practice and research are illustrated in Figure 10.2.

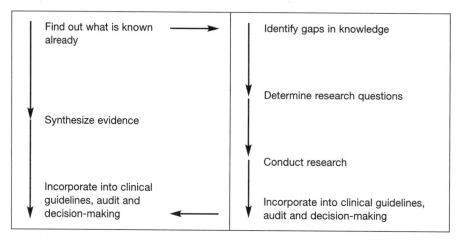

Figure 10.2 Links between evidence-based practice and research.

Several excellent texts are available to help occupational therapists adopt an evidence-based approach towards their work, for example Bury and Meade (1998). Some of the tools and processes developed to assist with evidence-based practice are outlined in brief below, with the reader being signposted towards further resources.

Searching for and appraising evidence

It is beyond the remit of this book to describe fully the process of finding and using the evidence base. Mountain and Lepley (1998) outlined the process of searching for evidence in an easily digested bulletin, and there are plenty of other resources available, particularly from information specialists in libraries.

Searching for evidence produces variable yields. For some topic areas, there is a wealth of evidence readily available, and in others there is little. The process of searching for literature is well supported by Internet knowledge sources and training programmes. One example is the CASP Initiative (Critical Appraisal Skills Programme, referenced in Appendix 3). This aims to help individuals and groups to identify and use quality evidence to support decisions in practice. Training and education are provided by CASP.

Once evidence has been located, the quality of that evidence, and therefore its reliability, has to be determined. There is a recognized hierarchy of research evidence to assist with this process, with the most reliable evidence considered to be the first two items on the list:

1. systematic reviews and meta-analyses of randomized controlled trials;
2. randomized controlled trials;
3. non-randomized experimental studies;
4. non-experimental studies;
5. descriptive studies;
6. respected opinion/expert discussion.

The hierarchy has recently been revised to introduce new levels for grading recommendations in evidence-based guidelines (Harbour and Miller, 2001), but in essence it remains the same.

Bowling (1997) described a systematic review as being prepared in a systematic manner to minimize biases and errors. This requires the adoption of stringent guidelines at every stage of the process. An identified set of search terms is used, documenting the databases used and the results of the search. A systematic review will often include literature from levels one and two of the hierarchy of evidence only, but this need not be the case. The most important aspect is the approach taken towards the review.

Published research literature embraces different types and quality of evidence. Various views have been expressed about the value of different forms of evidence. The evidence base for occupational therapy is limited in certain respects if this hierarchy is rigidly adhered to. Most of the evidence that exists tends to be small-scale and self-funded due to a long-standing lack of research investment. This has resulted in inadequate qualitative as well as quantitative evidence. It has also recently been acknowledged that selecting evidence solely in accord with the hierarchy of evidence can at times provide unhelpful, inconclusive results, as reported in Bandolier (see Appendix 3 for web address). A recent review of the documented evidence base regarding rehabilitation and people with dementia necessitated an exploratory rather than prescriptive approach to searching the literature. It also required an approach that included a wider variety of information, including that within the 'grey' or unpublished literature as well as the knowledge rooted in practice.

Despite limitations, it is still important to underpin decisions about services and interventions with the evidence base that exists (Muir Gray, 1997). This can require the adoption of a wide interpretation of evidence to include the results of analysis of routinely collected service data, reports of practice innovation and the views of service users and their carers, as well as published material. The quality of the evidence used in decision-making should subsequently be indicated; for example, the more robust evidence cited within this book has been emphasized.

In some cases the evidence base can promote the value of a particular intervention. However, the viability of implementation must be placed in the context of local circumstances. One example is the number of people who will potentially benefit from the intervention compared with the overall number of people to be treated. If the intervention is too expensive or time-consuming, or is only beneficial for a small minority, questions should be raised about how appropriate it is. This is the point at which evidence-based practice interfaces with clinical effectiveness.

Clinical guidelines

Clinical guidelines are developed out of the available evidence to assist practitioners in making the most appropriate treatment decision. The College of Occupational Therapists defines clinical guidelines thus:

> ... systematically developed statements, which assist occupational therapy practitioners and service users in making decisions about appropriate health and social care interventions. They outline the best known intervention or treatment for a specific condition and/or population. (Mountain and Sealey, 1999, p. 2)

As previously mentioned, NICE is producing national guidelines in a number of topic areas. Other bodies are also involved in guideline development. This book has drawn upon the National Clinical Guidelines for Stroke Rehabilitation, the development of which was led by the Royal College of Physicians, and the National Guidelines for Collaborative Rehabilitative Management of Older People who have Fallen, led by the Chartered Society of Physiotherapy. Additionally, staff can develop local guidelines for direct application in their workplace. These can be constructed from scratch or customized from national standards to include considerations for local implementation. The key feature of successful guidelines is that they are multi-disciplinary with key stakeholders being involved, including service users and their carers. Further details regarding the development of clinical guidelines and their application can be obtained from the College of Occupational Therapists (Mountain and Sealey, 1999).

Standards for practice

Unlike clinical guidelines, standards for practice can be uni-professional and, while they are evidence-based as far as possible, their development is not as rigorously grounded in the evidence base.

Standards for occupational therapy practice have been devised to guide the work of all occupational therapy staff. A range of standards can be obtained through the College of Occupational Therapists. There are a number of core standards that should underpin the work of all staff, as well as others for specialist areas of practice. Each standard is designed to be auditable, so they can be used to identify where improvements should be made as well as highlighting areas of excellence. A template can also be obtained to develop standards tailored to local practice and subsequently undertake an audit of the extent to which the standards are being met (College of Occupational Therapists, 2003).

Audit

Audit was first mandated in health care settings in the early 1990s with the aim being to improve the quality of care. This process involves the analysis of clinical care through the systematic collection and analysis of routinely collected service data, and has previously been mentioned in relation to standards for practice. Figure 10.3 shows the recognized audit cycle.

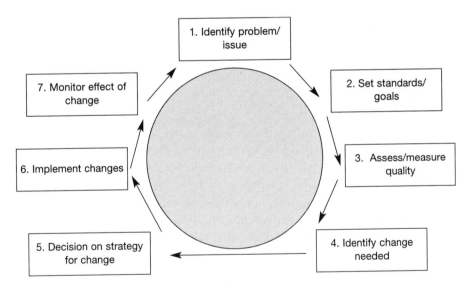

Figure 10.3 Clinical audit cycle.

Clinical audit is a provenly effective way of promoting and maintaining the quality of services, but only if the cycle shown in the above diagram is completed. Sealey (1998) provided a full description of clinical audit and how it can be applied by occupational therapists.

Outcome measurement

Outcome measures can be used to determine the effect of occupational intervention upon the individual, for example quality of life, function, attainment of treatment goals and user satisfaction. They can also be applied to determine service outcomes, for example length of stay and cost effectiveness. Therefore outcome measurement is an important dimension of clinical effectiveness.

Clarke et al. (2001) are unequivocal about why outcome measures should be used:

> Measuring outcomes means that occupational therapists are not using guesswork or inadvertently misleading themselves about the quality and effectiveness of their intervention. (Clarke et al., 2001, p. 6)

Outcome measurement can be undertaken from the perspectives of the service user and carer, practitioners, management or the government. These different uses of outcome measures are summarized in Table 10.1.

Table 10.1 Different applications of outcome measures

The user and/or their carer	• Quality of care received • Quality of life, post-intervention
Practitioners	• Effectiveness of the intervention • Allocation of time
Management	• Cost effectiveness • Effective throughput
Government	• Best use of public resources • Social inclusion

Some of the measures shown in Chapter 6 can also be used as outcomes, as well as assessments, if applied following treatment. Clarke et al. (2001) provide a diagram to illustrate the overlap between assessment and outcome measures (Figure 10.4).

It has been common practice for occupational therapists to devise their own methods of devising outcomes. As with the development of assessment measures, discussed in Chapter 6, the introduction of 'home grown' measures is not recommended practice. The creation of measures that will produce reliable and valid results when applied is a complex research procedure. The work of Clarke et al. (2001) includes a comprehensive list of outcome measures and is an invaluable resource for occupational therapists when selecting and applying outcomes.

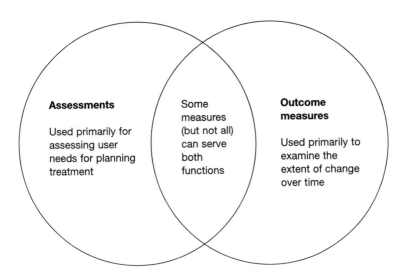

Figure 10.4 The relationship between assessment and outcome measures (Source: Clarke et al., 2001, p. 10).

Addressing the right research questions

Undertaking a review of the evidence in a specific topic area will confirm the extent of research that exists already and the quality of that evidence, and also indicate the evidence gaps that exist. (This relationship between research and evidence-based practice is shown in Figure 10.2.) Research gaps need to be identified in order to formulate the questions that need to be addressed.

A number of factors should be taken into account when identifying research questions regarding services and interventions for older people. These are illustrated in Figure 10.5.

Figure 10.5 indicates the need to consider four main factors. Two are concerned with governmentally led imperatives and how the identified goals are being actioned at local level. One example would be the standards within the National Service Framework for Older People (DoH, 2001a) and how they are being taken forward in localities. There is no doubt that research is more likely to attract funding if there are clear links to national government agendas. Long-standing policy neglect of older people until relatively recently led to research into ageing largely being set aside. However, the picture is now very different. The current emphasis upon meeting the needs of older people in the context of preventive strategies, healthy lifestyles, rehabilitation and strategies to help older

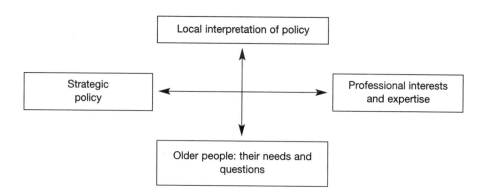

Figure 10.5 The dimensions to take into account when identifying research questions

people to remain living in the community mean that occupational therapists are well placed to raise and address relevant research questions. Therefore occupational therapists need to both understand national policy and be aware of local interpretation in order to engage with this agenda.

The third dimension shown in Figure 10.5 is the interests and concerns of the profession. Some commissioners of research are realizing the value of involving an occupational therapist owing to the skills they possess, for example in assessment, in exploring occupation and assisting individuals to make lifestyle changes and in provision of rehabilitative interventions. Examples of this interest are demonstrated through occupational therapy in the EQUAL (Extending Quality of Life of Older and Disabled People) programme funded by the Engineering and Physical Sciences Research Council, the funding for occupational therapy research provided through the Stroke Association and the recently established Department of Health awards for researchers from nursing and allied health professions.

The fourth and arguably the most important dimension is the questions and concerns being raised by older people themselves. As Chapters 1 and 5 described, the opinions of older people are now actively being sought. Additionally, the work of Consumer Involvement in NHS R&D (funded through the Department of Health) is creating the precedent of user involvement in all research activity. Again occupational therapists are in key positions to both hear and respond to those questions.

Questions raised at national level

The questions being raised at national level by researchers, policy-makers and national organizations advocating on behalf of older people provide important information for occupational therapists.

A strategic review of research into ageing (DoH, 1999b) identified the following needs for research, all of which fall into the interests of occupational therapy:

1. the appropriateness of care for older people and their carers and families across both health and social services;
2. promotion of autonomy and independence, and the appropriate interventions to maintain this;
3. prevention of functional limitations through both primary and secondary prevention and the identification of cost-effective practices;
4. quality of life and quality of care including the development of appropriate assessment tools and the appraisal of professional practice and the environments in which services are delivered.

The report drew out the need for more research into social care services, given their importance for older people. It also drew attention to the inadequacy of research into rehabilitation. The report highlighted a need for evidence into the cost-effectiveness of rehabilitative interventions and the optimum settings for rehabilitation.

Other reviews have drawn similar conclusions, for example the MRC strategic review of the health of older people in the UK, undertaken in 1994. A whole section within this review is devoted to rehabilitation, identifying four main research needs. These included the elements of packages of rehabilitation that seem to be effective, and psychosocial adjustment and integration as a component of rehabilitation. Further sections in the same document looked at prevention and reversibility of age-related disease and disability.

National initiatives to draw together research

A number of initiatives have been put in place to improve the remit and quality of research into ageing, and to draw together existing knowledge and expertise. One of the recommendations of the NHS strategic review (DoH, 1999b) was for the research effort to be drawn together so that work can be built upon.

The National Collaboration on Ageing Research (NCAR) is a partnership between four of the UK's research councils. It has been introduced in recognition of the need for concentrated effort to extend and improve research in this field. The remit of the NCAR includes the coordination and liaison between existing initiatives, the identification of key themes for research and the stimulation of multi-disciplinary research activity.

The EQUAL (Extending Quality of Life) initiative, managed by the Engineering and Physical Sciences Research Council (EPSRC) (one of the members of NCAR), aims to extend the active period of life through combining resources, expertise and capacity for innovation across a number of diverse constituencies. There is a growing body of researchers involved in EQUAL, together with older and disabled people and health and social care practitioners. A number of occupational therapists are already involved.

The Growing Older programme, funded by the Economic and Social Research Council (ESRC) exists to generate new knowledge on extending quality of life in older age and contribute towards policy development. Three examples of the 25 projects already funded through this initiative include evaluating the impact of reminiscence on quality of life of older people, public and private transport for older people, and older people and lifelong learning.

The need for a collaborative approach to research concerned with older people is an important message for the occupational therapy profession. There is no doubt that we are more likely to be successful if we make partnerships with others.

The research reported by Glass et al. in 1999 presented a strong case for occupational therapists to join forces with epidemiologists and public health physicians in determining the factors that facilitate healthy older age and help people to retain their independence.

Undertaking research concerned with older people

Only when the research questions have been identified and developed can the research methods by which the questions might most appropriately be addressed be considered. The research process is illustrated overleaf in Figure 10.6.

Research methods

Continuing debate continues between researchers as well as within health and social care practice regarding the optimum research methods to address certain questions. A common question concerns the value of qualitative as opposed to quantitative methodology. Arguments regarding the greater benefits of a qualitative as opposed to a quantitative approach can readily be located in the occupational therapy literature. However, these debates within the profession about the most 'valuable' methods obscure the real issue, which is the lack of research investment into occupational therapy and rehabilitation.

The Cochrane Library of Systematic Reviews consists of the most robust body of research, according to the hierarchy of evidence previously discussed in this chapter. Occupational therapy does have some evidence to

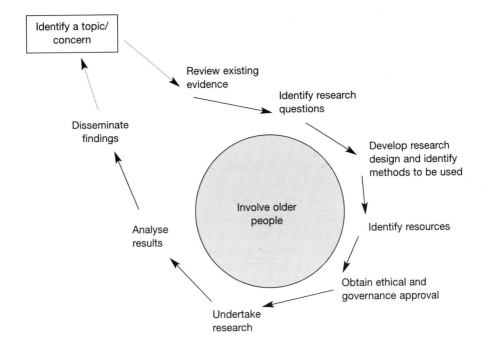

Figure 10.6 The research cycle

match the requirements of the Cochrane database. Examples of the 88 current reviews concerned with occupational therapy are a review of Snoezelen for dementia (Chung et al., 2003), a review of occupational therapy for patients with problems in activities of daily living after stroke (Legg and Drummond, 2003) and a meta-analysis of the effectiveness of occupational therapists with older people (Carlson et al., 1996).

There are a growing number of randomized controlled trials of occupational therapy. The work of Clark et al. (1997), Drummond and Walker (1995), Gilbertson et al. (2000) and Walker et al. (1999) has been cited within this book. We also have examples of research that has used a range of other methodologies.

The NHS strategic review of research into ageing and age-related disease and disability promoted the adoption of a wider paradigm within which to explore both population and individual outcomes:

> Large randomized controlled trials and overviews are valuable in the appraisal of the efficacy of treatments. However they do not provide information on the determinants of individual outcomes. Moreover their outcomes are often of uncertain generalizability, both in terms of the patients enrolled and the standards of care provided. (DoH, 1999b, p. 10)

Therefore the real consideration should be the question: Is it concerned with individual experience, as opposed to population benefit? Discussions should be taking place about whether the methods are informing what we need to know, particularly about the outcomes of therapeutic interventions. Often the application of a mix of methods is most appropriate.

Conducting ethical research

All health-conducted research must be ethically scrutinized by a Local Research Ethics Committee (LREC) if it involves human participants or material associated with people, for example case records and other data, and human tissues or fluids. If the intended research involves more than two fieldwork sites approval is required from a Multi-centre Research Ethics Committee (MREC). Examples of the requirements of ethics committees are patient and carer information sheets, clinician information, explanations about how consent for involvement will be obtained, details of how participants can withdraw from the study and how those involved will be kept informed of the progress and outputs of the study. At the time of writing, procedures to ensure the ethical approval of research projects involving social care were not in place. However, this is due to change imminently.

Research governance

Research governance is concerned with ensuring the quality of all research being undertaken in treatment and care settings. All trusts now have to ensure that governance arrangements are in place to monitor the quality of research being undertaken under the auspices of the organization. These new arrangements should take into account the views of users of services. Governance processes include:

- an independent peer review of the intended research to ensure its quality;
- agreement from the responsible clinicians if access to users of services is required;
- indemnity on the part of the individuals undertaking the project in case of any adverse event;
- necessary ethical approval, as described in the previous section.

The web links to information about ethics and governance for health are provided in Appendix 3.

Undertaking research with older people

The Department of Health Research and Development programme is heavily promoting the notion of user involvement in the research they fund. The Standing Group on Consumers in NHS Research was established on behalf of the Department of Health in 1996.

> Its aim: to ensure that consumer involvement in research and development improves the way that research is prioritized, commissioned and disseminated. (Standing Group on Consumers in NHS Research, 1999, p. 4)

To date the group has been involved in an exciting range of projects, for example involvement in the Cochrane database of systematic reviews, in the DoH-funded health technology assessment programme and in the production of guides for both users and researchers. Most recently, the group has extended its remit to social care and public health, accompanied by a forthcoming change of name.

The challenges of involving the lay public in research should not be underestimated, with a need for rigorous methods to ensure meaningful involvement (Entwistle et al., 1998). Bearing this in mind, older people can take on a variety of roles within the research process, and in so doing enrich both the process and the appropriateness of the findings. Some of these are described below.

Assisting with the identification of research agendas/questions

Setting priorities for research and development is a natural starting point for involving older people in research. This form of involvement is occurring more frequently with the drive to demonstrate the involvement of both the lay public and users of services in research. Older people and those using services are more frequently being asked to participate in identifying how resources for research should be targeted. This form of involvement has been fostered by the work of Consumer Involvement in NHS R&D.

As researchers

Older people can be active participants in the research process. Indeed, it would be very difficult to obtain government funding for research without demonstrating the involvement of older people or their advocates in the preparation of the proposal. Three models can be identified (Nuffield Institute for Health, 1997). These are:

- the older person as a research participant;
- the older person as a research adviser;
- the older person as a researcher.

All approaches demand enhanced communication between older people and researchers, between older people and service providers, and between researchers and those being researched. Researchers at the Nuffield Institute identified a number of considerations extending across all research endeavours with older people (Nuffield Institute for Health, 1997):

* Older people bring different views, derived from lived experience.
* Older people can feel more able to talk openly to other older people.
* The experience of being involved in the research process can enhance older people's feelings of confidence and self-worth.
* The involvement of older people in research is both costly and time-consuming.
* The process of user involvement can be demanding and difficult.
* If users are to be able to undertake their own research, funding has to be available.

Examples of studies involving older people are provided below.

Older people as research participants

The *Bulletin*, produced by the Nuffield Institute for Health (1997), cited a rapid appraisal study undertaken by the University of Hull and East Riding Health Authority to illustrate this type of involvement. This involved meeting older people, in groups and individually, over a six-month period to talk about their health needs and priorities, focusing upon the services available to them. Regular feedback was provided from the outset, with the Health Authority receiving regular reports of community views and feeding back their responses.

The work of Raynes (1999) and Barnes and Bennett (1998) has been discussed elsewhere in this book. These are further examples of older people taking the role of research participants.

Work to explore drug treatments for Parkinson's disease involved the Parkinson's Disease Society, with the role of the society being to help with the design of the trial and encourage participation. This involvement led Baker (2000) to conclude that patient groups need to support research of all types, from clinical trials to quality-of-life surveys.

Older people as research advisers

A study by Tozer and Thornton (1995) involved setting up a group of eight older people to advise on a research project undertaken by the Social Policy Research Unit at the University of York. The project was concerned with looking at ways of involving older people in providing their views about community care. The researchers found that keeping the advisers informed of the methods and progress of the research was demanding. However, while some of the members were initially suspicious of tokenism, this was overcome once specific tasks were set. These included designing questions for the fieldwork, devising questionnaires and topic guides and seeking literature on the recruitment of participants. Two members then volunteered to produce summaries of an interim research report. All advisers received payment for their time. Tozer and Thornton noted the positive effect of involvement upon the older people. They became advocates for user involvement and some went on to take an active role in user-led organizations for older people. Their involvement in the actual research process changed some of the emphasis of the work, particularly in the production of the final report.

Older people as researchers

Older people as researchers can involve the adoption of very different roles (Nuffield Institute for Health, 1997). A project to examine pensioners' living costs involved a volunteer group of older people undertaking a training programme over six months. It included sessions on questionnaire design, interviews and the ethics of social research. Following this the group conducted a pilot study. This resulted in the final questionnaire, to be applied as a semi-structured interview. The questionnaire included items identified by the older people as being important to quality of life, for example age, income, housing, fuel, food, health and social and domestic expenditure. Older people subsequently applied the interview. The academic researchers observed that, even though the process was a challenge, the involvement of older people as researchers greatly improved the quality of the data.

The European Older Women's Project (1991–94) spearheaded another example of a project described in the *Bulletin* (Nuffield Institute for Health, 1997). The Older Women's Project brought together older women from eight EU member states to celebrate older women's lives and debate action in order to influence policy. A group established in Lewisham involved around 40 older women from a variety of cultures. They were all interested in learning research skills, supported by paid staff from academic settings. The research question was concerned with older women living in Lewisham and their views of the NHS. A questionnaire was drafted, covering all aspects of health care. Sixteen women conducted interviews in the borough, with more subsequently being involved in coding the responses for analysis. Two members then entered the data using the SPSS statistical package, with analysis being conducted by the council IT analyst. The group then embarked on a second study of the housing situations of older women. One of the academics involved in the project reaffirmed the value of the acquisition and application of research skills by the group of older women.

Hollingbery (1999) reported the development of a proposal to develop mystery visits to hospitals to examine aspects of care in the same way that mystery shoppers test the system by shopping. The premise underpinning this idea was that, by conducting undercover visits, older people would overcome their compliance and reluctance to complain, and become empowered. Two focus groups of older people aged between 70 and 90 years old were conducted to explore the feasibility of this method. Participants were drawn from a database of older people willing to take part in research and questionnaires, called the Thousand Elders, held by the Centre for Applied Gerontology, University of Birmingham. The groups generally agreed that a mystery visitor scheme might work if there were good support available. Discussions also yielded a wealth of information about quality of hospital care and the experience of making complaints.

The work of Consumer Involvement in NHS R&D (soon to be Involve: promoting public involvement in NHS, public health and social care research) provides further examples of user involvement in projects (see Appendix 3 for web address).

Implications for occupational therapy

It is worth reinforcing that only a small proportion of the profession will become researchers. However, it is the responsibility of every occupational therapist to ensure that they are utilizing the existing evidence base in their work.

Use the existing evidence base

The College of Occupational Therapists has recently updated its research strategy. This acknowledges that most occupational therapists will be consumers of research rather than researchers, with only one per cent becoming research leaders. Therefore the essential task for the majority is to learn how to access and apply the existing evidence base in practice. Library services provide a range of services to assist with this.

Locate existing reviews

An increasing number of readily digested summaries of available research evidence are being produced to assist those working in health and social care to make informed treatment and commissioning decisions. Some of these reviews are being translated into clinical and practice guidelines. Additionally some research providers, such as the Joseph Rowntree

Foundation, have provided a search facility on their website, with short research digests being readily downloaded. A number of existing and new initiatives concerned with social care research are considering how research evidence can be most readily incorporated into practice. Occupational therapists are encouraged to search existing websites and use what exists already to inform practice, reserving time and resources to search for topics which have not been addressed.

Listen and respond to the questions being raised by older people

The opinions of those who use occupational therapy services are in themselves a valuable source of feedback about the effectiveness of services.

The different generations defined as older people have been examined throughout this book. For a variety of reasons 'younger older people' are more likely to question the services being provided and their efficacy. In common with other professionals, occupational therapists have to be ready to respond to queries from a variety of sources presented in a number of ways. Examples are the questions raised as a consequence of information downloaded from the Internet, concerns posed by relatives, and issues raised by other professionals on behalf of the older person. We need to be able to respond openly and honestly, backing up responses with evidence as far as possible. Furthermore, if the evidence to support a specific intervention is not available, its appropriateness should be reconsidered.

Identify those with the interest and ability to undertake research

In common with the majority of health and social care professions, occupational therapy has largely developed in the absence of a clearly defined evidence base. More research is required to examine the effectiveness of occupational therapy interventions, and the contribution of occupational therapy within specific service settings. Also there has been a lack of research funds to examine both occupational therapy interventions and services. This situation is now changing, with finance being made available through the DoH and HEFCE to stimulate research activity in nursing and allied health professions. This is due to the results of a study which unequivocally demonstrated the need for investment (HEFCE, 2001).

The generation of research evidence to support practice is beneficial for service users and for clinicians and managers. This being the case it is the responsibility of all members, and in particular service managers, to identify those who wish to further a career in occupational therapy research and assist them to achieve their goals.

Pointers for practice

- Introduce a culture of evidence-based practice into the workplace through engagement in a range of activities.

- Identify a departmental champion to assist with evidence-based practice.

- Learn how to use the Internet.

- Question the effectiveness of aspects of long-standing practice, and search for evidence to support or refute it.

- Use resources to assist with research and evidence-based practice available through the College of Occupational Therapists, and through your workplace library provision.

- Seek the participation of students on placement as they will be familiar with searching for evidence.

- Listen to the questions being raised by older people and their carers and always respond as fully and honestly as possible.

- Introduce clinical audit as a matter of routine, but ensure that the audit loop is complete.

CHAPTER 11

Working with older people: the challenges for occupational therapy

The previous chapters in this book have examined the concept of ageing as it is perceived by Western society (and in particular in the UK), and the implications for the individual of becoming old and in need of services. This is followed by a consideration of the occupational therapy interventions that can help an older person to acquire and retain the quality of life that they and their carers identify as being both appropriate and attainable.

One of the prime motivations for producing this work was to help practitioners and managers to prioritize the needs and wants of older people rather than those of services, of other professionals and of those charged with implementing policy. Given that health and social care services are frequently used as a barometer to determine the success or otherwise of the political party in power at the time, the influence of external agendas cannot be underestimated.

The specific challenge for occupational therapists is how to retain a balanced view of normal ageing and expectations of older age when working with older people who have become vulnerable. This challenge is enhanced in situations where it is not immediately clear (due to the effects of illness) what the lifestyle of that person has been, what aspirations they have had (and can still have) and what contribution they have made within their community. Each of the previous chapters in this book included the implications for occupational therapists of specific topic areas and suggested pointers for practice. This concluding chapter identifies a number of key principles that should underpin all occupational therapy interventions with older people, and the services within which those interventions are delivered.

The nature of professional confidence

To achieve best outcomes for older people and their carers, and for services, occupational therapists must be confident of their own professional skills and abilities.

The term 'professional confidence' has been used to describe the range of factors that can influence the judgements and subsequent clinical activity of occupational therapists. The inputs that lead to improved professional confidence and consequently to improved outcomes for older people and their carers were indicated through the research into the activity of health-employed occupational therapists working with older people with mental health problems (Mountain, 1998a). Figure 11.1 shows that the professional confidence of occupational therapists working with older people should be grounded in a specialist knowledge base, alongside a robust understanding of current policy requirements and a clear comprehension of the contributions of other workers across a range of agencies. This combination of skills and knowledge on the part of the individual occupational therapist is likely to lead to assessment and interventions that directly meet the needs of the user and their carer, involving other agencies as appropriate. If treatment is responsive to needs, it is likely that it will result in satisfactory experiences and outcomes for service users. This will command greater recognition from all stakeholders, thus reinforcing self-esteem and job satisfaction. The motivation provided through good job satisfaction is more likely to lead to the individual occupational therapist's building upon their knowledge base.

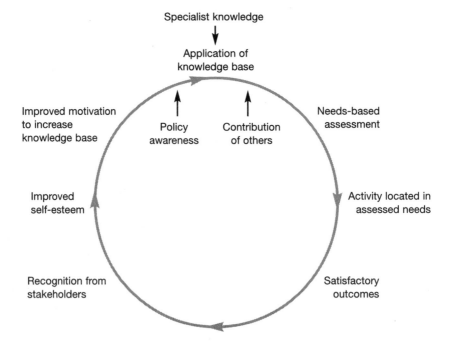

Figure 11.1 Factors leading to improved professional confidence.

While this hypothesis warrants further testing, it can be argued that its validity is confirmed through the literature cited throughout this book. The hypothesis, together with existing evidence, underpins the following nine key principles for occupational practice with older people, shown in Table 11.1. These principles pertain to all occupational therapists working in services for older people.

Table 11.1 Key principles for occupational therapy practice with older people

Key principle 1	Understand the history of the profession and its core purpose
Key principle 2	Maintain the quality of clinical work
Key principle 3	Listen to what older people want
Key principle 4	Follow assessment with interventions in response to assessed needs
Key principle 5	Undertake interventions in the most appropriate environment
Key principle 6	Develop professional maturity
Key principle 7	Use support staff effectively
Key principle 8	Work in partnership with other agencies and workers from other professions
Key principle 9	Look towards the needs of future generations of older people, including those of yourself and your family

Key principle 1: Understand the history of the profession and its core purpose

One of the main factors identified within professional confidence is clarity of role. This is necessary for sound judgement and the delivery of appropriate clinical activity. In recent years there has been a renaissance in the profession's view of the centrality of occupation and its value in creating meaning for life and maintaining health. The fundamental nature of this purpose should be sufficient for occupational therapists to confidently use it as a firm foundation for practice. Unfortunately the nature of the questions that are sometimes posed by occupational therapists about their specific contributions and value, particularly in multi-disciplinary team settings, suggests that this purpose is not always adequately grasped.

The history of the profession can go some way towards explaining the lack of clarity sometimes expressed by less experienced practitioners regarding the core aims of occupational therapy. Wilcock (2001, 2002) has recently documented this history. The arts and crafts movement shaped the early development of the recognized profession of occupational therapy in both the UK and the USA. This promoted the production of well-designed, hand-made goods. The process of craftsmanship in itself was believed to have a positive and curative effect. Later, in response to emerging needs, another ideology developed, which was concerned with a graded therapeutic purpose. The benefits of occupation were linked to improving function rather than the satisfaction gained from producing a polished artefact. The founders of occupational therapy had difficulty reconciling these two paradigms, with the undercurrents of this paradox remaining.

> Although Casson and American leaders remained dedicated to arts and crafts ideology (in the 1940s) they began to rely more heavily on patho-kinesiology and scientific reasoning to justify treatment. (Levine Schemm, 1993, p. 16)

These dilemmas remain, demonstrated by the move towards a focus on functional activity in the 1970s and the continued discussion to this day within the profession regarding the value of creative and other occupation-based interventions

Other factors external to profession ideologies have had a significant impact upon the directions taken by occupational therapy over the years. A key example is the introduction of occupational therapists into social service departments in response to the requirements of the Chronically Sick and Disabled Person's Act (1970). This led to occupational therapy involvement in assessment for, and provision of, disability equipment and housing adaptations. It has also resulted in an ongoing debate regarding whether occupational therapists are most appropriately employed by health or social services (Riley, 2002). Blom Cooper (1989) observed that the relationship with the medical profession in hospital settings, and to a lesser extent with social workers in social service settings, added to difficulties in exploiting the true potential of occupational therapy. In particular, the past requirement for medical prescription and supervision inevitably dictated the nature of the work undertaken. Paradoxically, the history of the profession as described by Wilcock (2001, 2002) demonstrates the true power of occupation and the ground-breaking work undertaken by the pioneers. As Riley (2002) concluded:

> As a profession it is important that we reflect upon the past in order to make mature and informed decisions about our future. (Riley, 2002, p. 507)

Furthermore, as described in previous chapters, there is little doubt now that individuals and bodies external to the profession are now more enlightened about the value of occupational-based interventions in promoting health and well-being. Now is definitely the time to assert the professional beliefs identified by the founders that are now being recognized by the wider health and social care community.

Key principle 2: Maintain the quality of clinical work

To promote quality work, located in the needs of service users and carers while at the same time obtaining recognition in the workplace and good job satisfaction, the following are required:

* an understanding of, and responsiveness to, policy;
* specialist knowledge;
* evidence-based practice.

Each of the above issues is now unpacked.

Understanding and responding to policy

Chapter 1 described how societal attitudes and prevailing policies shape the responses we all make to older people. Many references have been made in other chapters to policy initiatives that impact upon the nature of public services received by older people. In the past, some policy decisions have been ill-founded and not led to positive outcomes for services or for the people they were designed for. However, the comparatively recent high-level acknowledgement of the value of rehabilitation and prevention in enabling older people to remain at home and experience continued quality of life continues to present a range of possibilities for occupational therapy; for example:

* community care policy, implemented in 1993, requiring that all people should be enabled to stay at home should they choose to do so;
* the prevention agenda, introduced in the late-1990s and leading to grants to social services to develop services, and most recently as a target for service development identified in the National Service Framework for Older People (Standard 8);
* the new policy requirements for cross-boundary service delivery legislated through the NHS Plan in 2000, presenting a golden opportunity for occupational therapists working for both health and social services to promote their true value through the pooling of expertise and resources;
* the requirement to introduce intermediate care services, coordinated by intermediate care coordinators in all localities by April 2001;

- the requirement to provide quality, integrated community equipment services, largely in response to the Audit Commission's reports of their parlous state in 2000 and again in 2002;
- the policy foci upon the value of rehabilitation and provision of quality, user-focused services.

As well as directing the nature of service provision, politicians can also be extremely influential in shaping the manner in which interventions are delivered within services, as described in Chapter 5. The conclusions that can be drawn from this is that we have to work with the government agenda in order to maximize the effectiveness of our contributions. Occupational therapists in all service settings and at any level of seniority have to be able to comprehend current policy and understand how it is being interpreted and implemented at a local level. This includes developing a complete understanding of current policy-led jargon. This knowledge is necessary to ensure that practice both complements and capitalizes upon current policy initiatives.

As well as helping occupational therapists to deliver interventions in line with current thinking, policy knowledge can be empowering in that it can help both practitioners and service managers to anticipate changes that will occur, and develop proactive rather than reactive strategies. More senior members of the profession should ensure that they are in positions of influence at national and local levels whenever the opportunity presents itself. Recent examples would be through membership of local implementation groups for the National Service Framework for Older People.

Development of a specialist body of knowledge

It is only comparatively recently that the need for an expert health and social care workforce for older people has received general recognition. Care of older people used to be a 'Cinderella specialty', attracting little funding and interest, and frequently viewed by practitioners as being one of the least desirable options. Furthermore, in the past, unskilled, undesirable staff (from all professional groups) might be allocated to work with older people, particularly in the old institutional social and health care settings. It is now realized that working with older people who have become vulnerable is both complex and demanding, involving risk assessment, service provision and protection. The co-existence of several factors described in Chapter 3, for example physical and/or mental ill health and frailty due to ageing, combined with a less-than-ideal living environment, requires skilled assessment and intervention from practitioners from a range of disciplines working closely together. Furthermore, problems can be exacerbated for those older people for whom a condition has remained undetected over a protracted period of time and for those who live alone without an informal care network. The specific circumstances of each individual have to be taken into account, including cultural and ethnic origins and socio-economic circumstances. Working with older people also necessitates working with their carers. Moreover, for some older people, interventions are more likely to maintain the status quo than provide a cure. The work of Perrin and May (2000) eloquently described the mix of expertise and care required to maintain a quality service with people with severe dementia.

Working with older people requires all occupational therapists to constantly extend and refine their skill base. We need to be able to draw upon a specific body of professionally based expertise as well as being equipped to undertake roles of a more generic nature. Membership of the specialist section of the College of Occupational Therapists is an ideal way of supporting the development and extension of specialist knowledge.

Ensuring that practice is located in best evidence

The responsibility of ensuring that practice is underpinned by evidence of effectiveness is something that we owe to the older people referred to us for occupational therapy. Producing this book would have been unethical without references to research and other forms of evidence. As described in Chapter 10, practising in an evidence-based manner is challenging. It not only requires information-retrieval skills and knowledge, but also can highlight the need to abandon aspects of ingrained practice shown to be of little or no value. The benefits do, however, exceed the drawbacks. As well as being a policy and professional imperative, it can direct resources to where they can be of most value, and assist individual occupational therapists to build upon a proven body of knowledge.

Key principle 3: Listening to what older people want

Over the years many research projects (several of which have been referred to in this book) have demonstrated the importance of listening carefully to the older person and their carer, and taking their views into account. Practitioners also need to ensure that they provide full and accurate information so that the individual is able to make informed choices about their treatment and care. Evers et al. (1994) demonstrated that a number of factors are associated with beneficial experiences on the part of older service users and their carers. These included longer-term relationships with professionals and the development of shared understanding and strategies for problem solving. The time pressure within service settings can make this difficult. However, research and clinical experience has also shown that time can be wasted pursuing goals that are not shared by the older person. Needs-based assessment and identification of services to meet assessed needs necessitates spending more time with the older person, accepting their views of their care networks and needs (Godfrey and Moore, 1996).

Key principle 4: Follow assessment with interventions in response to assessed needs

Figure 11.1 indicates that assessment located in needs is more likely to lead to appropriate interventions and good outcomes. Moreover, the prime determinant of service quality for older people and their carers is the clinical interventions they experience. In the study by Mountain (1998a) those service users and carers who received longer-term treatment were more satisfied than those who experienced short-term assessment, substantiating the view that short-term assessment (often undertaken to meet the information needs of other professionals) does not usually serve the interests of older people. Despite this knowledge, a preoccupation with assessment rather than treatment is a conspicuous feature of the occupational therapy service still received by many older people (Mountain, 1998a; Perrin, 2001).

> Are we breeding a generation of occupational therapists who do not know how to use occupations therapeutically? (Perrin, 2001, p. 12)

At its most extreme, this has led to reluctance to follow assessment with any form of intervention. It is also evident that in certain settings, occupational therapists are compromised to such an extent by the demands of functional assessment that they are unable to provide interventions. However, it is also apparent that interventions have been devalued by occupational therapists themselves. Service users are either assessed and recommendations forwarded to other professions, or the treatment process has been handed over to support staff. The role of support staff is important in the delivery of interventions, but it is also important for occupational therapists themselves to remain involved and responsive to the full range of needs of the older person throughout the treatment process, particularly when needs are complex. The case for understanding and responding to older people as occupational rather than functional beings, each with a rich history, has been eloquently illustrated by the individual citations from older people themselves within the previous chapters.

Key principle 5: Undertake interventions in the most appropriate environment

All occupational therapists will be able to reflect upon situations where the environment has affected their work. The treatment environment is a highly influential factor in that it can either contribute towards, or conversely erode, the quality of clinical work, as described in Chapter 9.

Policy-led changes have resulted in many services that used to be provided within institutional settings now being delivered in the community. Mountain (1998a) found that the process of occupational therapy was most likely to be viewed favourably by a variety of stakeholders (including older people themselves) when delivered in community settings. Working in the community presented new challenges for occupational therapists. These included the application of skills, maintaining an up to date knowledge and development of networks with a range of services. The study also found that occupational therapists working in hospital settings had to manage a different set of challenges. These were located in power battles with other professionals, and traditional views of role maintained by other disciplines.

The development of new styles of service for older people is an opportunity for occupational therapists to work in settings that support, rather than erode, what they are trying to achieve.

Key principle 6: Develop professional maturity

In 1989 the Commission of Enquiry into Occupational Therapy (Blom Cooper, 1989) observed that reliance for referral upon others, medicine and social work in particular, was hindering the development of the profession. This dependency, combined with allowing other disciplines to direct our work in some instances, was preventing occupational therapists from demonstrating their true worth.

The fact that relationships with other disciplines have to be maintained to ensure referral routes is self-evident. Overall clinical responsibility must lie with the responsible medical officer. However, recent policy is now enabling the development of practice that acknowledges medical priorities but is not dictated to by doctors. It also promotes the value of rehabilitation in the community, a skill that complements but cannot be replicated by the skill base of social workers. Now is the time to assert the value of the profession and set aside those aspects of practice, referred to in previous chapters, that have become part of the expected repertoire of occupational therapists, and which should be abandoned, questioned more often or passed onto other, less-qualified individuals. There are several examples, including:

• a continuing preoccupation with pre-discharge home visits, which do not predict the ability of the older person to cope in the longer term at home and should be undertaken with far greater consideration (Mountain and Pighills, 2003);

- assessing and providing simple, readily obtainable pieces of equipment – a process that could be managed by support staff in many situations (Mountain, 2000);
- undertaking assessment of function and failing to provide any interventions (Clarke et al., 1996).

Key principle 7: Use support staff effectively

Occupational therapy as a profession has been accustomed to employing support staff such as helpers and technical instructors to enhance the workforce. Traditionally, these groups of staff have been accountable to occupational therapists only. While this arrangement has worked well in many situations, in others occupational therapists themselves have limited the potential of the support worker role. The result has been that some qualified staff have spent too much time undertaking simple tasks that do not match a skill base requiring three-year pre-registration training.

This pattern is now rapidly changing, stimulated by the growth in intermediate care services alongside the requirement for a flexible workforce able to work across established service and professional boundaries (Nancarrow and Mountain, 2002). For the qualified workforce, this is leading to demands for involvement in areas of work that were previously considered to be the domain of specific professional groups. Additionally, new and enhanced rehabilitation services for older people mean that there are insufficient numbers of occupational and physiotherapists to meet demand both now and in the future. Consequently, these developments are leading to a proliferation of generic workers, able to undertake a range of tasks without the constraints of professional line management; for example, some social service departments are training their home care staff to undertake simple rehabilitative interventions. A generic approach can meet needs more appropriately in community settings, in that one worker is able to provide a range of interventions, for example nursing, occupation-based and mobility.

Instead of being a threat to the profession, occupational therapists should view these developments as presenting real opportunities. New workers can enable the devolvement of simple rehabilitative tasks to a generic workforce, thus releasing time to target and apply expertise to greatest effect in situations where needs are complex. An essential but frequently neglected requirement is the involvement of trained occupational therapists in the design and implementation of appropriate training programmes for generic workers.

Key principle 8: Work in partnership with other agencies and workers from other professions

Few readers will challenge the following statement:

> It is clear that professional isolationism is neither acceptable nor appropriate and if maintained will not meet the challenges that health and social care continue to face. (Cole and Perides, 1995, p. 62)

Recent policy goals are demanding that workers, previously separated by professional and organizational divides, work closely together to benefit the people in receipt of their services (DoH, 2000a). These requirements are underpinned by the perceived desirability of interdisciplinary and cross-agency working, especially for services for older people. Consequently, uni-disciplinary, uni-agency practice is rapidly becoming a thing of the past. This is a prime opportunity to create a more effective working environment. Effective patterns of integrated working demand close partnerships with other professional groups, and a shift away from rigid task demarcation within services concerned with the health and social care of the same group of people.

However, it is evident that interdisciplinary, cross-agency working is not an automatic process but one that has to be continually worked at for success. All professions have to cope with the demands of working with each other as well as with the older people referred to them. A common philosophy of care and the use of universally understood terminology have to develop. This requires team building and training on the part of all workers. In common with other disciplines, occupational therapists have to continue to work at this. Even when considering working with colleagues from the same profession but employed by different organizations, there are many challenges (Mountain, 2001a). The extent of the cultural divide across health and social care cannot be underestimated. It is underpinned by different belief systems and illustrated through the use of different jargon, for example medical and social rehabilitation. One of the ways is for occupational therapists working for different organizations serving the same locality to meet together on a regular basis to establish a dialogue. Joint training programmes are also provenly effective in helping to promote a common approach.

Working in true partnership also requires professional confidence and maturity, described in key principle 1. Dependence upon the 'good will' of other professional groups is a very different matter to working in partnership, described through key principle 2.

Key principle 9: Look towards the needs of future generations of older people, including those of yourself and your family

This is perhaps the most important principle both for individual occupational therapists and for the profession as a whole. Proactive responsiveness to change will secure the future of occupational therapy and ensure that our services remain both needed and appropriate. Increasing numbers of older people in our society mean that the involvement of occupational therapy will continue to be sought. Demands for services are certain to shift from those promulgated by an illness model to one with health promotion and prevention at its core. Re-investment in occupation as the main theoretical and practical construct underpinning practice, alongside new opportunities presented by policy initiatives, technological advances and inclusive design, is creating the optimal climate for the profession to demonstrate its true worth. Chapter 9 discussed the use of devices to promote active rehabilitation, drawing a distinction between this use of new technologies and other devices marketed to promote care and independence. This is an area where there has been some progress, but solutions have been neither accepted nor mainstreamed as yet. The profession must be ready to accept new methods of working that the use of technology will create.

Conclusions

These are exciting times for occupational therapists working with older people. Decision-makers are increasingly aware of the value of the contributions of occupational therapists. This is leading to increasing demand that we must ensure we are adequately equipped to meet. This book has tried to confirm where efforts might be most appropriately directed in light of current evidence and expectations. Some of the views expressed are contentious and open to discussion. This was deliberate, as it is only by having the debate within the profession that we can examine our practice and ensure that it remains relevant throughout the twenty-first century.

References

Abrams M (1980) Transitions in middle and later life. In: Johnson ML (ed.), Transitions in Middle and Later Life. London: British Society of Gerontology.

Adams A, Wilson D (1996) Accommodation for Older People with Mental Health Problems. York: Joseph Rowntree Foundation Findings, Social Care Research 87.

Age Concern (2000) Turning Your Back on Us: Older People and the NHS. London: Age Concern England.

Agree E (1999) The influence of personal care and assistive devices on the measurement of disability. Social Science and Medicine 48: 427–43.

Allan K (2001) Communication and consultation: exploring ways for staff to involve people with dementia in developing services. York: Policy Press and Joseph Rowntree Foundation.

Alzheimer's Disease Society (1992) The Alzheimer's Disease Report: Caring for Dementia Today and Tomorrow. London: ADS.

Alzheimer's Disease Society (1995) Right from the Start; Primary Health Care and Dementia. London: ADS.

Ameratunga SN, Brown PM (2000) Commentary: older people's perspective on life after hip fractures. British Medical Journal 320: 345.

American Association of Occupational Therapists (1995) Position paper: purposeful activity. American Journal of Occupational Therapy 49: 1081–82.

Aminazadeh F, Edwards N, Lockett D, Nair RC (2000) Utilization of bathroom safety devices, patterns of bathing and toileting, and bathroom falls in a sample of community living older adults. Technology and Disability 13: 95–103.

Appleton NJW (2002) The Needs and Aspirations of Older People Living in General Housing. York: Joseph Rowntree Foundation Findings ref N32.

Arber S, Ginn J (1993) Gender and Later Life: A Sociological Analysis of Resources and Constraints. London: Sage Publications.

Ashburn A (2001) Screening people with Parkinson's disease to identify those at risk of falling. National Research Register. www.tap.ccta.gov.uk

Audit Commission (1997) The coming of age: improving care services for older people. Oxon: Audit Commission.

Audit Commission (2000a) Fully Equipped. London: Audit Commission.

Audit Commission (2000b) The Way to Go Home. London: Audit Commission & DoH.

Audit Commission (2002a) Fully Equipped 2002. London: Audit Commission.

Audit Commission (2002b) Forget Me Not 2002: Developing Mental Health Services for Older People in England. London: Audit Commission.

Audit Commission (2002c) Integrated Services for Older People: Building a Whole System Approach in England. London: Audit Commission.

Baker M (2000) Patient care (empowerment): the view from a national society. British Medical Journal 320: 1660–62.

Ballinger C, Payne S (2000) Falling from grace or into expert hands? Alternative accounts about falling in older people. British Journal of Occupational Therapy 63(12): 573–79.

Banerjee S (1993) Prevalence and recognition rates of psychiatric disorder in the elderly clients of community care service. International Journal of Geriatric Psychiatry 8: 121–31.

Barlett H, Burnip S (1999) Improving care in residential and nursing homes. Generations Review 9(1): 8–10.

Barnes D (1997) Older people with mental health problems living alone: anybody's priority? London: Social Services Inspectorate and Department of Health.

Barnes M (1997) Care, Communities and citizens. Essex: Longman Press.

Barnes M, Bennett G (1998) Frail bodies, courageous voices: older people influencing community care. Health and Social Care in the Community 6(2): 102–11.

Bath P, Philp P, Boydell L et al. (2000) Standardized health check data from community-dwelling elderly people: the potential for comparing populations and estimating need. Health and Social Care in the Community 8(1): 17–21.

Benjamin J (1976) The Northwick Park ADL Index. British Journal of Occupational Therapy 39(12): 301–6.

Benson S (ed.) (2000) Creative approaches to individualised care for people with dementia. Journal of Dementia Care. Person Centred series.

Better Care; Higher Standards (2002) London: DoH.

Better Government for Older People (2000) All Our Futures. Wolverhampton Science Park: Better Government for Older People Programme.

Blom Cooper L (1989) Occupational Therapy; An Emerging Profession in Health Care. London: Duckworth Press.

Bond J, Farrow G, Gregson BA et al. (1999) Informal caregiving for frail older people at home and in long term care institutions: who are the key supporters? Health and Social Care in the Community 7(6): 434–4.

Bore J (1994) Occupational therapy home visits: a satisfactory service? British Journal of Occupational Therapy 57(3): 85–8.

Bowie P, Mountain G (1993) Life on a long stay ward: extracts from the diary of an observing researcher. International Journal of Geriatric Psychiatry 8: 1001–7.

Bowie P, Mountain G, Clayden D (1992) Assessing the environmental quality of long-stay wards for the confused elderly. International Journal of Geriatric Psychiatry 7: 95–104.

Bowling A (1991) Measuring Health: A Review of Quality of Life Measurement Scales. Milton Keynes: Open University Press.

Bowling A (1995) Measuring Disease. Milton Keynes: Open University Press.

Bowling A (1997) Research Methods in Health. Milton Keynes: Open University Press.

Bowling A (1999) Ageism in cardiology. British Medical Journal 319: 1353–55.

Brayman SJ, Kirby T (1982) The comprehensive occupational therapy evaluation (COTE) scale. In: BJ Hemphill (ed.), The Evaluative Process in Psychiatric Occupational Therapy. New Jersey: Slack Inc.

British Geriatric Society (1988) Joint Statement of Professional Associations: Discharge to the Community of Elderly Patients in Hospitals. London: BGS.

British Thoracic Society (1997) COPD guidelines summary. Thorax 52(Supp 5): S1–28.

Brody EM, Saperstein AR, Lawton MP (1989) A multi-service respite program for caregivers of Alzheimer's patients. Journal of Gerontological Social Work 14: 41–74.

Brown AR, Mulley GP (1997) Injuries sustained by caregivers of disabled people. Age and Ageing 26: 21–3.

Burch S, Borland C (2001) Collaboration, facilities and communities in day care services for older people. Health and Social Care in the Community 9(1): 11–18.

Burton JE (1989) The model of human occupation and occupational therapy practice with elderly patients Part 1: Application. British Journal of Occupational Therapy 52(6): 219–21.

Bury T, Meade J (1998) Evidence Based Health Care for Therapists. Oxford: Butterworth Heinemann.

Cabinet Office (2000a) Older people have their say. MORI with the Cabinet Office. London: Service First Publications.

Cabinet Office (2000b) Winning the generation game. Performance and Innovation Unit report. London: Cabinet Office.

Caldock K, Nolan M (1994) Assessment and community care: are the reforms working? Generations Review 4(4): 2–4.

Cancerbacup (2003) Cancer and Older People. London: Cancerbacup.

Care & Repair England (2001) Making the links: developing services which address the housing, health and care needs of older people. Leeds: Design Box.

Carers and Disabled Children Act (2000) London.

Carers (Recognition and Services) Act (1995) London.

Care Standards Act (2000) London.

Carlill G, Gash E, Hawkins G (2000) Preventing unnecessary hospital admissions: an occupational therapy and social work service in an accident and emergency department. British Journal of Occupational Therapy 65(10): 440–5.

Carlson M, Fanchiang S, Zemke R, Clark F (1996) A meta analysis of the effectiveness of occupational therapy for older persons. American Journal of Occupational Therapy 50: 89–98.

Carlson M, Clark F, Young B (1998) Practical contributions of occupational science to the art of successful ageing: how to sculpt a meaningful life in older adulthood. Journal of Occupational Science 5(3): 107–18.

Challis D (1998) Integrating health and social care: problems, opportunities and possibilities. Research, Policy and Planning 16(2): 7–11.

Challis D, Darton R, Johnson L et al. (1991) An evaluation of an alternative to long stay hospital care for frail elderly patients: 1 the model of care. Age and Ageing 20: 236–44.

Challis D, von Abendoff R, Brown P, Chesterman J (1996) Care management and dementia: an evaluation of the Lewisham Intensive Case Management Scheme. PSSRU Discussion Paper 1242, University of Kent, London School of Economics and University of Manchester.

Challis D, Darton R, Hughes J et al. (2001) Intensive care management at home: an alternative to institutional care? Age and Ageing 30: 409–13.

Challis T (1996) Purposeful activity and elderly mentally ill people: why? British Journal of Occupational Therapy 1996: 183–4.

Chambers P (1994) A biographical approach to widowhood. Generations Review 4(3): 8–12.

Chartered Society of Physiotherapists, College of Occupational Therapists and Royal College of Speech and Language Therapists (1997) Partnership in the Manual Handling of Patients. British Journal of Occupational Therapy 60(9): 406.

Chenoweth B, Spencer B (1986) Dementia: the experience of family caregivers. The Gerontologist 26(3): 267–72.

Chesterman J, Bauld L, Judge K (2000) Satisfaction with the care-managed support of older people: an empirical analysis. Health and Social Care in the Community 9(1): 19–30.

Christiansen C (1994) Classification and study in occupation: a review and discussion of taxonomies. Journal of Occupational Science 1(3): 3–21.

Chronically Sick and Disabled Persons Act (1970) London: HMSO.

Chung JCC, Lai CKY, Chung PMB, French HP (2003) Snoezelen for dementia (Cochrane Review). In: The Cochrane Library, Issue 1, 2003. Oxford: update software.

Clark CA, Corcoran M, Gitlin LN (1995) An exploratory study of how occupational therapists develop therapeutic relationships with family caregivers. American Journal of Occupational Therapy 49(7): 587–94.

Clark FA, Carlson M, Zemke R et al. (1996) Life domains and adaptive strategies of low-income, well older adults. American Journal of Occupational Therapy 50(2): 99–108.

Clark FA, Azen SP, Zemke R et al. (1997) Occupational Therapy for independent living older adults. Journal of the American Medical Association 278: 1321–6.

Clark FA, Azen SP, Carlson M et al. (2001) Embedding health-promoting changes into the daily lives of independent-living older adults; long term follow up of occupational therapy intervention. Journal of Gerontology (Psychological Sciences) 56B: 60–3.

Clark H, Spatford J (2001) Piloting Choice and Control for Older People: An Evaluation. York: Policy Press and Joseph Rowntree Foundation, Findings, Ref 431.

Clark M, Steinburg M, Bischoff, N (1997) Patient readiness to return home: discord between expectations and reality. Australian Journal of Occupational Therapy 44(3): 132–41.

Clarke C, Sealey-Lapes C, Kotsch L (2001) Outcome Measures: Information Pack for Occupational Therapists. London: College of Occupational Therapists.

Clarke H, Dyer H, Hartman L (1996) Going Home; Older People Leaving Hospital. Bristol: Policy Press and Joseph Rowntree Foundation.

Clarke H, Dyer S, Horwood A (1998) That Bit of Help. York: Policy Press and Joseph Rowntree Foundation.

Clemson L, Roland M, Cumming R (1992) Occupational therapy assessment of potential hazards in the homes of elderly people: an inter-rater reliability study. Australian Occupational Therapy Journal 39(3): 23–6.

Clemson L, Fitzgerald MH, Heard R (1999) Content validity of an assessment tool to identify home fall hazards: the Westmead Home Safety Assessment. British Journal of Occupational Therapy 62(4): 171–9.

Close J, Ellis M, Hooper R et al. (1999) Prevention of falls in the elderly trial (PRO-FET). The Lancet 353: 93–7.

Closs J (1997) Discharge communications between hospital and community health care staff: a selective review. Health and Social Care in the Community 5(3): 181–97.

Closs SJ, Stewart LSP, Brand E, Currie CT (1995) A scheme of early supported discharge for elderly trauma patients: the views of patients, carers and community staff. British Journal of Occupational Therapy 58(9): 373–6.

Cointet S (2000) Joint proposal: model for occupational therapy services, Strathkelvin. Project report: East Dumbartonshire Council, Greater Glasgow Primary Care NHS Trust, Strathkelvin LHCC and North Glasgow University Hospitals NHS Trust.

Cole R, Perides M (1995) Managing values and organizational climate in a multi-professional setting. In: L Mackay, K Soothill, C Webb (eds), Interprofessional Relations in Health Care. London: Edward Arnold.

Coleman J (1990) Psychological ageing. In: J Bond, P Coleman (eds), Ageing in Society. London: Sage Publications.

Coleman PG (2002) Spiritual Beliefs and Existential Meaning in Later Life. http://www.esrc.ac.uk/esrcontent/ourresearch/growing_older.asap

College of Occupational Therapists (1997) Interprofessional Curriculum Framework for Health Care Advisers. London: COT.

College of Occupational Therapists (2000) Code of Ethics and Professional Conduct for Occupational Therapists. London: COT

College of Occupational Therapists (2001) A Strategy for the Delivery of Occupational Therapy in Local Health and Social Care Communities: From Interface to Integration. London: COT.

College of Occupational Therapists (2003) Professional Standards for Occupational Therapy Practice. London: COT.

College of Occupational Therapists and Association of Directors of Social Services (1999) Meeting the Challenge; Occupational Therapy for the Community. London: COT.

Connelly AL (1998) The impact of the manual handling operations regulations 1992 on the use of hoists at home; the patient's perspective. British Journal of Occupational Therapy 61(1): 17–21.

Cooper SA (1997) High prevalence of dementia among people with learning disabilities not attributable to Down's syndrome. Psychological Medicine 27: 609–16.

Craddock J (1996a) Perspectives of the occupational therapy profession to the perspective of the disability movement, part 1. British Journal of Occupational Therapy 59(1): 17–22.

Craddock J (1996b) Perspectives of the occupational therapy profession to the perspective of the disability movement, part 2. British Journal of Occupational Therapy 59(2): 73–8.

Csikszentmihalyi M (1993) Activity and happiness: towards a science of occupation. Journal of Occupational Science: Australia 1(1): 38–42.

Cullen M, Blizzard R, Livingston G, Mann A (1993) The Gospel Oak project 1987–1990: provision and use of community services. Health Trends 25(4): 142–5.

Cumming E, Henry W (1961) The Process of Disengagement. New York: Basic.

Cunningham S (2000) Disability, oppression and public policy: disabled people and the professionals' interpretation of the manual handling operations 1992. Keighley: Independent Living Ltd.

Curry (2001) The Use of Information and Communication Technology (ICT) in Assistive Technology for Older and Disabled People: an Overview of Current UK Activity. rcurry@dialin.net

Cvitkovitch Y, Wister A (2001) The importance of transportation and prioritisation of environmental needs to sustain well being among older adults. Environment and Behaviour 33(6): 809–29.

Davies ADM, Smith C, Gargaro P, Dodd A, Newton BA (1990) A method for assessing dressing skills in elderly patients. British Journal of Occupational Therapy 53(7): 272–4.

Davis A, Ellis K, Rummery K (1997) Access to assessment. London: Joseph Rowntree Foundation with Policy Press.

Deane KHO, Ellis-Hill C, Playford ED et al. (2001) Occupational therapy for Parkinson's disease. (Cochrane Review) In: The Cochrane Library, Issue 4, 2001. Oxford: Update Software.

Deeming C (2001) A Fair Deal for Older People: Public Views on the Funding of Long-term Care. London: King's Fund.

Deipen E, Baillon SF, Redman J et al. (2002) A pilot study of the physiological and behavioural effects of Snoezelen. British Journal of Occupational Therapy 65(2): 61–6.

de Jong-Gierveld J, van Solinge H (1995) Ageing and Its Consequences for the Socio-medical System. Strasbourg: Council of Europe Press.

Department for Education and Employment (1998) The Learning Age: A Renaissance for Britain. London: HMSO.

Department for Transport, Local Government and the Regions (2000) Quality and Choice: A Decent Home for All, Housing Green Paper. London: DTLR.

Department for Transport, Local Government and the Regions (2001) Quality and Choice in Older People's Housing: A Strategic Framework. London: DTLR.

Department for Transport, Local Government and the Regions and Department of Health (2001) Supporting People: Policy into Practice. London: DTLR and DoH.

Department of Health (1989a) Discharge of Patients from Hospital; Circulars LAC (89)7 and HC (89)5. London: DoH.

Department of Health (1989b) Working for Patients. London: HMSO.

Department of Health (1989c) Caring for People: Community Care in the Next Decade and Beyond [Griffiths Report]. London: HMSO.

Department of Health (1990) The Community Care Act. London: HMSO

Department of Health (1992) The Health of the Nation. London: DoH.

Department of Health (1994) Hospital Discharge Workbook. London: DoH.

Department of Health (1995) Responsibilities for Meeting Continuing Healthcare Needs. HSG(95)8/LAC(95)5.

Department of Health (1997a) The Health of the Nation: A Handbook on the Mental Health of Older People. London: DoH.

Department of Health (1997b) The New NHS: Modern, Dependable. London: DoH.

Department of Health (1997c) EL(97)62, Better Services for Vulnerable People. London: DoH.

Department of Health (1998a) A First-Class Service: Quality in the New NHS. London: DoH.

Department of Health (1998b) Modernising Social Services. London: DoH.

Department of Health (1998c) Saving our Lives: Our Healthier Nation. London: Stationery Office.

Department of Health (1999a) National Service Framework for Coronary Heart Disease. London: DoH.

Department of Health (1999b) NHS R&D Strategic Review: Ageing and Age-associated Disease and Disability. London: DoH.

Department of Health (1999c) National Service Framework for Mental Health. London: DoH.

Department of Health (1999d) Caring about Carers: A National Strategy. London: DoH.

Department of Health (1999e) Community Occupational Therapy Services: Report of a Conference Programme Linking the Thinking – Integrated Practices. Wetherby: DoH.

Department of Health (1999f) Service Action Teams: Summary of Action Plans. London: DoH.

Department of Health (2000a) The NHS Plan. London: HMSO.

Department of Health (2000b) National Beds Enquiry – Shaping the Future NHS. London: DoH.

Department of Health (2000c) The NHS Cancer Plan. London: DoH.

Department of Health (2001a) The National Service Framework for Older People. London: DoH.

Department of Health (2001b) The Expert Patient: A New Approach to Chronic Disease Management for the 21st Century. London: DoH.

Department of Health (2001c) Better Care Higher Standards. LAC (2001)6: HSC 2001/006. London: DoH.

Department of Health (2001d) Continuing Care: NHS and Local Councils' Responsibilities. HSC2001/015:LAC(2001).

Department of Health (2001e) Shifting the Balance of Power. London: DoH.

Department of Health (2001f) Intermediate Care. London: HSC 2001/01: LAC (2001)1.

Department of Health (2001g) The 2000 Health Survey for England. London: DoH.

Department of Health (2002a) National Service Framework for Diabetes. London: DoH.

Department of Health (2002b) Supporting the Implementation of Patient Advice and Liaison Services Resource Pack. London: DoH.

Department of Health (2002c) The Single Assessment Process for Older People. London: DoH.

Department of Health (2002d) HSC 2002/001; LAC (2002)1 Guidance on the Single Assessment Process for Older People. www.doh.gov.uk/sap/hsc200201.htm

Department of Health (2003) LAC(2003)8) The Financial Assessment for Residential Accommodation. www.doh.gov.uk/scg/crag

Department of Health and Department of the Environment (1997) Housing and Community Care: Establishing a Strategic Framework. Wetherby: DoH.

Department of Health and Social Services Inspectorate (1998) They Look After Their Own, Don't They? Inspection of Community Care Services for Black and Minority Ethnic Older People. Wetherby: DoH.

Department of Health, Social Services Inspectorate and Scottish Office Social Work Services Group (1991) Care Management and Assessment: Summary of Practice Guidance. London: HMSO.

Department of Social Security (1998) Supporting People: A New Policy and Funding Framework for Support Services. London: DSS.

Department of Trade and Industry (2000a) Ageing Population Panel: The Age Shift; a Consultation Document. London: DTI.

Department of Trade and Industry (2000b) The Age Shift: Priorities for Action. London: DTI.

Dickie VA (1998) Clinical interpretation of the unpackaging of routine in older women. American Journal of Occupational Therapy 52(3): 176–8.

Dimond B (1997) Legal Aspects of Care in the Community. Basingstoke: Macmillan.

Drummond EAR, Walker MF (1995) A randomized controlled trial of leisure therapy after stroke. Clinical Rehabilitation 9: 283–90.

Eakin P (1989) Assessments of activities of daily living: a critical review. British Journal of Occupational Therapy 52(1): 11–15.

Eakin P, Baird H (1995) The Community Dependency Index: a standardised assessment of need and measure of outcome for community occupational therapy. British Journal of Occupational Therapy 58: 17–21.

Easterbrook L (1999) When We Are Very Old: Reflections on Treatment, Care and Support of Older People. London: King's Fund.

Easterbrook L (2002) Healthy Homes, Healthier Lives. Nottingham: Care and Repair England.

Edwards NI, Jones DA (1998) Ownership and use of assistive devices amongst older people in the community. Age and Ageing 27(4): 463–8.

Effective Health Care Bulletin (1996) Preventing falls and subsequent injury in older people. NHS Centre for Reviews and Dissemination 2(4): 16.

Egan M, Warren SA, Hessel PA, Gilewich G (1992) Activities of daily living after hip fracture; pre and post discharge. Occupational Therapy Journal of Research 12(6): 345–56.

Elkan R, Kendrick D, Dewey M et al. (2001) Effectiveness of home based support for older people: a systematic review and meta-analysis. British Medical Journal 323: 719.

Ellis K (1993) Squaring the Circle: User and Carer Participation in Needs Assessment. York: Joseph Rowntree Foundation.

Enderby P, Stevenson J (2000) What is intermediate care? Looking at needs. Managing Community Care 8(6): 35–40.

Entwistle VA, Renfrew MJ, Yearly S et al. (1998) Lay perspectives: advantages for health research. British Medical Journal 316: 463–6.

Etan (1998) The Ageing Population and Technology: Challenges and Opportunities. European Commission, the Etan Expert Working Group.

Evans E (1990) Who is the Client? The Community Occupational Therapy Support to Elderly Dementia Patients and Their Carers in West Dorset. British Journal of Occupational Therapy 53(7): 280–84.

Evers H, Cameron E, Badger F (1994) Interprofessional work with old and disabled people. In: Leathard A (ed.) Going Interprofessional: Working Together for Health and Social Care. London: Routledge.

Fillenbaum CG (1988) Multidimensional Functional Assessment of Older Adults: The Duke Older Americans Resources and Services Procedures. Lawrence Erlbaum Associates.

Finch J (1995) Responsibilities, obligations and commitments. In: I Allen, E Perkins (eds), The Future of Family Care for Older People. London: HMSO.

Fine J (2000) The effect of leisure activity on depression in the elderly: implications for the field of occupational therapy. Occupational Therapy in Health Care 13(1): 45–59.

Finlay L (1997) The practice of psychosocial occupational therapy. Cheltenham: Stanley Thornes Press.

Finlayson M, Havixbeck K (1992) A post discharge study on the use of assistive devices. Canadian Journal of Occupational Therapy 59(4): 202–7.

Fisher AG (2003) Assessment of Motor and Process Skills: Development, Standardization and Administration Manual, 5th edn (vol. 1). Colorado: 3 Star Press Inc.

Fisher M (1998) Knowledge Based Practice. London: NISW Noticeboard.

Fiske J, Griffiths J, Jamieson R, Manger D (2000) Guidelines for oral health care for long stay patients and residents. London: British Society for Disability and Oral Health.

Flanagan SR, Ragnnarsson KT, Ross MK, Wong DK (1995) Rehabilitation of the geriatric orthopaedic patient. Clinical Orthopaedics and Related Research 316: 80–92.

Fontana A (1977) The Last Frontier: The Social Meaning of Growing Old. Sage: Beverley Hills.

Foresight – Ageing Population Panel (2000) Healthcare in 2020: Healthcare Panel Consultation Document. London: DTI.

Forster A, Young J (2002) Clinical and cost effectiveness of physiotherapy in the management of elderly people following stroke. London: Chartered Society of Physiotherapists.

Forster A, Young J, Langhorne P (1999) Systematic review of day hospital care for elderly people. British Medical Journal 318: 837–41.

Franklin B (1998) Forms and functions; assessing housing need in a community care context. Health and Social Care in the Community 6(6): 420–8.

Frankum JL, Bray J, Ell MS, Philp I (1995) Predicting post-discharge outcome. British Journal of Occupational Therapy 58(9): 370–2.

Gaber I (2003) Saga of satisfaction. Guardian Society, 12 February 2003. See also www.esrc.ac.uk

Gautam P, Macduff C, Brown I, Squair J (1996) Unplanned readmissions of elderly patients. Health Bulletin 56(6): 449–57.

George LK, Bearon LB (1980) Quality of Life in Older Persons: Meaning and Measurement. New York: Human Sciences Press.

George LK, Gwyther LP (1986) Caregiver wellbeing: a multidimensional examination of family caregivers of demented adults. Gerontologist 26(3): 253–9.

Gilbertson L, Langhorne P, Walker A et al. (2000) Domiciliary occupational therapy for patients with stroke discharged from hospital: randomised controlled trial. British Medical Journal 320: 603–6.

Gilchrist C (1999) Turning Your Back on Us. London: Age Concern England.

Gilhooly ML (1984) The impact of caring on care-givers: factors associated with the psychological well-being of people supporting a demented relative in the community. British Journal of Medical Psychology 57: 35–44.

Gill TM, Williams CS, Robison JT, Tinetti ME (1999) A population based study of environmental hazards in the homes of older persons. American Journal of Public Health 89(4): 553–6.

Gillespie LD, Gillespie WJ, Cumming R et al. (2000) Interventions to reduce incidence of falling in the elderly (Cochrane Review). In: the Cochrane Library, Issue 1. Oxford: Update Software.

Gitlin LN, Burgh D (1994) Issuing assistive devices to older patients in rehabilitation: an exploratory study. American Journal of Occupational Therapy 49(10): 994–1000.

Gitlin LN, Mann W, Tomita M, Marcus S (2001) Factors associated with home environmental problems among community-living older people. Disability and Rehabilitation 23(7): 777–87.

Glass TA, Mendes de Leon C, Marottoli RA, Berkman LF (1999) Population based study of social and productive activities as predictors of survival among elderly Americans. British Medical Journal 319: 478–83.

Glendenning C, Coleman A, Rummery K (2002) Partnerships, performance and primary care: developing integrated services for older people in England. Ageing and Society 22(2): 185–208.

Glyn Thomas T, Stevens RS (1974) Social effects of fractures of the neck of the femur. British Medical Journal 3: 456–8.

Godfrey M (1998) Older People with Mental Health Problems: A Literature Review. Leeds: Nuffield Institute for Health.

Godfrey M (1999) Preventive Strategies for Older People: Mapping the Literature on Effectiveness and Outcomes. York: Joseph Rowntree Foundation and Anchor Trust.

Godfrey M, Moore J (1996) Hospital Discharge: User, Carer and Professional Perspectives. University of Leeds: Nuffield Institute for Health.

Godfrey M, Wistow G (1997) The user perspective on managing for health outcomes: the case of mental health. Health and Social Care in the Community 5(5): 325–32.

Goldberg D, Williams P (1988) General Health Questionnaire. Windsor: NFER-Nelson.

Goldthorpe SB, Lloyd N (1993) The awareness of and need for occupational therapy equipment and adaptations for elderly people. British Journal of Occupational Therapy 56(7): 243–6.

Golledge J (1988) Distinguishing between occupation, purposeful activity and activity, part 1: review and explanation. British Journal of Occupational Therapy 61(3): 100–5.

Great Britain (1995) Disability Discrimination Act. London: HMSO.

Green S (1995) Elderly mentally ill people and quality of life: who wants activities? British Journal of Occupational Therapy 58: 377–82.

Green S, Acheson Cooper B (2000) Occupation as a quality of life constituent: a nursing home perspective. British Journal of Occupational Therapy 63(1): 17–24.

Greene JG, Smith R, Gardiner M, Tinbury BC (1982) Measuring behavioural disturbance of elderly demented patients in the community and its effects on relatives: a factor analytic study. Age and Ageing 11: 121–6.

Grundy E (1995) Demographic influences on the future of family care. In: I Allen, E Perkins (eds), The Future of Family Care for Older People. London: HMSO.

Hambly M, Adams S (2003) Should I stay or should I go? Developing housing options for older people. Nottingham: Care and Repair England.

Hannan D (1997) More than a cup of tea: meaning construction in an everyday occupation. Journal of Occupational Science, Australia 4(2): 69–74.

Hanson EJ, Clarke A (2000) The role of telematics in assisting family carers and frail older people at home. Health and Social Care in the Community 8(2): 129–37.

Harbour R, Miller J (2001) A new system for grading recommendations in evidence based guidelines. British Medical Journal 323: 334–6.

Harrison S, Politt C (1994) Controlling Health Professionals; The Future of Work and Organisation in the NHS. Milton Keynes: Open University Press.

Hassall J (1993) Why do hospital based occupational therapists carry out post discharge home visits with elderly people? British Journal of Occupational Therapy 56(9): 325–9.

Hasselkus BR (1992) The meaning of activity; day care for persons with Alzheimer disease. American Journal of Occupational Therapy 46(3): 199–206.

Havighurst RJ, Albrecht R (1953) Older People. New York: Longman Press.

Hayward C, Ashlee P (1999) A study of the Provision of Adaptations Funded by Disabled Facilities Grants by a Social Services Occupational Therapy Department within one London Borough. Location unknown.

Health Act (1999) London: DoH.

Health Advisory Service (1982) The Rising Tide. London: HMSO.

Health Advisory Service (2000) Not because they are very old: an independent enquiry into the care of older people on acute wards in district general hospitals. London: HAS 2000.

Health and Safety Commission (1999) Manual Handling in the Health Services. Sudbury: HSE.

Health and Safety Executive (1992) S1 1992/2793 Manual Handling Operations Regulations. London: HMSO.

Healy J, Yarrow S (1997) Parents Living with Children in Old Age. Joseph Rowntree Foundation, Findings, Social Care Research 100.

Henwood M (1999) The Future of Health and Care of Older People: The Best Is Yet to Come. London: Age Concern England.

Herbert G, Mort M (1996) Thinking Across Boundaries: Integration of Occupational Therapy Services. Leeds: Nuffield Institute for Health.

Herbert G, Townsend J, Ryan T et al. (2000) Rehabilitation Pathways for Older People after Fractured Neck of Femur. Leeds: Nuffield Institute for Health and York Health Economics Consortium.

Heywood F (2001) The Effectiveness of Housing Adaptations. York: Joseph Rowntree Foundation, Findings, Ref 811.

Heywood F, Smart G (1996) Funding Adaptations: The Need to Cooperate. Findings: housing research 186. York: Policy Press with Joseph Rowntree Foundation.

Higher Education Funding Council for England (2001) Research in nursing and the allied health professions. Report of Task Group 3 to HEFCE and the Department of Health. Bristol: HEFCE. www.hefce.ac.uk/Pubs/hefce/2001/01_63.htm

Hoad P (2002) Drawing the Line: The Boundaries of Volunteering in the Community Care of Older People. Health and Social Care in the Community 10(4): 239–46.

Hobson JP, Edwards NI, Meara RJ (2001) The Parkinson's disease activities of daily living scale: a new and brief subjective measure of disability in Parkinson's disease. Clinical Rehabilitation 15: 241–46.

Hockey J, James A (1993) Growing up and growing old: a discussion of ageing and dependency in the life course. Generations Review 3(4): 2–4.

Hodgson C, Higginson I, Jefferys P (1998) Carer's checklist – an outcome measure for people with dementia and their carers. London: Mental Health Foundation.

Hollingbery R (1999) You can't ring the bell! Generations Review 9(1): 17–19.

Horne D (1998) Getting better? Inspection of hospital discharge arrangements for older people. Wetherby: Social Care Group, DoH.

Hornstein Z (2001) Age Discrimination Legislation: Choices for the UK. York: Joseph Rowntree Foundation and Policy Press Findings.

Hughes-Roberts J, Redfern Jones T (1990) A novel remit. Nursing Times, 27 March, 87(13): 226–28.

Human Rights Act (1999) London: Stationery Office.

Hunt A (1978) The Elderly at Home: A Study of People Aged 65 and Over Living in the Community in 1976. London: OPCS.

Hunt SM, McEwen J, McKenna SP (1985) Measuring health status: a new tool for clinicians and epidemiologists. Journal of the Royal College of General Practitioners 35: 185–8.

Hurst K (1996) The managerial and clinical implications of patient-focussed care. Journal of Management in Medicine 10(3): 59–77.

Huusko TM, Karppi P, Avikainen V et al. (2000) Randomised, clinically controlled trial of intensive geriatric rehabilitation in patients with hip fracture: subgroup analysis of patients with dementia. British Medical Journal 321: 1107–11.

Ilott I, Mounter C (2000) Occupational science: an impossible dream or agenda for action. British Journal of Occupational Therapy 63(5): 238–40.

Ilott I, White E (2001) 2001 College of Occupational Therapists' research and development strategic vision and action plan. British Journal of Occupational Therapy 64(6): 270–7.

Improvement and Development Agency for Local Government (2000) Local Authority Occupational Therapy Workload Survey, 1999. London: I&DEA.

Intercollegiate Working Party for Stroke (1999) National Clinical Guidelines for Stroke. London: Royal College of Physicians.

Iwarsson S (1999) The housing enabler: an objective tool for assessing accessibility. British Journal of Occupational Therapy 62(11): 491–5.

Iwarsson S, Isacsson I (1998) ADL independence in the elderly population living in the community: the influence of functional limitations and physical environmental demand. Occupational Therapy International 5(3): 173–93.

Jackson J (1996) Living a meaningful existence in old age. In: R Zemke, F Clarke (eds), Occupational Science: The Evolving Discipline. Philadelphia: FA Davies.

Jackson J, Carlson M, Mandel D et al. (1998) Occupation in Lifestyle Redesign: The Well Elderly Study Occupational Therapy Programme. American Journal of Occupational Therapy 52(5): 326–36.

Jackson J, Mandel DR, Zemke R, Clarke FA (2001) Promoting quality of life in elders: an occupation-based occupational therapy program. WFOT Bulletin 43: 5–12.

James F (2002) The OT in A&E experience. Occupational Therapy News, Jan 2002, 10/1, 25.

Jeffers B (1995) Structuring time in retirement. Generations Review 5(2): 9–11.

Jeffrys M (1996) Bradeley retirement village: a good or bad thing? Generations Review 6(1): 1997.

Jenkins J, Felce D, Lunt B, Powell L (1977) Increasing engagement in activity of residents in old people's homes by providing recreational materials. Behaviour Therapy Research 15: 429–34.

Jonsson H, Kielhofner G, Borell L (1997) Anticipating retirement: the formation of narratives concerning an occupational transition. American Journal of Occupational Therapy 51(1): 49–56.

Jonsson H, Borell L, Sadlo G (2000) Retirement: an occupational transition with consequences for temporality, balance and the meaning of occupations. Journal of Occupational Science 7(1): 29–37.

Jorm AF, Korten AE, Henderson AS (1987) The prevalence of dementia: a quantitative integration of the literature. Acta Psychiatrica Scandanavica 76: 465–79.

Jorm AF, Henderson S, Mackinnon AJ et al. (1993) The disabled elderly living in the community: care received from family and formal services. Medical Journal of Australia 158: 383–8.

Kemp B, Kleinplatz F (1985) Vocational rehabilitation of the older worker. American Journal of Occupational Therapy 39(5): 322–6.

Kendall A (1996) Preparation for retirement: the occupational perspective. Journal of Occupational Science: Australia 3(1): 35–8.

Khaw K-T (1997) Healthy aging. British Medical Journal 315: 1090–6.

Khaw K-T (1999) How many, how old, how soon? British Medical Journal 319: 1350–2.

Kielhofner G (1985) A Model of Human Occupation: Theory and Application. Baltimore, MD: Williams & Wilkins; 2nd edn, 1995.

Kielhofner G, Nicol M (1989) The model of human occupation: a developing conceptual tool for clinicians. British Journal of Occupational Therapy 60(3): 103–10.

Kielhofner G, Forsythe K (1997) The model of human occupation: an overview of current concepts. British Journal of Occupational Therapy 52: 210–14.

Kielhofner G, Henry AD (1988) Development and investigation of the Occupational Performance Interview. American Journal of Occupational Therapy 42: 489–98.

Kielhofner G, Henry AD, Whalens D (1989) A User's Guide to the Occupational Performance History Interview. Bethesda, MD: American Occupational Therapy Association.

King's Fund (2001) Rehabilitation Services Provided in Residential Care Homes: Information Pack. London: King's Fund rehabilitation programme.

Kirkland S, Mitchell T (1995) Occupational therapy in an orthopaedic early discharge programme. Australian Occupational Therapy Journal 42: 31–4.

Kitwood T (1997) Dementia Reconsidered. Buckingham: Open University Press.

Klein SI, Rosage L, Shaw G (1999) The role of occupational therapists in home modification programs at an area agency on aging. Physical and Occupational Therapy in Geriatrics 16(3/4): 19–37.

Kneebone I, Harrop A (1996) Patient confidence in return home: development of a measurement instrument. Australian Occupational Therapy Journal 43: 19–23.

Knipscheer CPM, Broese van Groenou MI, Leene GJF et al. (2000) The effects of environmental context and personal resources on depressive symptomatology in older age: a test of the Lawton model. Ageing and Society 20: 183–202.

Kogan M, Redfern S (1995) Making Use of Clinical Audit: A Guide to Practice in the Health Professions. Buckingham: Open University Press.

Kreibich N, Todd B, Holt G, Smith T (1991) Care of the elderly patient following surgery for a fracture of the proximal femur. Health Trends 27(2): 43–5.

Lambert R (1998) Occupation and lifestyle: implications for mental health practice. British Journal of Occupational Therapy 61(5): 193–7.

Landes R, Popay J (1993) 'My sight is poor but I'm getting on now'; the health and social care needs of older people with vision problems. Health and Social Care in the Community 7(3): 325–35.

Lau A, Chi I, McKenna K (1998) Occupational Therapy International 5(2): 118–39.

Law M, Baptiste S, Carswell A et al. (1994) Canadian Occupational Performance Measure, 2nd edn. Hamilton, Ontario: Canadian Association of Occupational Therapists.

Law M, Cooper B, Strong S et al. (1996) The person-environment-occupation model; a transactive approach to occupational performance. Canadian Journal of Occupational Therapy 63(1): 9–23.

Law M, Stewart D, Letts L et al. (1999) Effectiveness of Activity Programmes for Older Persons with Dementia: A Critical Review of the Evidence. McMaster University, Hamilton, Ontario: Occupational Therapy Evidence-Based Practice Research Group.

Lawton MP (1975) Philadelphia Geriatric Center Morale scale: a revision. Journal of Gerontology 30: 85–9.

Leather P, Sykes R (undated) The Future of Community Care: A Consumer Perspective. Oxford: Anchor Housing Trust.

Lee V, Ross B, Tracy B (2001) Functional assessment of older adults in an emergency department. Canadian Journal of Occupational Therapy, April: 121–9.

Legg L, Drummond AE (2003) Occupational therapy for patients with problems in activities of daily living after stroke (Cochrane Review). In: The Cochrane Library, Issue 1, 2003. Oxford: Update Software.

Letts L, Law M, Rigby P et al. (1994) Person-environment assessments in occupational therapists. American Journal of Occupational Therapy 48(7): 608–18.

Letts L, Scott S, Burtney J et al. (1998) The reliability and validity of the safety assessment of function and the environment for rehabilitation (SAFER tool). British Journal of Occupational Therapy 61(3): 127–32.

Levin E, Sinclair I, Gorbach P (1994) Better for the Break. London: NISW.

Levin RE, Gitlin LN (1992) A model to promote activity competence in elders. American Journal of Occupational Therapy 4(2): 147–53.

Lewis H, Fletcher P, Hardy B et al. (1999) Developing a Preventive Approach with Older People. London: Anchor Trust.

Lindesay J, Marudkar M, van Diepen E, Wilcock G (2002) The second Leicester survey of memory clinics in the British Isles. International Journal of Geriatric Psychiatry 17: 41–7.

Lister R (1999) Loss of ability to drive following stroke: the early experiences of three elderly people on discharge from hospital. British Journal of Occupational Therapy 62(11): 514–20.

Logan PA, Ahern J, Gladman JRF, Lincoln NB (1997) A randomised controlled trial of enhanced occupational therapy for stroke patients. Clinical Rehabilitation 11(2): 107–13.

Lothian K, Philp I (2001) Maintaining the dignity and autonomy of older people in the healthcare setting. British Medical Journal 322: 668–70.

Luce A, McKeith I, Swann A et al. (2001) How do memory clinics compare with traditional old age psychiatry services? International Journal of Geriatric Psychiatry 16(9): 837–45.

Ludwig FM (1997) How routine facilitates well being in elderly women. Occupational Therapy International 4: 213–28.

Lysack CL, MacNeill SE, Neufield SW, Lichtenberg PA (2002) Elderly inner city women who return home to live alone. Occupational Therapy Journal of Rehabilitation 22(2): 59–69.

McCloughry H, Murphy A (1998) Disabled and older people in the community: issues of dependency – an occupational therapy project. Nottingham: Nottingham Social Services.

McCreadie C (1996) Elder Abuse: Update on Research. London: Age Concern Institute of Gerontology.

McCreadie C, Seale J, Tinker A, Turner-Smith A (2002) Older people and mobility in the home: in search of useful assistive technologies. British Journal of Occupational Therapy 65(2): 54–60.

MacDonald AJD (1997) ABC of mental health in old age. British Medical Journal 315: 413–17.

Mace NL (1990) Management of problem behaviours. In: NL Mace (ed.), Dementia Care: Patient, Family and Community. Baltimore: Johns Hopkins University Press.

McInnes E, Powell J (1994) Drug and alcohol referrals: are elderly substance abuse diagnoses and referrals being missed out? British Medical Journal 308: 444–6.

McIntyre A (1999) Elderly fallers: a baseline audit of admissions to a day hospital for elderly people. British Journal of Occupational Therapy 62(6): 244–8.

McKee KJ (1998) The body drop: a framework for understanding recovery from falls in older people. Generations Review 8(4): 11–14.

McKenna SP, Hunt SM (1991) Elderly patients and the National Health Service. Journal of the Royal Society of Health 111(4): 126–30.

Mackenzie L (2001) Falls amongst older people in the community: a snapshot of research and practice. WFOT Bulletin 43: 13–17.

Mackintosh SA, Leather P (1994) Funding and managing the adaptation of owner occupied homes for people with physical disabilities. Health and Social Care in the Community 2(4): 229–39.

McLean D, Lord S (1996) Falling in older people at home: transfer limitations and environmental risk factors. Australian Occupational Therapy Journal 43: 13–18.

McWalter G, Toner T, McWalter A et al. (1998) A community needs assessment; the CarenapD. International Journal of Geriatric Psychiatry 13: 16–22.

Mahoney FI, Barthel DW (1965) Functional evaluation: the Barthel Index. Maryland State Medical Journal 14: 61–5.

Mandel D, Jackson J, Zemke R et al. (1999) Lifestyle Redesign: Implementing the Well Elderly Program. Bethesda: American Occupational Therapy Association.

Mandelstam M (1993) How to Get Equipment for Disability. London: Disabled Living Foundation.

Mandelstam M (1997) Equipment for Older and Disabled People. London: Jessica Kingsley.

Mandelstam M (2001) Safe use of disability equipment and manual handling: legal aspects – part 2, manual handling. British Journal of Occupational Therapy 64(2): 73–80.

Mann A, Graham N, Ashby D (1984) Psychiatric illness in residential homes for the elderly: a survey in one London Borough. Age and Ageing 13: 257–65.

Mann WC, Hurren D, Tomita M et al. (1994) Environmental problems in homes of elders with disabilities. Occupational Therapy Journal of Research 14(3): 191–211.

Marshall M (ed.) (2000) Astrid: A Social and Technological Response to Meeting the Needs of Individuals with Dementia and Their Carers. Stirling: Dementia Services Development Centre. http://www/ASTRIDGuide.org

Marshall T (1997) Infected and affected: HIV, AIDS and the older adult. Generations Review 7(4): 9–11.

Martin J, Meltzer H, Elliot D (1988) The Prevalence of Disability among Adults. London: OPCS Surveys of Disability in Great Britain, HMSO.

Mayers CA (1998) An evaluation of the use of the Mayers' lifestyle questionnaire. British Journal of Occupational Therapy 61(9): 393–8.

Means R (2002) History lessons for the 'modernisers' of health and welfare. Generations Review 12(2): 10–12.

Medical Research Council (1994) The Health of the UK's Elderly People. London: MRC.

Medical Research Council Cognitive Function and Ageing Study (MRC CFAS) and Resource Implications Study (RIS MRC CFAS) (2000) Profile of disability in elderly people: estimates from a longitudinal implications study. British Medical Journal 318: 1108–11.

Meetham K, Thompson C (1992) Setting up the Scarcroft project – the problems of joint working. Caring for People 9: 6–7.

Metitieri T, Zanetti O, Geroldi C et al. (2001) Reality orientation therapy to delay outcomes of progression in patients with dementia. A retrospective study. Clinical Rehabilitation 15: 471–8.

Metz D (2000) Innovation to prevent dependency in old age. British Medical Journal 320: 460–1.

Miller JA (1991) Community Based Long Term Care: Innovative Models. London: Sage Publications.

Minkler M, Estes CA (eds) (2000) Critical Perspectives on Ageing; The Political and Moral Economy of Growing Old. New York: Baywood Publishing Co.

Mistiaen P, Duijnhower E, Wijkel D et al. (1997) The problems of elderly people at home one week after discharge from an acute care setting. Journal of Advanced Nursing 25: 1233–40.

Mitchell E (2000) Managing carer stress: an evaluation of a stress management programme for carers of people with dementia. British Journal of Occupational Therapy 63(4): 179–83.

Mountain G (1997) Services for Physically Frail Older People: Developing a Total Service Approach within an Intermediate Care Framework. Leeds: Nuffield Institute for Health.

Mountain G (1998a) An Investigation into the Activity of Occupational Therapists Working with the Elderly Mentally Ill. University of Leeds, unpublished PhD thesis.

Mountain G (1998b) Rehabilitation of Vulnerable Older People: Nature of the Evidence Base and Implications for Occupational Therapists. London: College of Occupational Therapists.

Mountain G (1998c) The delivery of community mental health services to older people. Mental Health Review 3(1): 7–15.

Mountain G (2000) Occupational Therapy in Social Services Departments: A Review of the Literature. London: College of Occupational Therapists and Centre for Evidence Based Social Services.

Mountain G (2001a) United we stand, divided we fall! British Journal of Occupational Therapy 64(3): 153–4.

Mountain G (2001b) The contribution of the occupational therapist to the diagnosis, assessment and treatment of depression in old age. In: S Curran, JP Wattis, S Lynch (eds), Practical management of depression in older people. London: Hodder Headline.

Mountain G (2002) Integrating health and social care: the experience of occupational therapy. Managing Community Care 10(2): 44–8.

Mountain G (forthcoming) Rehabilitation for people with dementia: pointers for practice from the evidence base. In: M Marshall (ed.), Think Rehab. London: Jessica Kingsley.

Mountain G, Bowie P (1992) The possessions owned by long stay psychogeriatric patients. International Journal of Geriatric Psychiatry 7: 285–90.

Mountain G, Bowie P (1995) The quality of long-term care for dementia: a survey of ward environments. International Journal of Geriatric Psychiatry 10: 1029–35.

Mountain G, Godfrey M (1995) Respite care provision for older people with dementia: a review of the literature. Leeds: Nuffield Institute for Health.

Mountain G, Moore J (1995) Quality of Life of Older People. University of Leeds, unpublished study.

Mountain G, Moore J (1996) What Do Occupational Therapists Working with Older People Do? Leeds: Nuffield Institute for Health.

Mountain G, Lepley D (1998) Finding and Using the Evidence Base: General Principles. London: College of Occupational Therapists.

Mountain G, Sealey C (1999) Developing Clinical Guidelines for Occupational Therapy Practice. London: College of Occupational Therapists.

Mountain G, Pighills A (2003) Pre-discharge visits with older people: time to review practice. Health and Social Care in the Community 11(20): 146–54.

Mountain GA, Bowie PCW, Dabbs AR (1990) Preliminary report on nurse job satisfaction on wards for the elderly mentally ill. Health Services Management Research 3(1): 22–30.

Mountain G, Bowie P, Dabbs A (1994) The relationship between well-being and job satisfaction for staff working on long stay wards for the elderly confused. Health Services Management Research 7(4): 229–34.

Mountain G, Carman S, Ilott I (2001) Work Rehabilitation and Occupational Therapy: A Review of the Literature. London: College of Occupational Therapists.

Muir Gray JA (1997) Evidence Based Health Care: How to Make Policy and Management Decisions. London: Churchill Livingstone.

Mulley GP (1995) Preparing for the late years. The Lancet 345: 1409–13.

Murphy E (1986) Dementia and Mental Illness in the Old. London: Papermac.

Murphy E (1999) With respect to old age. British Medical Journal 318: 681–2.

Murray SA, Manktelow K, Clifford C (2000) The interplay between social and cultural context and perceptions of cardiovascular disease. Journal of Advanced Nursing 32(5): 1224–34.

Mynatt ED, Rogers WA (Winter 2001/2002) Developing technology to support the functional independence of older adults. Ageing International 27(1): 24–41.

Nancarrow S, Mountain G (2002) Staffing Intermediate Care Services: A Review of the Literature to Inform Workforce Planning. Sheffield: Sheffield Hallam University.

National Association of Neurological Occupational Therapists (2000) National Clinical Guidelines for Stroke: Impact on Occupational Therapy Practice. London: NANOT (College of Occupational Therapists).

National Audit Office (1994) National Health Service Day Hospitals for Elderly People in England: Report by the Comptroller and Auditor General. London: HMSO.

National Back Exchange, Royal College of Nursing, Ergonomics Society, College of Occupational Therapists Chartered Society of Physiotherapists (1998) The Inter-Professional Curriculum Framework for Back Care Advisors. London: HSE.

National Coordinating Centre for Health Technology Assessment (2000) Disability Equipment and Adaptations to Facilitate Early Discharge from Hospital. Health Technology Brief, 030, Southampton, NCCHTA.

National Health Service Executive (1996) Promoting Clinical Effectiveness: A Framework for Action in and through the NHS. Leeds: DoH.

National Health Service Executive South West Regional Office, Social Services Inspectorate & Older Persons Modernisation Team (2001) Intermediate Care Classification of Terms. Bristol: Older Persons Modernisation Team.

National Institute for Social Work (1988) Residential Care – A Positive Choice. Report of the Independent Review of Residential Care. London: HMSO.

Naylor MD, Brooten D, Campbell R et al. (1999) Comprehensive discharge planning and home follow-up of hospitalized elders: a randomized controlled trial. Journal of the American Medical Association 281(7): 613–20.

Neal M, Briggs M (1999) Validation therapy for dementia (Cochrane Review). In: The Cochrane Library, Issue 1, 2000. Oxford: Update Software.

Neill J, Williams J (1992) Leaving Hospital: Elderly People and Their Discharge to Community Care. London: National Institute for Social Work.

Nelson DL (1988) Occupation: form and function. American Journal of Occupational Therapy 42(10): 633–41.

Nelson DL (1997) Why the profession of occupational therapy will flourish in the 21st century. American Journal of Occupational Therapy 51(1): 13–24.

Netten A, Smith P, Healey A et al. (2002) OPUS: a measure of social care outcome for older people. PSSRU: research summary 23.

Neville-Jan A, Verrier Piersol C, Kielhofner G (1993) Adaptive equipment: a study of utilization after discharge. Occupational Therapy in Health Care 8(4): 3–14.

Nocon A (1993) GPs' assessment of people aged 75 and over: identifying the need for occupational therapy services. British Journal of Occupational Therapy 56(4): 123–6.

Nocon A, Baldwin S (1998) Trends in Rehabilitation Policy: A Review of the Literature. London: Audit Commission and King's Fund.

Nolan MR, Caldock K (1996) Assessment: identifying the barriers to good practice. Health and Social Care in the Community 4(2): 77–85.

Nolan MR, Grant G (1991) Respite care: factors influencing consumer perceptions of quality and acceptability. In: F Laczko, C Victor (eds) Social Policy and Elderly People. Aldershot: Avebury.

Nolan MR, Grant G (1993) Service evaluation: time to open both eyes. Journal of Advanced Nursing 18: 1434–42.

Nolan MR, Grant G, Ellis NC (1990) Stress is in the eye of the beholder: reconceptualising the measurement of carer burden. Journal of Advanced Nursing 15: 544–55.

Nuffield Institute for Health (1997) Involving older people in research. Bulletin of the Collaborative Centre for Priority Services Research 4, Spring.

Nuffield Institute for Health (2000) Meeting the Standard? Analysis of the First Round of Local 'Better Care Higher Standards' Charters. University of Leeds: Nuffield Institute for Health.

Nuffield Institute for Health (2002) Exclusivity or Inclusion? Meeting Mental Health Needs in Intermediate Care. Leeds: Nuffield Institute for Health with the Joseph Rowntree Foundation.

O'Caithan A (1994) Evaluation of a hospital at home scheme for the early discharge of patients with fractured neck of femur. Public Health Medicine 16(2): 205–10.

Oldman C (2000) Is Enhanced Sheltered Housing an Effective Replacement for Residential Care for Older People? York: Joseph Rowntree Foundation, Findings Ref D30.

Oliver R, Blathway J, Brackley C, Tamaki T (1993) Safety assessment of function and the environment for rehabilitation (SAFER). Canadian Journal of Occupational Therapy 60: 127–32.

Opinion Leader Research (2001) A report on the Findings of a Listening Exercise Conducted with People from Socially Excluded Groups Evaluating the Discussion Documents: 'Reforming the NHS Complaints Procedure' and 'Involving Patients and the Public in Health Care'. London: Prepared for the DoH.

Opit L, Pahl J (1993) Institutional care for elderly people; can we predict admissions? Research, Policy and Planning 10(2): 2–5.

Packham G (1999) Quality assurance and clinical audit: information and equipment provision. British Journal of Occupational Therapy 62(6): 278–82.

Parker CJ, Gladman JRF, Drummond AER et al. (2001) A multicentre randomized controlled trial of leisure therapy and conventional occupational therapy after stroke. Clinical Rehabilitation 15: 42–52.

Parker G, Lawton D (1994) Different Types of Care, Different Types of Carer: Evidence from the General Household Survey. London: HMSO.

Parker MG, Thorslund M (1991) The use of technical aids among community based elderly. American Journal of Occupational Therapy 45(8): 712–18.

Parker S (2002) Rehabilitation of Older Patients: Day Hospital Compared to Rehabilitation at Home. National Research Register. www.tap.ccta.gov.uk

Parkes J, Shepperd S (2001) Discharge Planning from Hospital to Home (Cochrane Review). In: The Cochrane Library, 4. Oxford: Update Software.

Patterson CJ, Mulley GP (1999) The effectiveness of predischarge home assessment visits: a systematic review. Clinical Rehabilitation 15: 291–5.

Pattie AH, Gilleard CJ (1979) Manual of Clifton Assessment Procedures for the Elderly (CAPE). Sevenoaks: Hodder & Stoughton Educational.

Payne S, Hanley M, Coleman P (2000) Interactions between nurses during handovers in elderly care. Journal of Advanced Nursing 32(2): 277–85.

Peace S, Kellaher L, Willcocks D (1997) Re-evaluating Residential Care. Buckingham: Open University Press.

Perrin T (1996) The role and value of occupation in dementia care. Generations Review 6(1): 12.

Perrin T (1997) Occupational needs in severe dementia: a descriptive study. Journal of Advanced Nursing 25: 934–41.

Perrin, T (2001) Don't despise the fluffy bunny: a reflection from practice. British Journal of Occupational Therapy 64(3): 129–34.

Perrin T, May H (2000) Wellbeing in Dementia: An Occupational Approach for Therapists and Carers. London: Churchill Livingstone.

Peter A (1994) Glenrothes geriatric day hospital: role clarification and its implications. Health Bulletin 52(1): 4–11.

Phillips N, Renton L (1995) Is assessment of function the core of occupational therapy. British Journal of Occupational Therapy 58(2): 72–4.

Pointon S (1997) Myths and negative attitudes about sexuality in older people. Generations Review 7(4): 6–8.

Pound P, Gompertez P (1999) A patient-centred study of the consequences of stroke. Clinical Rehabilitation 12: 338–47.

Pound P, Gompertez P, Ebrahim S (1993) Development and results of a questionnaire to measure carer satisfaction after stroke. Journal of Epidemiology and Community Health 47(6): 500–5.

Powell Lawton M (1983) Environment and other determinants of well-being in older people. Gerontologist 23: 349–57.

Prasher V (1995) Age specific prevalence, thyroid dysfunction and depressive symptomatology in adults with Down's syndrome and dementia. International Journal of Geriatric Psychiatry 19: 25–31.

Primrose CS, Primrose WR (1992) Geriatric respite care: present practice and potential for improvement. Health Bulletin 50(5): 399–405.

Provence MA, Hadley EC, Hornbrook MC et al. (1995) The effects of exercise on falls in elderly patients: a preplanned meta-analysis of the FICSIT trials. Journal of the American Medical Association 273(17): 1341–7.

Qureshi H, Walker A (1989) The Caring Relationship: Elderly People and Their Families. Basingstoke: Macmillan.

Rai GS, Kinirons M, Wientjes H (1995) Falls handicap inventory: an instrument used to measure handicaps associated with repeated falls. Journal of the American Geriatrics Society 43: 723–4.

Ramsay D, Coid DR (1994) Home Treatment Team: Operational Policy. London: Riverside Mental Health Trust, Elderly Care Services.

Raynes N (1999) Older residents' participation in specifying quality in nursing and residential care homes. Generations Review 9(2): 10–12.

Raynes N, Temple B, Glenister C, Coulthard L (2001) Involving service users in defining home care specifications. York: Joseph Rowntree Foundation, Findings 2001, no 611.

Reddy S, Pitt B (1993) What becomes of demented patients referred to a psychogeriatric unit? An approach to audit. International Journal of Geriatric Society 8: 175–80.

Reich S, Tilling K, Hopper A (1998) Clinical decision making, risk and occupational therapy. Health and Social Care in the Community 6(1): 47–54.

Reynolds T, Thornicroft G, Abas M et al. (2000) The Camberwell assessment of need for the elderly (CANE). Development, validity and reliability. British Journal of Psychiatry 176: 444–52.

Richards SH, Coast J, Gunnell DJ et al. (1998) Randomised controlled trial comparing effectiveness and acceptability of an early discharge, hospital at home scheme with acute hospital care. British Medical Journal 316: 1796–1801.

Rickard W (1995) HIV/AIDS and older people. Generations Review 5(3): 2–6.

Riley J (2002) Occupational therapy in social services: a missed opportunity? British Journal of Occupational Therapy 65(11): 502–8.

Robb B (1967) Sans Everything. London: Thomas Nelson.

Robertson MC, Devlin N, Gardner MM, Campbell AJ (2001) Effectiveness and economic evaluation of a nurse delivered home exercise programme to prevent falls. 1: randomised controlled trial. British Medical Journal 322: 697–701.

Robinson BC (1983) Validation of a caregiver strain index. Journal of Gerontology 38(3): 344–8.

Robinson J, Batstone G (1996) Rehabilitation: A Development Challenge. London: King's Fund Publishing.

Robinson RA (1961) Some problems of clinical trials in elderly people. Gerontologia Clinical 3: 247–57.

Royal College of Physicians (1989) Fractured Neck of Femur: Prevention and Management. London: Royal College of Physicians.

Royal College of Psychiatrists (1998) Health of the Nation Outcome Scales for Older Adults (HoNOS 65+). London: Royal College of Psychiatrists.

Royal Commission on Long Term Care (1999) With Respect to Old Age: Long Term Care – Rights and Responsibilities. London: Stationery Office.

Rudd AG, Irwin P, Rutledge Z et al. (2001) Regional variations in stroke care in England, Wales and Northern Ireland: results from the National Sentinel Audit of Stroke. Clinical Rehabilitation 15: 562–72.

Sacket DL, Richardson WS, Rosenberg W (1997) Evidence-based Medicine: How to Practise and Teach Evidence-Based Medicine. Edinburgh: Churchill Livingstone.

Sainty M (1990) Effective identification of elderly patients requiring occupational therapy. British Journal of Occupational Therapy 53(2): 57–60.

Salkeld G, Cameron ID, Cumming RG et al. (2000) Quality of life related to fear of falling and hip fracture in older women: a time trade off study. British Medical Journal 320: 341–6.

Sanford RA (1975) Tolerance of debility in elderly dependents by supporters at home: its significance for hospital practice. British Medical Journal 3: 471–3.

Schemm R (1993) Bridging conflicting ideologies: the origins of American and British occupational therapy. American Journal of Occupational Therapy 48(11): 1082–8.

Schemm RL, Gitlin L (1998) How occupational therapists teach older people to use bathing and dressing devices in rehabilitation. American Journal of Occupational Therapy 25(4): 276–81.

Schweitzer JA, Mann WC, Nochajski S, Tomita M (1999) Patterns of engagement in leisure activity by older adults using assistive devices. Technology and Disability 11: 103–17.

Scott I (1999) Optimising care of the hospitalised elderly: a literature review and suggestions for future research. Australian and New Zealand Journal of Medicine 29(2): 254–64.

Scottish Centre for the Promotion of the Older Person's Agenda (2003) Update no. 3. Edinburgh: Queen Margaret University College.

Scottish Executive Health Department (2000) Our National Health: A Plan for Action, a Plan for Change. Edinburgh: Scottish Executive.

Scottish Executive Health Department (2001) Better Care for All Our Futures. Edinburgh: Scottish Executive.

Scrutton S (1992) Ageing, Healthy and in Control. London: Chapman & Hall.

Scrutton S (1999) Counselling Older People. London: Arnold.

Sealey C (1998) Clinical Audit Information Pack. London: College of Occupational Therapists.

Sealey C (1999) Clinical Governance: An Information Guide for Occupational Therapists. London: College of Occupational Therapists.

Seddon D, Robinson CA (2001) Carers of older people with dementia: assessment and the Carers Act. Health and Social Care in the Community 9(3): 151–8.

Sheffield Institute for Studies on Ageing (1997) EASY-Care: Elderly Assessment Instrument UK version 1999–2002. Sheffield: Community Sciences Centre, Northern General Hospital.

Sheill A, Kenny P, Farnworth MG (1993) The role of the clinical nurse coordinator in the provision of cost effective orthopaedic services for older people. Journal of Advanced Nursing 18: 1424–8.

Sheldon B (1995) Cognitive Behavioural Therapy: Research, Practice and Philosophy. London: Routledge.

Sihto M (1999) Increasing older persons' employment in Finland: in search of a new strategy. Journal of Ageing and Social Policy 10(3): 65–81.

Simpson JM, Marsh N, Harrington R (1998) Guidelines for managing falls among elderly people. British Journal of Occupational Therapy 61(4): 165–8.

Sinclair A, Dickinson E (1998) Effective Practice in Rehabilitation. London: Audit Commission and King's Fund.

Sinclair I, Parker R, Leat D, Williams, J (1990) The Kaleidoscope of Care: Review of Research on Welfare Provision for Elderly People. London: NISW, HMSO.

Smith RD, Widiatmoko D (1998) The cost effectiveness of home assessment and modification to reduce falls in the elderly. New England Journal of Public Health 22(4): 436–40.

Smith RO (1992) The science of occupational therapy assessment. Occupational Therapy Journal of Research 12(1): 3–15.

Social Policy Ageing Information Network (SPAIN) (2001) The Underfunding of Social Care and its Consequences for Older People. London: Help the Aged and Age Concern.

Social Services Inspectorate and Department of Health (1993) Guidance on Standards for Short Term Breaks. London: HMSO.

Social Services Inspectorate and Department of Health (1995) Social Service Departments and the Care Programme Approach: An Inspection. London: DoH.

Social Services Inspectorate and Department of Health (1997a) At Home with Dementia. London: DoH.

Social Services Inspectorate and Department of Health (1997b) Assessing Older People with Dementia Living in the Community. London: DoH.

Sopp L, Wood L (2001) Consumer and industry views of lifetime homes. JRF Findings, ref. 371.

South and East Belfast Trust (undated) ITHACA: Telematics for Integrated, Client Centred Community Care. Belfast: S&E Trust.

Spector A, Orrell M, Davies S, Woods RT (1998a) Reminiscence therapy for dementia (Cochrane Review). In: The Cochrane Library, Issue 1, 2000. Oxford: Update Software.

Spector A, Orrell M, Davies S, Woods RT (1998b) Reality orientation for dementia (Cochrane Review). In: The Cochrane Library, Issue 1, 2000. Oxford: Update Software.

Spence JC, Davidson HA (1998) The community adaptive planning assessment: a clinical tool for documenting future planning with clients. American Journal of Occupational Therapy 52(1): 19–29.

Spence JC, Hersch G, Eschenfelder V, Fournet J, Murray-Gerzik M (1998) Outcomes of protocol-based and adaptation-based occupational therapy interventions for low income elderly persons on a transitional unit. American Journal of Occupational Therapy 53(2): 159–70.

Standing Group on Consumers in NHS Research (1999) Involvement Works: Second Report of the Standing Group on Consumers in NHS Research. Winchester: Consumers in NHS Research Support Unit.

Stanhle A, Linquist I, Mattson E (2000) Important factors for physical activity among elderly patients one year after an acute myocardial infarction. Scandinavian Journal of Rehabilitation Medicine 32: 111–16.

Stanley M (1995) An investigation into the relationship between engagement in valued occupations and life satisfaction for elderly south Australians. Journal of Occupational Science, Australia 2(3): 100–14.

Steiner A (2001) Intermediate care: more than a nursing thing. Age and Ageing 30: 433–5.

Steiner A, Vaughan B (1997) Intermediate care: a discussion paper arising from a King's Fund seminar held on 30 October 1996. London: King's Fund.

Stewart LSP, McMillan (1998) Rehabilitation schemes for elderly people with a hip fracture. British Journal of Occupational Therapy 61(8): 367–70.

Stewart S (1999) Use of standardised and non-standardised assessments in a social services setting: implications for practice. British Journal of Occupational Therapy 62(9): 417–23.

Stroke Association (2001) Speaking Out About Stroke Services. London: Stroke Association.

Stroke Unit Trialists' Collaboration (2003) Organised inpatient (stroke unit) care for stroke (Cochrane Review). In: The Cochrane Library, Issue 1, 2003. Oxford: Update Software.

Strudwicke AM, Gillespie CR, Sever ED (1991) Using attitudes to predict daily living independence in stroke patients. British Journal of Occupational Therapy 54(3): 101–4.

Styrborn K (1995) Early discharge planning for elderly patients in acute hospitals: an intervention study. Scandinavian Journal of Social Medicine 23(4): 234–85.

Swift C (2001) Falls in later life and their consequences – implementing effective services. British Medical Journal 322: 855–7.

Tamm M (1999) What does a home mean and when does it cease to be a home? Home as a setting for rehabilitation and care. Disability and Rehabilitation 21(2): 49–55.

Tennant A (2001) Continuing care of adults with a physical and complex disability: identifying eligibility criteria and funding responsibility. National Research Register. www.tap.ccta.gov.uk

Tinker A (1995) Housing and older people. In: I Allen, E Perkins (eds), The Future of Family Care for Older People. London: HMSO.

Tinker A (1997) Older People in Modern Society, 4th edn. London: Longman.

Thornely G, Chamberlain MA, Wright V (1977) Evaluation of aids and equipment for the bath and toilet. British Journal of Occupational Therapy 40(10): 243–6.

Thornton P (1989) Creating a Break: A Home Relief Scheme for Elderly People and Their Carers. Mitcham: Age Concern England.

Thornton P, Mountain G (1992) A Positive Response: Developing Community Alarm Services for Older People. York: Joseph Rowntree Foundation and Community Care.

Townsend P (1962) The Last Refuge: A Survey of Residential Institutions and Homes for the Aged in England and Wales. London: Routledge & Kegan Paul.

Townsend J, Dyer S, Cooper J et al. (1992) Emergency admissions and readmissions of patients aged over 75 years and the effects of a community based discharge scheme. Health Trends 24(4): 136–9.

Tozer R, Thornton P (1995) A meeting of minds: older people as research advisers. University of York: Social Policy Research Unit, Social Policy Report No. 3.

Tullis A, Nicol M (1999) A systematic review of the evidence for the value of functional assessments of older people with dementia. British Journal of Occupational Therapy 62(12): 554–63.

Twigg J (1992) Carers in the service system. In: Twigg J (ed.), Carers: Research and Practice. London: HMSO.

Twigg J, Atkin K (1994) Carers Perceived: Policy and Practice in Informal Care. Milton Keynes: Open University Press.

Twigg J, Atkin K (1995) Carers and services: factors mediating service provision. Journal of Social Policy 24(1): 5–30.

Twigg J, Atkin K, Perring C (1990) Carers and Services: A Review of Research. London: HMSO.

Tyson S, Turner G (2000) Discharge and follow-up for people with stroke: what happens and why. Clinical Rehabilitation 14: 381–92.

van Diepen E, Baillon S, Redman J et al. (2002) A pilot study of the physiological and behavioural effects of Snoezelen in dementia. British Journal of Occupational Therapy 65(2): 61–6.

van Haastregt JCM, Dierderiks M, van Rossum E et al. (2000) Effects of preventive home visits to elderly people in the community: systematic review. British Medical Journal 320: 754–8.

Vaughan B, Lathlean J (1999) Intermediate Care: Models in Practice. London: King's Fund.

Venable E, Hanson C, Shechtman O, Dasler P (2000) The effects of exercise on occupational functioning in the well elderly. Physical and Occupational Therapy in Geriatrics 17(4): 29–42.

Verbrugge LM, Rennert C, Madans JH (1997) The greater efficacy of personal and equipment assistance in reducing disability. American Journal of Public Health 87(3): 384–92.

Victor CR, Healey J, Thomas A, Seargant J (2000) Older patients and delayed discharge from hospital. Health and Social Care in the Community 8(6): 443–52.

Vincent C, Drouin G, Routhier F (1999) Environmental control systems for disabled and older adults: a challenge on the threshold of a new millennium. Germany: Proceedings of the AAATE Conference 1999.

Wade DT, Legh-Smith J, Hewer RL (1985) Social activities after stroke. International Journal of Rehabilitation Medicine 7(4): 176–81.

Walker MF, Gladman JRF, Lincoln NB et al. (1999) Occupational therapy for stroke patients not admitted to hospital. The Lancet 354: 278–80.

Ward G, Macaulay F, Jagger C, Harper W (1998) Standardised assessment: a comparison of the community dependency index and the Barthel Index with an elderly hip fracture population. British Journal of Occupational Therapy 61(3): 121–6.

Ware JE, Sherbourne CD (1992) The MOS 36-item short-form health survey (SF-36). Medical Care 30(6): 473–81.

Waterman K, Waters K, Awenat Y (1996) The introduction of case management on a rehabilitation floor. Journal of Advanced Nursing 24: 960–7.

Welsh Assembly Government (2003) The Strategy for Older People in Wales. Cardiff: Welsh Assembly.

Wenger C (1984) The Supportive Network: Coping with Old Age. London: NISW.

Wenger C (1992) Help in Old Age: Facing Up to Change. Liverpool: Liverpool University Press.

White VK (1998) Ethnic differences in the wellness of elderly persons. Occupational Therapy in Health Care 11(3): 1–15.

Whiteford G (1997) Occupational deprivation and incarceration. Journal of Occupational Science 4(3): 126–30.

Whiteford G, Townsend E, Hocking C (2000) Reflections on a renaissance of occupation. Canadian Journal of Occupational Therapy 67(1): 61–9.

Wielandt T, Strong J (2000) Compliance with prescribed adaptive equipment: a literature review. British Journal of Occupational Therapy 62(6): 269–71.

Wilcock AA (1993) A theory of human need for occupation. Occupational Science, Australia 1(1): 17–24.

Wilcock AA (1998) Occupation for Health. British Journal of Occupational Therapy 61: 340–50.

Wilcock AA (1999) Reflections in doing, being and becoming. Australian Occupational Therapy Journal 46: 1–11.

Wilcock AA (2001) Occupation for Health, Volume 1: A Journey from Self Help to Prescription. London: British Association and College of Occupational Therapists.

Wilcock AA (2002) Occupation for Health, Volume 2: A Journey from Prescription to Self Health. London: British Association and College of Occupational Therapists.

Wilkin D, Jolley DJ (1979) The modified Crichton Royal Behavioural rating scale. Behavioural Problems among Old People in Geriatric Wards and Residential Homes. Research Report no. 1, Manchester University.

Wilkin D, Thompson C (1989) Crichton Royal behavioural rating scale. In: User's Guide to Dependency Measures in Elderly People. Sheffield: University of Sheffield, social services monograph.

Wilkinson P, Armstrong B, Landon M (2001) The Impact of Housing Conditions on Excess Winter Deaths. York: Joseph Rowntree Foundation Findings, ref N11.

Willcocks D, Peace S, Kellagher L (1987) Private Lives in Public Places. London: Tavistock.

Williams EI, Fitton F (1998) Factors affecting early unplanned admission of elderly patients to hospital. British Medical Journal 297: 784–7.

Williamson SL, Holmes SP, McCleod CA (1995) Health Gain Investment Programme for People with Mental Health Problems (Part Three): Elderly People with Mental Health Problems. NHS Executive (Trent) and Centre for Mental Health Services Development (London).

Wilson D, Aspinall P, Murie A (1995) Older People's Satisfaction with their Housing. York: Joseph Rowntree Foundation, Findings No. 146.

Winchcombe, M (1998) Community Equipment Services: Why Should We Care? London: Disabled Centres Living Council.

Wood W (1996) Delivering occupational therapy's fullest promise: clinical interpretation of 'life domains and adaptive strategies of a group of low-income well older adults'. American Journal of Occupational Therapy 50(2): 109–12.

Woolham J, Frisby B (2002) Building a local infrastructure that supports the use of assistive technology in the care of people with dementia. Research, Policy and Planning 20(1): 11–24.

World Health Organization (2001) International Classification of Functioning, Disability and Health (ICF-2). Geneva: WHO.

World Health Organization, Health and Welfare Canada and Canadian Public Health Association (1986) Ottowa Charter for Health Promotion. Ottowa, ON: Department of National Health and Welfare.

Wormald RPL, Wright LA, Courtney P et al. (1992) Visual problems in the elderly population and implications for services. British Medical Journal 304: 1226–9.

Wright FD (1986) Left to Care Alone. Aldershot: Gower.

Wynne-Hartley D (1991) Living Dangerously: Risk Taking, Safety and Older People. London: Centre for Policy on Ageing.

Yerxa EJ (1992) Some implications of occupational therapy's history for its epistemology, values and relation to medicine. American Journal of Occupational Therapy 46(1): 79–83.

Yerxa EJ, Clark F, Frank G et al. (1990) Occupational therapy in the 20th century: a great idea whose time has come. Occupational Therapy in Health Care 6: 1–15.

Ziv N, Roitman DM, Katz N (1999) Problem solving, sense of coherence and instrumental ADL of elderly people with depression and normal control group. Occupational Therapy International 6(4): 243–56.

Appendices

Appendix 1: Studies from which quotes from older people have been cited

Mountain G (1998) An investigation into the activity of occupational therapists working with the elderly mentally ill. University of Leeds, unpublished PhD thesis.

This thesis sought to investigate the purpose, nature and efficacy of occupational therapy in health service settings. The research design consisted of four empirical studies, each testing different aspects of a hypothesized model of occupational therapy activity. A total of 14 older people with mental health problems were interviewed in depth about their perceptions and experiences of occupational therapy. Pilot interviews with four day hospital attendees were undertaken prior to interviewing the main cohort of service users. This was to highlight any problems in undertaking such interviews and to enable the topic guide to be checked and modified. As well as substantiating the methodology for further interviews, several questions emerged through the undertaking of the pilot:

- What are the reasons for older people opting into or out of treatment?
- When should help be offered at the expense of independence?
- What are the reasons for lack of patient involvement in planning overall treatment?
- What are the outcomes of day hospital attendance?

Following the pilot interviews, nine older women who had recently or were still receiving occupational therapy in a selected location were invited for interview. All had a diagnosis of mental health problems of sufficient severity to have warranted hospital admission. Additionally, they had a range of other problems spanning physical disability, illness and frailty.

Mountain G (1997) Mental health services for older people: development of a community approach to treatment and care. University of Leeds: Nuffield Institute for Health.

This work was concerned with examining the nature of services that might be introduced for older people with mental health problems in line with the move towards community provision. It incorporated an examination of the evidence base and a country-wide mapping of services that existed at the time. The project also involved interviewing a number of service users and carers about their perception of services, and what would be the optimum range of provision to meet their needs. A total of seven current service users were interviewed: five women and two men. We did not seek information about the nature of their mental health problems. However, it was clear from the discussion that the majority, if not all, had a depressive illness. Additionally, four carers were interviewed with the assistance of the local carers' centre.

Mountain G, Moore J (1995) Quality of life of older people. University of Leeds, unpublished study.

This work involved group interviews with older people from a range of circumstances and settings about perceptions of quality of life in retirement. The intention was to contact a diverse cross-section of groups so that as much information as possible would be collected across the whole sample. Therefore selection was made on the basis of culture, social and personal circumstances and extent of disability. The following groups participated:

- attendees of a day centre for older Jewish people;
- attendees of a day centre for Sikh elders;
- a group for people who had been bereaved;
- a day setting for those who were housebound;
- two groups of voluntary advisors to services providing community support to older people;
- a luncheon club on a large council estate;
- a friendship club sited in an inner city area with a predominant population of students.

Two researchers facilitated each of the groups, with each of the interviews being taped and transcribed. The group with Sikh elders was conducted through an interpreter.

Appendix 2: Methodological underpinning

This book sought to use evidence to describe best practice in occupational therapy with older people, in the belief that the views of the authors in themselves are not an adequate foundation to support the clinical work of occupational therapists. It was necessary to access diverse sources of information. These have included the professional, medical and sociological research evidence as well as policy documents and guidance, and descriptions of practice innovation.

The following sources of evidence were used:

1. electronic databases to identify necessary references: Cinhal, Amed, HMIC;
2. the Cochrane Library of Systematic Reviews;
3. searches of electronic journals, *The Lancet* and *British Medical Journal*;
4. searches of websites for relevant publications: see list in Appendix 3;
5. hand searches of the following journals: *British Journal of Occupational Therapy*, *American Journal of Occupational Therapy*, *Health and Social Care in the Community*, *Ageing and Society*, *Generations Review*.
6. grey literature in the form of theses and reports.

Given the wide remit of occupational therapy with older people, specific search terms were not adopted. Literature relevant to each chapter heading was sought.

The final work includes a range of evidence, including the views of older people cited during interviews undertaken as part of the research studies described in Chapter 1, as well as published research, grey literature and accounts of practice innovation.

In the context of the established hierarchy of evidence, some of the cited examples of research are more robust than others. An explanation of the nature and rigour of studies has been provided for the reader. The requirement to use the strongest evidence as defined by the established hierarchy had to be balanced with the importance of the topic area under discussion and the extent of the current evidence base. A key example is that of intermediate care, where policy implementation has promoted the wide-scale development of services. However, the evidence base to support this range of services remains inconclusive at the time of writing. Another example is the application of technology to care and rehabilitation. This is an area where we need to learn far more about what works and for whom, but we also need to be alert to the fact that developments will have a huge impact in the near future.

Appendix 3: Relevant organizations, networks and sources of advice

Action on Elder Abuse   www.elderabuse.org.uk

Age Concern England   www.ace.org.uk

Alzheimer's Society   www.alzheimers.org

Alzheimer's Society (UK)   www.alzheimers.org.uk

American Well Elderly study   www.usc.edu/assets/ot/faculty/
                                               research/2.html

Arthritis Research Campaign   www.arc.org

Bandolier (evidence-based health care)   www.jr2.ox.ac.uk/bandolier

Bradford Dementia Group   www.brad.ac.uk/acad/health/bdg

British Heart Foundation   www.bhf.org.uk

British Society of Gerontology   www.britishgerontology.org

CancerBACUP   www.cancerbacup.org.uk

Care and Repair England   www.careandrepairengland.org.uk

Carers UK   www.carersuk.demon.co.uk

Casp (Critical Appraisal Skills Programme)   www.phru.nhs.uk/casp/casp.htm

College of Occupational Therapists   www.cot.co.uk

Counsel and Care   www.counselandcare.org.uk

Crossroads carers   www.crossroads.org.uk

Equal Network (EPSRC)   www.equal.ac.uk

Foundation for Assistive Technology   www.fastuk.org
  (FASTUK)

Growing Older Programme (ESRC)   www.shef.ac.uk/uni/projects/gop

Help the Aged   www.helptheaged.org.uk

Housing Options for Older   www.housingcare.org/choice/
  People   decision/tools/hoop

Involve   www.invo.org.uk

National Electronic Library for Health	www.nelh.nhs.uk
National Institute for Clinical Excellence	www.nice.org.uk
National Osteoporosis Society	www.nos.org.uk
Occupational Therapy for Older People (OTOP) (specialist section of the College of Occupational Therapists)	www.cot.co.uk/specialist/intro.html
Parkinson's Disease Society	www.parkinsons.org.uk
Princess Royal Trust for Carers	www.carers.org/home
Research ethics	www.corec.org.uk
Research governance	www.doh.gov.uk/research
Scottish Intercollegiate Guidelines (SIGN)	www.sign.ac.uk
Single assessment process	www.doh.gov.uk/scg/sap
Social Care Institute for Excellence	www.scie.org.uk
Tools and scales (single assessment process)	www.doh.uk/scg/sap/toolsandscales

Index